With Compliments

TESTING THE LIMITS

Number Fifteen:
Centennial of Flight Series

Roger D. Launius, General Editor

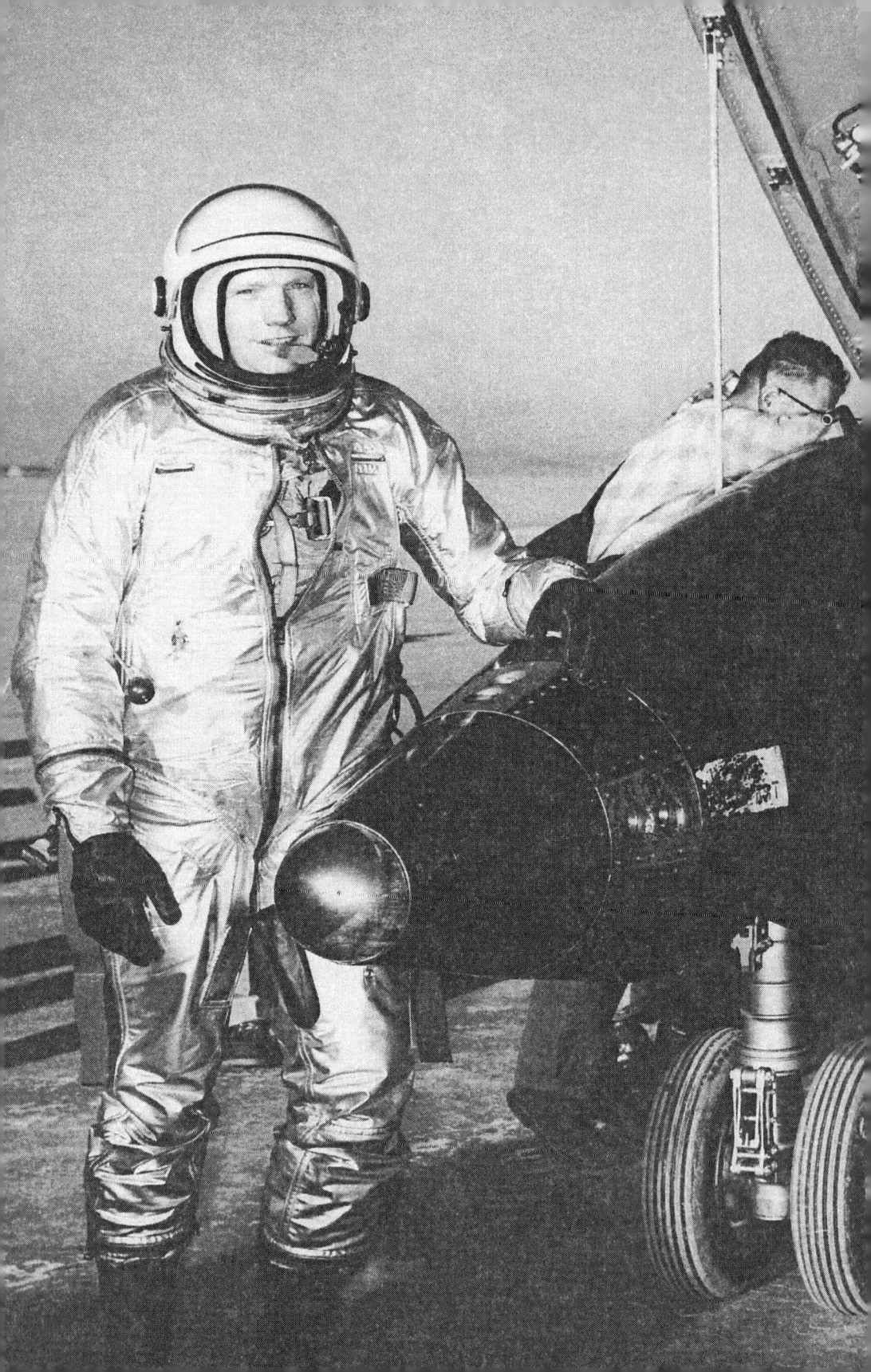

TESTING THE LIMITS

*Aviation Medicine
and the Origins of
Manned Space Flight*

MAURA PHILLIPS MACKOWSKI

Texas A&M University Press • *College Station*

Library of Congress Cataloging-in-Publication Data

Mackowski, Maura Phillips.
  Testing the limits : aviation medicine and the origins of manned
space flight / Maura Phillips Mackowski.— 1st ed.
    p. cm. — (Centennial of flight series ; no. 15)
  Includes bibliographical references and index.
  ISBN 1-58544-439-1 (cloth : alk. paper)
    1. Aviation medicine—United States—History.   2. Space
medicine—United States—History.   I. Title.   II. Series.
RC1054.U5M33 2005
616.9'80213—dc22   2005002910

To my family

and to those whose mission

it has been, is, and will be

to make flight as safe as possible.

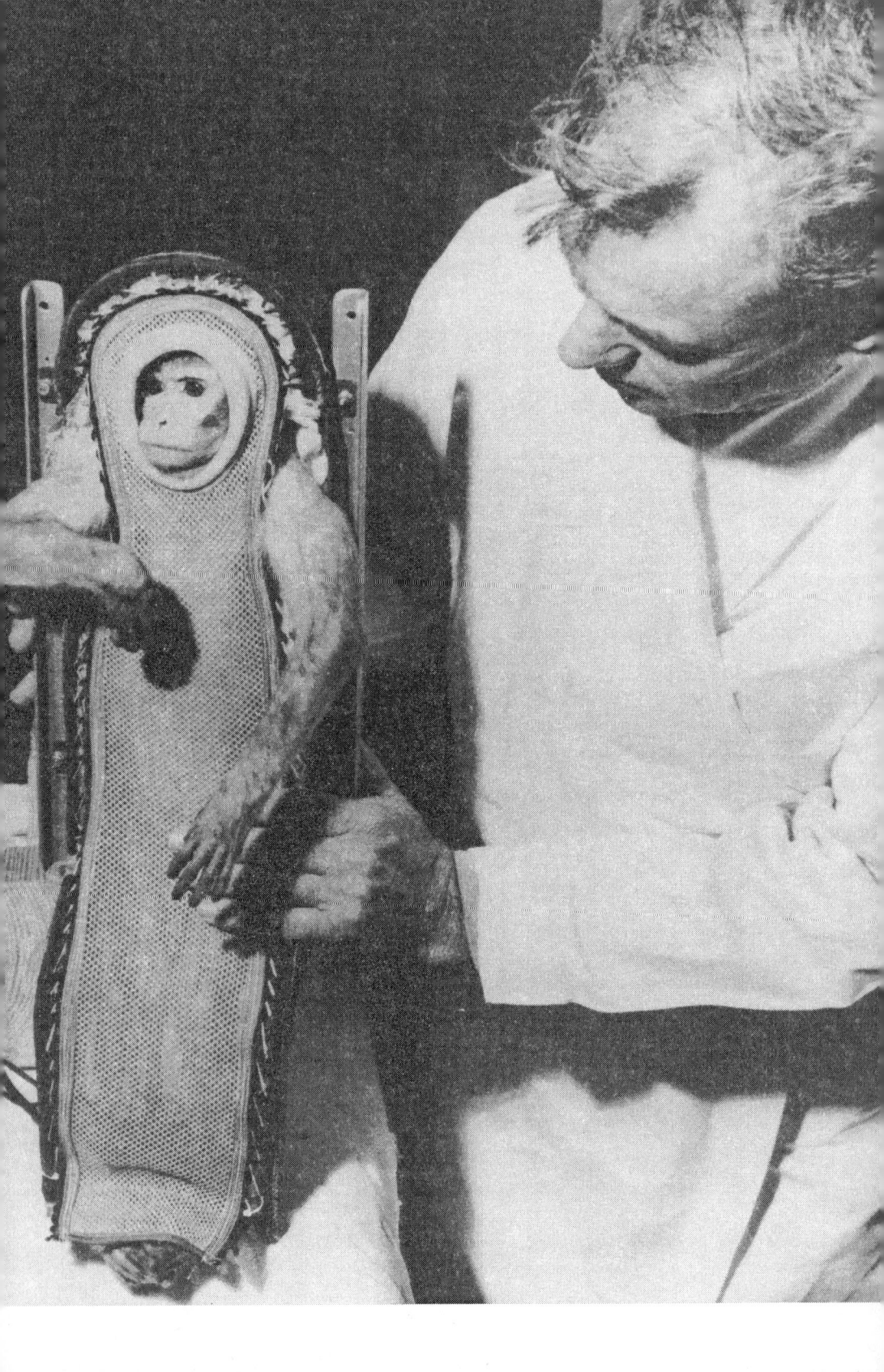

CONTENTS

Acknowledgments   IX

Introduction   3

PART I: Aviation Medicine   9

   Chapter 1. The Americans   11

   Chapter 2. The Germans   39

   Chapter 3. World War II   69

PART II: Space Medicine   103

   Chapter 4. The Paperclips   105

   Chapter 5. The Fastest Man Alive   137

   Chapter 6. Organizing for Space   173

   Chapter 7. "Detailed to NASA"   199

Epilogue: Out in the Cold   214

Notes   218

Nomenclature and Sources   259

Bibliography   267

Index   275

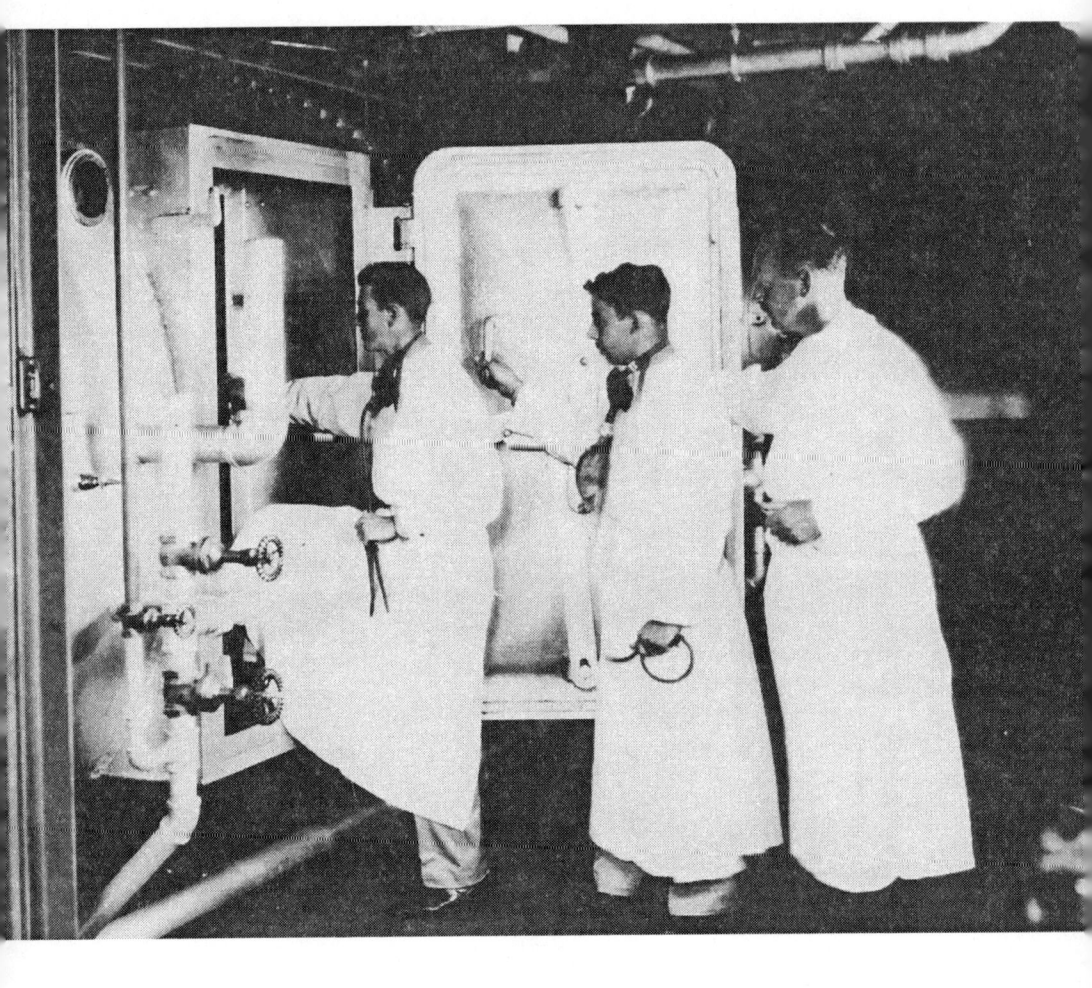

ACKNOWLEDGMENTS

This book started out a number of years ago as a freelance magazine assignment and evolved from there. Consequently, lots of debts have accumulated along the way, and there are many people and institutions I wish to thank.

I start with the hardworking, dedicated, and knowledgeable historians who work for the federal repositories that hold much of the documentary and photographic evidence I have studied for this endeavor. These include in particular the historians of the Eisenhower, Johnson, and Truman presidential libraries, where I researched the papers of Jacqueline Cochran, Lyndon Johnson, and James Webb, respectively. The Air Force Historical Research Agency at Maxwell AFB is an excellent source of oral histories, photos, and unit histories, and, at Brooks AFB in San Antonio, historian S.Sgt. Patrick Longe, librarian Joe Franzello, and Hangar Nine museum historian Shelia Klein accommodated my requests to look through the uncataloged papers, old photos, and rare books. Former Smithsonian National Air and Space Museum historian Lillian Kozloski wrote the academic paper that became the original magazine piece, an article on a group of women who attempted to become astronauts during the Mercury program years. The NASA Headquarters History Office has been consistently helpful since I first contacted them in search of documents for that article.

Several private and university-sponsored archives also provided assistance and documentation. These include the Lowell Observatory in Flagstaff, Arizona, where librarian Antoinette Beiser, archivist Marty Hecht, and astronomer emeritus Henry Giclas helped me to date certain events from the 1950s and gave me full access to Percival Lowell's own books and the observatory's uncataloged records. The Lilly Library at Indiana University in Bloomington allowed me to use the copious notes, multiple transcripts, and many sound recordings in the Shirley Thomas Collection, which contains the material she used for her *Men of Space* book series. Wright State University has a very large collection on the subject of aerospace medicine and made copies for me of several rare films from early high-altitude and aviation-medicine research. The University of California–San Diego library has a collection devoted to high-altitude medicine, including the Ulrich C. Luft and Bruno Balke papers as well as those of John B. West, mountaineer and professor emeritus of medicine. The Luft Papers are housed there thanks to the efforts of John West and Fred Luft, and they are an excellent source of information about German mountaineering in the 1930s, the research in aviation medicine that took place in Germany during the 1930s and 1940s, the relationship among the scientists mentioned in this book, and the experience of the Project Paperclip scientists and their families in America. The archives of the Rensselaer Polytechnic Institute in Troy, New York, contain the very well-organized and cataloged papers of George M. Low, an Austrian immigrant and NACA engineer who directed the Mercury manned space effort for NASA. The staff members at the Rockefeller Foundation archives were very cooperative and helpful during my search for the records of Hubertus Strughold's fellowship year in the United States in the late 1920s, which include the insightful assessments made by his American hosts a decade later, when he was working under the Hitler regime.

The medical library at the University of New Mexico sent me transcripts of oral-history interviews with members of the Lovelace Foundation, including key people in space medicine during the 1950s. The Health Sciences Center Library at the University of Arizona in Tucson has a good collection of medical journals, and the main library there has the full set of the National Archives and Records Administration's microfilmed accounts of the physicians' trials at Nuremberg after World War II. These records are an invaluable source of information on the education, ethics, and professional practices of doctors and scientists who were active during the Nazi years, the work done by Germany's many aviation-medicine research institutions, and, of course, the deadly experiments carried out at Dachau. At the Arizona State University library, the government documents librarians were quite helpful in locating a variety of federal publications and information, and I extend a very special thanks to the Interlibrary Loan department. I was their best customer.

Many museums were also a source of information and assistance. In the United States, the International Women's Air and Space Museum, now in Columbus, Ohio, has a small but very helpful collection on the Mercury women. In Germany, Tassi Römisch of the Space Museum Mittweida and Raumfahrt Service did some research on my behalf, locating resources that were both useful and accessible by long distance. In Munich, the staff of the Deutsche Alpenverein's museum was very helpful with photos, as were the personnel of the Deutsches Museum.

Without financial assistance, travel would have been impossible. I extend my thanks to the Johnson Library, the Truman Library, and the Lilly Library, all of which provided travel grants to use their collections. The American Historical Association and the Southwest Oral History Association both gave grants for travel, equipment, and supplies. The Max Millett Family Fund of Arizona State University (ASU) supported my research in the Southwest, and the Associated Students of ASU provided a stipend that covered my travel to Alabama. My parents, Gladys and Carl Phillips, and my sister, Gina Phillips, either wrote checks or slipped cash into my pocket, while my husband, Michael, brought home the paychecks. Our Lady of the Lake University archivist Eva Maria Flores; Auburn University instructor Bert Frandsen; my sister, Gina; and my brother, John Phillips, all provided a place to stay, food to eat, and transportation during my research visits to California, Texas, and Alabama. John also gave me a special tour of the Johnson Space Center, supplied useful information about current practices in astronaut selection and training, and provided VIP accommodations at a launch—his flight aboard STS-100 in April 2001. Thank you, everyone!

Many other people also aided my efforts. Environmental historian Stephen J. Pyne of Arizona State University and fellow History of Science Society members James Strick of Franklin and Marshall College and Mark Solovey of ASU–West actively supported my intellectual endeavors, as did ASU's Noel Stowe, Jannelle Warren-Findley, and Robert Trennert. Sam Schmieding, a friend and former photojournalist, shared driving expenses with me on research trips to Tucson and Flagstaff. My father, who learned to fly at Randolph Field courtesy of the Army Air Corps and is still an active pilot, has a photographic mind when it comes to airplanes. His identification of vintage aircraft and descriptions of their capabilities and construction were invaluable, and his knowledge of uniforms, medals, campaign ribbons, and military protocol was of great help in dating undocumented images, "reading" service records from old photos of officers in uniform, and understanding the machinations of the military. My daughters, Sarah and Katie, helped proofread and assemble the manuscript. I also extend heartfelt thanks to my husband, Michael, our son, Benjamin, and my extended family and friends for their material and moral support.

Joseph N. Tatarewicz at the University of Maryland–Baltimore County deserves special thanks for pointing me toward the Shirley Thomas Collection. Other fellow members of the Society for the History of Technology, in particular historian Andrew Butrica and Roger Launius, chair of the Department of Space History at the National Air and Space Museum (NASM), offered much insight from their own experience in researching and writing space history. Independent film producer Jim Cross arranged for me to meet all of the surviving Mercury women at a filming of an NBC *Dateline* segment at the NASM in December 1994. Author Dana Kilanowski took time out from writing a biography of John Paul Stapp to help me locate sources. I am grateful to Tony Reichardt and Les Dorr Jr., then of *Final Frontier* magazine, for assigning me the story on the Mercury women, and I am indebted to St. Louis editor and publisher Ellen Sherberg for giving me a start in journalism, my career for eleven years. Thanks also go to attorneys Keith Jenkins and Marty Stoneman for their legal advice and to Rob Speers of OSAM, Inc., for his help in capturing vintage photos from microfilm.

I extend my appreciation to retired master craftsman Roland Dornes, who shared photos and served as a Brooks AFB guinea pig himself. I am, of course, also very grateful to the many people who spoke to me of their own work in aviation and aerospace medicine, their experiences in Germany and as immigrants to America, their interactions with the military and NASA, and their own or their family members' lives and careers under Hitler, in the United States, or in the Soviet Union. Most of their memories are proud and happy ones, but a few are sad or painful, and I value their openness and generosity. The words "thank you" hardly say enough.

Any errors in this work are mine.

TESTING THE LIMITS

INTRODUCTION

One impression that nearly everyone who reads Tom Wolfe's 1979 best-seller *The Right Stuff* comes away with is that doctors and pilots are mortal enemies. The aggressive and courageous fliers want only to get up there and do their job, which, in the case of Wolfe's test pilots, is protecting the country while expanding the boundaries of aeronautical knowledge. Flight surgeons, on the other hand, are desk-bound eggheads who frown on risk taking and think of aviators as king-sized guinea pigs for some trivial experiment. Their medical tests are pure voodoo, and when a pilot is done, there's a good chance of being grounded, maybe for life.

For the sake of entertainment, making physicians the comic foil worked well for Wolfe. As history, however, it is dead wrong. The flight surgeon was often the military pilot's closest, even *only*, ally. Furthermore, the pilots that Wolfe wrote about, the sixty-nine men being screened for the Mercury astronaut program, owe a particular debt to the military aviation medicine specialists. They ensured that only those most fit to fly were considered for the job; that the evaluation process was done fairly and anonymously; and that, from the start, consideration was given to the astronaut as pilot rather than merely passenger. Finally, they determined whether human beings could even survive in the space environment and live through the ordeals of takeoff and reentry. This they often did at the risk of their own necks and reputations.

The knowledge needed to safely put a human being into orbit was not self-evident or easily obtained. Space medicine as a discipline evolved from several factors. Primary was the development of aviation medicine into a recognized professional specialty. Then came the establishment of dedicated organizations and research facilities. Finally, physiological, psychological, and human-factors research (the study of the pilot-machine interface) had to align with advances in engineering and physics so that vehicle and pilot could work together and function in the space environment. Both world wars served to boost national interest in, and consequently spending for, research in human-factors engineering and high-altitude medicine, aeronautics, and physics. Vital, too, was the melding of two scientific cultures at the end of World War II, as émigré German aeromedical specialists, premier in the field, came to work in U.S. military labs.

American or German, the people who brought the United States to a position of space readiness invariably took a calculated risk. They insisted on testing everything the pilot might use or experience—and always on themselves first. They believed in education, scientific openness, and cooperation among disciplines and across national boundaries. All had the outlook of the true visionary; they knew that someday humankind would travel well beyond the speed of sound and far past the boundaries of the atmosphere.

The research that would place Americans in space in 1961 was carried out in military, not civilian, medical laboratories. Today their story is little known by a public that has witnessed the many spectacular successes of America's civilian space agency, the National Aeronautics and Space Administration (NASA). However glorious NASA's work in human factors and medicine, though, it was built on the shoulders of military giants.

This book is roughly chronological but largely character driven. It opens with the tale of an aeromedical naif who was the best the United States had to offer in 1929, then moves on to his counterpart in Nazi Germany. Finally, it depicts the hybridization of American and German talent that proved necessary for the United States to achieve manned space flight just thirty-two years later.

One physician is credited with single-handedly resuscitating aviation medicine in the United States, moribund after World War I. Capt. Harry G. Armstrong founded the country's key aeromedical research laboratory at what was then Wright Field, in Dayton, Ohio, and brought it from the primitive stage to professional preeminence. He also reintroduced research at the U.S. Army's School of Aviation Medicine, which had dropped science in favor of pedagogy. Armstrong took research and training functions overseas in 1942, organizing a lab and school in England, where Eighth Air Force flight surgeons worked to reduce combat deaths among air crews. He became a leading figure in the Aero Medical Association, the only professional organization dedicated to aviation (and later space) medicine and still struggling for recognition as a specialty. Armstrong cofounded the first Department of Space Medicine just four years and four months after witnessing the first V-2 attack on London and realizing that it was a portent of transportation modes to come.

Armstrong lacked credentials as a researcher and scientist, but as an air corps flight surgeon he had seen an appalling number of deaths and crippling injuries. Unafraid to admit his own shortcomings, he surrounded himself with qualified personnel from whom he could learn the profession of science and with whom he could accomplish the most good for aviators. Armstrong had never before written professionally, but his personal style suited itself to articles and books that were helpful, explanatory, clear, and never over the heads of readers, enlisted personnel, or Ph.D.'s. His reputation preceded him; he became known worldwide for his research skill and respected for his integrity, empathy, modesty, leadership, and a work ethic that consistently put him in harm's way.

In spite of Armstrong's endeavors, the leader then in aviation medicine was not the United States but Hitler's Germany, which also set the pace in aeronautical-engineering research. One reason for that country's lead was the accessibility of the Alps for high-altitude research. Another was that German medical schools and graduate science programs were the best in the world in the late-nineteenth and early-twentieth centuries, attracting students from all over the world. During the interwar years, Germany had also begun to rebuild its air force and quietly established a number of engineering test stations and aeromedical research labs.

By the time America entered the war, Germany was a good decade ahead of anyone in vehicle design, with jet aircraft, ejection seats, rocket-powered airplanes, helicopters, and missiles. Armstrong's counterpart in Germany, Hubertus Strughold, also a physician, had a large staff with hugely superior scientific training. Strughold, for example, held a Ph.D. in physiology, had studied under a world leader in sensory physiology, and had spent a year in the United States on a Rockefeller Fellowship. He had been appointed to the directorship of a new research lab in Berlin and given carte blanche by the Luftwaffe to hire staff, acquire equipment, and carry out research. Like the Americans, the German doctors field-tested every theory and every piece of equipment on themselves.

The Second World War served as a watershed for aviation medicine in both nations. The United States had to gear up massively to field air forces that could operate in disparate regions: northern Europe, the Mediterranean, North Africa, and Asia. An enormous number of flight surgeons were required to screen and train pilots and air crew who would be flying faster, more powerful aircraft at altitudes that were three times those of the previous conflict. Germany's war covered a much smaller geographic area but relied heavily on technological advances, which in turn posed new medical challenges. On top of the scientific tasks, there was also the personal challenge of functioning under a dictatorship that favored their professional work but, in the case of Strughold and most of his staff, was anathema to their personal views.

After the war, Armstrong and others recognized their counterparts' reduced circumstances as an opportunity not to be missed. V-2 rocket designer Wernher von Braun and his team had already left Soviet-held Peenemünde to surrender themselves to the United States in hope of finding a home in a well-funded American research facility. Under the clandestine Project Paperclip, U.S. Army Air Force (USAAF) medical corps leaders recruited former Third Reich science and engineering personnel. Strughold and most of his former employees accepted their offer and came to the army's School of Aviation Medicine (SAM) in San Antonio, Texas.

Thoughts of actually going to the moon and Mars were the stuff of science fiction, and neither the Paperclips nor the Americans at the school were ever promoters of von Braun's plans for colonizing the planets. Only a few astronomers and life scientists (including Strughold) spent time in the study of exobiology, the existence of life beyond Earth. Strughold carried his interest a step further, getting Armstrong's approval to establish the Department of Space Medicine at the School of Aviation Medicine, part of the U.S. Air Force after July 1, 1949.

The army began to evaluate captured German technology, in particular the rocket plane, jet aircraft, and ejection seat. As a result, Chuck Yeager broke through the sound barrier in a rocket-powered vehicle. His flight surgeon, John Paul Stapp, rode a rocket-propelled sled to study the effects of extreme acceleration and deceleration. Germans had already found out that their great speeds meant that pilots could not bail out and live, and Stapp did not want that to happen when jets became standard issue in the new air force.

Even as he labored in the California desert and the Germans settled in for what was originally a one-year stay in the United States, a group of academics had already seized the scientific moment, experimenting with captured V-2s in the New Mexico barrens. Energized by the strides that physics had made during the war, they turned to the challenge of creating new instrumentation and finding ways to launch and recover live payloads. Both the school and the Wright lab took part, conducting nearly all of the life-sciences experiments.

The Wright laboratory opened a field station in New Mexico to carry out additional human-factors research under Paul Stapp, this time making the administrators' interest in outer space more explicit. They worked at the edges of the atmosphere with high-altitude balloons and on the ground continued to test human endurance against extreme acceleration and deceleration. By late 1958 they had formed an idea of the composition of the upper atmosphere and space. Increasingly, the air force envisioned vehicles that could take off and land like aircraft but also negotiate the strange environment of space. Weightless research began in all three test facilities.

In 1957, the Soviet Union's electrifying success with the *Sputnik* satellite had shifted the playing field for the aeromedical specialists. The political response, including the formation of the new NASA, was led by Sen. Lyndon Johnson from Texas, a frequent visitor to the School of Aviation Medicine. It also generated research funding for the school and the labs and made "space" a word one could now use in proper air force company.

Leading-edge USAF aeromedical and human-factors projects, including the X-15 research aircraft, became dry runs for developing methods to screen and select candidates for NASA's first project, the Mercury astronaut program. The initial medical tests were carried out by a civilian, W. Randolph Lovelace II, former chief of Armstrong's laboratory at Wright Field during World War II. He had since consulted for the National Advisory Committee for Aeronautics (NACA), the X-15 project, and the airlines. From there, the candidates went to the Wright lab, now under Paul Stapp, for more medical and extensive psychological tests. These were the models for the infamous *Right Stuff* tests, but they were hardly meaningless exercises conjured up by a group of dreamy-eyed intellectuals or pilot-hating sadists. The tests were necessary and accurate, and the staff demonstrated true concern for the pilots who would be venturing out beyond Earth. In April 1961, Alan Shepard became America's first man in space.

One unique story offers insight into a critical NASA decision of the period: to allow only military-jet test pilots to pilot their spacecraft. A study from 1959 to 1961 by Lovelace, then NASA's chief medical-science consultant, evaluated females as astronaut candidates. In 1961, however, President Kennedy committed the nation to a moon race. Inserting a civilian woman into the Mercury program to score propaganda points (as the USSR would do in 1963 with Valentina Tereshkova) was absolutely out of the question to the White House and to NASA's gung-ho administrator, James Webb. Setting aside the favorable medical evidence and popular sentiment, NASA chose to go with the proven article: male military-jet test pilots. Ultimately the official policy became one of detailing active-duty military fliers to NASA, allowing it to continue calling itself a civilian space agency while exploiting the military's aeromedical expertise and flight-training resources.

Ultimately, the original visionaries of the air force's aerospace-medicine laboratories would collectively become the Moses of the space age: They were not allowed to enter the promised land. The small manned space program the air force kept when NASA was formed was later aborted. The medical teams that had assumed they would handle screening and selection for the new space agency were told there was no need for their services, and in the adrenaline rush of the moon race, the Kennedy administration approved a brand-new space-medicine facility for NASA, just two hours east of San Antonio. Today, little evidence remains at the Johnson Space Center (or at air force facilities) of the role that the military's aviation laboratories and the Paperclip immigrants played in making possible everything that human beings have accomplished in space.

PART I

Aviation Medicine

Chapter 1

THE AMERICANS

The 1920s and 1930s marked the emergence of the airplane as a major component of the nation's transportation system and of aircraft manufacturing as an important industry in the United States. Despite drastic cutbacks in military spending after World War I, the federal government was from the start the driving force in this growth. It organized the airmail service and in contracting it out to private carriers kicked off the growth of the airline industry. Its National Advisory Committee for Aeronautics (NACA) served as aeroengineering consultants for manufacturing. The army's advanced design group led with crucial improvements that transferred to commercial aviation. Its military personnel taught men to fly, and the Department of Commerce's new Aeronautics Branch set up the licensing requirements that determined who in this burgeoning field was qualified to step into the cockpit and who was not.

This last function, matching human with machine, could not be left to the flier alone. Plainly the airplane was a much touchier machine than the automobile and posed greater risks to its driver, passengers, and others on the ground. Furthermore, its place in the nation's armory as a platform for observation and bombing, as well as its role in military transportation, dictated that only the fittest be entrusted with its use. It would take a specially trained physician to determine who was medically qualified to fly, to approve a request for a license, or to ground an unfit pilot.

Regardless of whether anyone knew it, with that decision the government in effect solidified the existence of what had been a catch-as-catch-can field of applied research and learning: aviation medicine. Special knowledge was needed to determine the physical, mental, and emotional faculties required to pilot existing aircraft, particularly for military applications. Much more research would prove necessary to keep up with rapid technological advances that would take aircraft much higher and allow them to travel at significantly faster speeds than ever before. Human-factors studies would be important to provide enough comfort and efficiency for effective piloting. Air crews would need to be trained in the proper use of safety equipment, and, of course, someone would have to train the doctors.

The knowledge that existed at the time could be found only among a small group of physicians who were part of the U.S. Army Air Corps. They were indoctrinated at various army medical schools, chiefly its School of Aviation Medicine (SAM) in San Antonio, Texas, and officially called "flight surgeons." The education the army provided was insufficient and already obsolete, however. In 1929, learning to ride a horse and drive a six-mule ambulance was still a required part of the curriculum.[1] Worse, the school itself had abandoned its modest research effort, which would only put safety and efficiency that much further behind.

Within the civilian aviation community, things were no better. There were no guidelines on who could call themselves aviation medical examiners, and although some motivated people at a few hospitals and clinics performed research of personal interest, no civilian entity existed to conduct or coordinate long-term scientific studies. At the Mayo Clinic in Minnesota, a former SAM doctor, Walter Boothby, was doing the only real investigative work, looking for new treatments for lung patients.[2]

Historians of science, technology, and medicine have defined science as the quest for knowledge for the sake of enhancing understanding and engineering as the search for the best design of artifacts. Medicine, physiology, and human factors are all considered "applied sciences," meaning they use the intellectual and material tools of science to develop or improve existing objects, processes, and systems. All three seek the best methods to improve the functioning of the human body.

At that time, aviation medicine was simply too new and too fragmented to exist as a bona fide medical specialty or applied science in the United States. Such was the case in Britain, Canada, and most other nations, too. No country was ready in any way for the massive wartime buildup of aviation capability they would need in a few short years, either in materiel or human talent.

A group of air-minded American physicians banded together in 1929 to create a professional organization that could at least lend some cohesion to their efforts. The Aero Medical Association gave flight surgeons and civilian doctors a place for open communication about and exchange of information. At the same time, it also fostered a collegial dialogue between civilians and the military.

One person more than any other, though, can be credited for turning the specialty around. Harry George Armstrong, a Minneapolis physician with no previous flying experience, went through the School of Aviation Medicine in 1929 and came out committed to a career as a military flight surgeon. His outspokenness landed him a chance to work at the leading military design shop of its day—Wright Field, in Dayton, Ohio. Partly to educate himself but chiefly to stop the carnage he had seen as a line medical officer, he began to research problems in aviation medicine, to assemble a team of professional scientists, and to build a functioning laboratory. By the time the United States went to war in 1941, Armstrong had nearly single-handedly brought aviation-medicine research from the biplane era to a point at which America could compete with the world's leader in the field—Nazi Germany.

HARRY ARMSTRONG

The open-cockpit P-16 fast-attack plane roared along just two thousand feet above snow-covered Minnesota towns and farms, now and then passing over the bends of the ice-choked upper Mississippi. It was an odd-looking bird, built for speed, with small lower wings affixed behind a larger upper pair. Both sets were aft of the engine but in front of tandem seats, with the top pair meeting the fuselage gull-fashion to form a V through which the pilot could aim a weapon. The gunner normally sat in a swivel chair, ready to shoot at foes coming from any direction. The occupants' heads stuck up above the fuselage and wings and were completely unprotected from the cold or the airstream.

To Capt. Harry Armstrong, a physician, the man in the backseat that February morning, installing a windshield would have been sound medical advice. Not that he was an aeronautical engineer; he just knew that the machine was no more efficient than the pilot who operated it, and this operator was *cold*. Officially, Armstrong's job as squadron flight surgeon for the First Pursuit Group at Selfridge Field, near Detroit, was to screen pilot applicants and tend to their medical needs, grounding the pilots when necessary, and to pass along to the fliers what he had learned at the SAM. Too bad he couldn't do anything about the weather.

The P-16 was heading into a twenty-mile-an-hour wind, and the temperature at the Minneapolis airport had registered minus forty at takeoff, producing a windchill of ninety-six degrees below zero. The cold had already knifed right through both pairs of Armstrong's long underwear, and ice had formed where his breath condensed on the portion of his wool-lined flying helmet that covered the nose and mouth. The army's leather pants, leather jacket, and huge leather gloves, all lined with sheep's wool, were nearly ineffective at this temperature. Armstrong couldn't feel his hands or his feet, and the numbness in his face and thighs told him that he would have to check for frostbite when they landed in Chicago.

Even if they had not been wearing helmets, the numbing vibration of the metal tubing skeleton of the fabric-covered biplane and the drone of its engine would have made verbal contact between pilot and passenger impossible. So when the control stick between Armstrong's legs shook suddenly, it got his attention. They were only fifteen minutes into the two-and-a-half-hour flight, but the pilot was gesturing at Armstrong to take the controls. The army had given Armstrong two weeks of flight training, and he had done a little bit of passenger-seat flying when he was out on check rides. He ought to be able to keep them both out of trouble while the pilot scratched his itch. The flight surgeon took the stick and, putting his feet on the rudder pedals, held the aircraft in steady flight.

As he flew, he could see the man in front pull his goggles off over his helmet and scrape the lenses with his gloved hands. They were nearly covered with frost. Armstrong's were taking on a glaze as well. He saw the pilot attempting to rub some warmth into his face and the stiffness out of his fingers, even as his own hands began to freeze around the control stick. Damn, this was cold! He couldn't feel his feet but tried flexing his toes inside the boots to get the blood flowing. His eyes were starting to burn and tear even with goggles, and his vision began to blur. Finally, Armstrong shook his own stick to get the pilot's attention, and he resumed control.

The sky was a brilliant blue above them, and, looking down, he could see the snow-crusted ice that was the river, banked by the tall bare branches of the ash and maple trees. The river wound its way past sparkling, snow-blanketed fields, here and there cross-hatched with long white "caterpillars" made by snowplows forging along the main farm roads between Minneapolis and La Crosse. Dark streaks marked spots where the plow had scraped the surface and the bright sunshine had caused the ice and snow to sublimate. Armstrong was a farm boy from South Dakota, where winter had always meant an abundance of snow and ice, raw chapped skin, fingers and toes with no feeling left in them, and clothing that never completely dried between the time you hung it up in the class cloakroom and donned it again when it was time to trudge home. That kind of weather had been cold; up here, however, it was indescribably, unbelievably, absolutely impossibly *arctic*.

A short time later Armstrong's stick shook again. They were still three hundred miles from Chicago. He lasted just a few minutes at the controls, then had to shake the stick himself to ask the pilot to give up trying to clear his goggles and fly the P-16 once more. The stick shook yet again; he took hold and flew the plane on an even course until he thought the other man had had time to perform his ice-removal task, shift his feet around, and maybe put his hands inside his jacket to pick up a bit of body heat. Then it was Armstrong's turn. He shook the stick and waited for the pilot to take the controls, then took off his goggles once more and scraped off the ice. Wait; the stick was shaking again. Would this go on all the way to Chicago?

It did, but somehow the two men made it. When they landed, both Armstrong and the pilot had frostbite down the fronts of their thighs, and in the morning Armstrong discovered that he had lost half of his vision. His corneas had frozen during the flight and then swollen while he was asleep.[3]

Back in the warmth of his office, Armstrong calculated that a pilot working at zero degrees was only half as effective as one at seventy, and that forty below induced a drop to less than fifteen percent of normal efficiency. Multiplying the number of days below zero and the number of pilots based at cold-weather locations, Armstrong knew that it was insanity to expect anything like preparedness should there ever be a winter war. Granted, the last conflict had been fifteen years ago, and, judging by their tightness with military budgets, Congress seemed to have decided that America was never going to get involved in a global nightmare like World War I again. Still, the army ought to be able to equip its aircraft with windshields and, for those with cockpits, heaters that would bring the temperature inside at least to zero.[4]

Armstrong wrote an urgent, on-the-record letter to the army air surgeon in Washington, telling him about the trip and its hazards and commenting bluntly that, in combat, "I would have been delighted if someone had shot me down and put me out of my misery." He went on to suggest a course of action. "[S]omething has to be done about giving better protection to our airmen against cold and things like goggles freezing over," he wrote. "[T]he unit responsible for development of that equipment . . . [ought to] be told to get busy and do something about this."[5]

Two weeks later he got his answer: a set of orders sending him to Wright Field, the army's incubator for new aircraft designs, as a consultant to the equipment branch. Instead, Armstrong flew to Washington and confronted the air surgeon, then Maj. Coleridge L. Beaven. Armstrong did not mince words, regardless of Beaven's superior rank. "What the hell is the idea of sending me?" he asked. "I've never in my life been in a research laboratory. I don't know a damn thing about it. If you send me down there I'm going to make a fool out of myself and be absolutely ineffective." He added a colorful description of what such an assignment would do for his career, then waited for his superior's response. It was pithy—and without pity. "You're the guy who complained, aren't you?"[6]

In spite of his protests, Armstrong took the job. He was, after all, as qualified as the next person, a specialist in industrial medicine with a post-graduate education in aviation medicine and three years of doctoring the pilots at Fort Snelling, Minnesota; Camp Custer, Michigan; and the First Pursuit Group at Selfridge.[7] He had done plenty of hands-on medical work there and had accumulated some flying time in several models of military aircraft, mainly the Curtiss C-14, an open-cockpit cargo aircraft with a single engine and big cantilevered wings, and the large C-4, a metal-skinned trimotor that carried passengers and cargo. There was also the chilly P-16.[8]

Armstrong also had a keenly empathetic and compassionate outlook toward his pilots, and it was that attitude more than the extra flight pay that moved him to take his bedside manner skyward. Those under him would find that his professional modesty made him the boss that everyone wanted to work for—taking every risk himself first, facilitating his employees' research, and ensuring that everyone got full credit for their accomplishments. His knowledge and character had already led him to take chances on behalf of his men and to spend significant time getting to know them on their own terms as aviators.

One testimony to Armstrong's affinity for and his belief in aviation medicine as a separate discipline is a study he carried out while at Selfridge. It was one of the first analyses of the psychological stresses of *peacetime* aviators. The author evidently spent a significant amount of time in the air and in the company of pilots because he wrote not only with compassion but also with great frankness, reflecting a close personal understanding of the fliers' experiences. It was penned more in practical than scientific language, but it attempted to make observations that were in line with the accepted professional protocols of the day.

Armstrong actually wrote the article after being sent to Dayton and used the pseudonym "Freud Jung." He may never have sent the paper to a journal for publication, but it ended up ultimately in the air force's archives. Its style reveals an author as yet unskilled at writing pieces for professional journals, but it has the ring of first-person authenticity.

In the article, Armstrong related that he had surveyed 163 army air corps pilots to find out what motivated them in their work and what problems they encountered in carrying it out. It is a credit to Armstrong's approachability as a flight surgeon that he apparently had almost one-hundred-percent co-operation from the pilots in answering his questions about stress, fear, and other personal difficulties.

The informants were between the ages of twenty-two and fifty and had anywhere from one to eighteen years of service and from zero to nearly six thousand hours of flight time. Personality traits that were common to the group, he found, were extroversion, "a great amount of courage, alertness, energy, and vitality[,] . . . intensity, generosity, warmheartedness, friendliness, and devotion to duty and family. Their actions were frank and vigorous, their feelings ruled the intellect more than good judgment, and [these] feelings were devoted to those around them."

The medical problems that the men reported, he concluded, were "organic, due to working conditions. Carbon monoxide poisoning and oxygen [deprivation] both cause nerve damage, as does inhalation of pure oxygen, centrifugal and centripetal forces and head trauma. The worst is emotional strain." This last observation is both insightful and noteworthy for its mention of psychiatric ailments as being on a par, medically, with accidents and illness.

The personal details in the report demonstrate the level of trust Armstrong's pilots placed in him. The population under study, after all, might have worried that he would ground them for the slightest evidence of imperfection. Also, as an officer, a military aviator was not likely to whine about emotional upset or minor unpleasantness on the job. In any event, such complaints were not typically uttered in the early 1930s, when jobs were scarce and when voicing fear outside of combat was considered unmanly. Armstrong found that the pilots worried about age-related changes in eyesight costing them their jobs, reporting minor illnesses for fear of being grounded, and, more poignantly, "the constant attempt to regain face, to reclaim and hold a fading dream" as aviation became commonplace and pilots became "humans instead of gods."

Death comes not only in wartime but also in peace, and for the military flier it is too close and happens far too often. Armstrong pulled no rhetorical punches in describing the numerous gruesome ends that he and the pilots had witnessed:

Military pilots, due to their formation flying, are usually the witnesses to the crashes of fellow officers. The crashes undoubtedly produce the most violent known deaths. Not only do these individuals frequently witness a friend . . . and companion hurtle to destruction, but hurrying to the rescue usually find a mangled corpse with brain tissue spattered over the instrument board, naked bones projecting through flesh, and the body a jelly-like mass conforming to its shape only by the clothing. Frequently, gallons of spilled gasoline turn the twisted mass of wreckage into a concentrated hell of searing flame while the victim writhes and curls amid the stench of burning flesh.

To witness one of these scenes is never to forget it. To witness one and fly, one must forget it, repress it, and thereby a new conflict arises.

To Armstrong, a flying career in the army meant years of stuffing the usual fears of loud noises, high places, and falling somewhere into the back corner of one's psyche, then making more room for new fears: of being unable to undo a stuck canopy, of a parachute's failing to open, of being trapped in flaming wreckage, and of causing another person's death. Over the three years that he conducted his study, ten deaths occurred, one natural and nine from accidents. The pilots made nineteen emergency parachute jumps, had seven midair collisions, and sustained seventy-seven accidents overall, with injuries to thirty-nine people.[9]

WRIGHT FIELD, 1934

In August 1934, Armstrong and his family arrived at Wright Field in Dayton, Ohio. For the U.S. military, this was the mecca for leading-edge aviation enthusiasts, those who were passionate about not only powered flight but lighter-than-air craft as well. The Goodyear-Zeppelin Corporation, an American-German joint venture, built balloons and dirigibles for the army and navy in Akron. The army, which controlled essentially all of the scientific ballooning in the United States, was competing with the Soviet Union to set world records for altitude while carrying out upper-atmospheric research. Expedition organizers came to Wright Field for help in planning the human-factors and operational components of these ventures.[10]

The airplane had put the city on the map, however, and Wright Field was the center for the army's modest program of aircraft design and test engineering. Jimmy Doolittle worked at nearby McCook Field but buzzed in and out of Wright periodically. He had earned the first doctorate in aeronautical engineering, flown for the army in WWI, and as a civilian pioneered in "blind" flying. He had been the first to perform the high-G, outside-loop maneuver and had set a transcontinental speed record. In short, he was easily the country's foremost test pilot. Unbeknownst to Armstrong, aviator Wiley Post had come to Wright to test his own homemade pressure suit two months earlier. Air racer Jacqueline Cochran would come to know Armstrong and the Wright team in the course of evaluating a prototype oxygen mask that would allow her to fly higher (and thus faster) during races. Even Orville Wright still came by on occasion. Because of the amount and nature of this activity, Wright Field was the natural place to which any individual or group working on human factors in aviation and high-altitude physiology would gravitate.

When Armstrong came to Dayton, the problems of aviation medicine were fairly limited by today's standards. A heavily armed pursuit plane (fighter aircraft) was likely to be a biplane, whose ceiling, or altitude limit, was about eighteen thousand feet and whose speed was less than two hundred miles per hour. Even aircraft on the drawing board did not hint that noticeable improvements in either speed or range were on the way. Pilots were concerned with the cold, exposure to the elements, onboard fires, and bailouts. At very high altitudes they faced the additional danger of anoxia—lack of oxygen. Above ten thousand feet a person would become disoriented, sluggish, and forgetful in the thin atmosphere. Beyond fifteen thousand feet, lack of oxygen brought unconsciousness and death. No one knew for sure how many lives anoxia had cost in the three decades since the Wright brothers had flown, but the army suspected that many accidents that had been considered pilot error might actually have been the result of oxygen deprivation.

Part of Armstrong's challenge was to convince pilots of that danger. Many of them, however, chose to believe they were less sensitive to oxygen deficiency than the next flier and refused to use breathing gear. Others disdained the equipment because it was uncomfortable, which it was. Pilots had to fly with a pipe stem clenched in their teeth. That, in turn, was connected to a hose that fed oxygen from a tank into the pilot's mouth. At high altitudes the stem froze to the user's lips. On the warmer days pilots joked that they were "smoking" the oxygen.[11]

Consequently, when Armstrong reported to the equipment branch at Wright Field, he was not sure what to expect. The official army position on medical research was that most of the problems associated with flying had already been solved during World War I. Furthermore, piloting was something one could do only during daylight hours and in fairly clement weather. However, Armstrong suspected that the engineers at Wright would always be looking for ways to make airplanes fly faster, higher, and farther. That implied a need for a ready supply of pilots—test pilots, specifically. It also meant that the field was still the engineers' turf and that machines got most of the attention, not the pilots who flew them.

Building 16 was to be Armstrong's new workplace, but, entering on his first day, he saw only a large open space with many desks. His own desk, it turned out, constituted his entire "office." It was hardly the place for a private doctor-patient chat. Armstrong soon learned that he was not particularly welcome in the equipment branch, either. He was the only doctor in an all-engineer group and was to be treated as an outside consultant of sorts, but no one sought his advice.

One day Armstrong's gaze fell on the floor next to his desk, where he noticed what looked like a trap door. He had been told that there was no basement in the building, so he wondered where a trap door would lead. Opening the door, he peered inside and saw a staircase receding into the darkness. Gingerly he climbed down it. The basement was anything but nonexistent; it held a machine shop and areas for photography and drafting, and—something else.[12] Armstrong spotted an immense white cylinder with a door, three windows that resembled portholes, and some pipes and dials. Several feet taller than Armstrong's own five-foot, eleven-inch frame, the object was made of iron and obviously extremely heavy. The seams of the big container were studded with numerous rivets. Armstrong knew enough about boilers and industrial equipment to realize that the compartment was designed to withstand enormous pressure.[13] Putting two and two together, he figured out what the device was used for: It was the high-altitude chamber from the army's original flight-surgeon school at Mineola, Long Island.[14]

Organized in 1918, the school had originally been used only for instruction, not research. An adjacent laboratory was operated by the same personnel, however, and organizationally the two were considered a single unit. Both had burned down in 1921, and when the facility was rebuilt, it no longer housed a

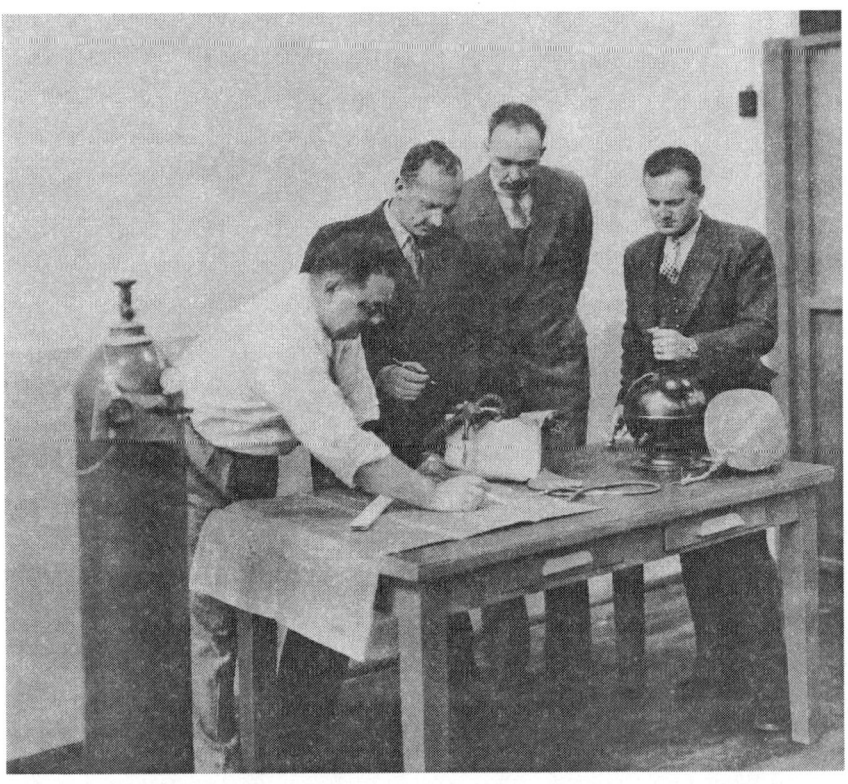

Designing an early oxygen system at Wright Field. Armstrong is second from left. USAF *photo.*

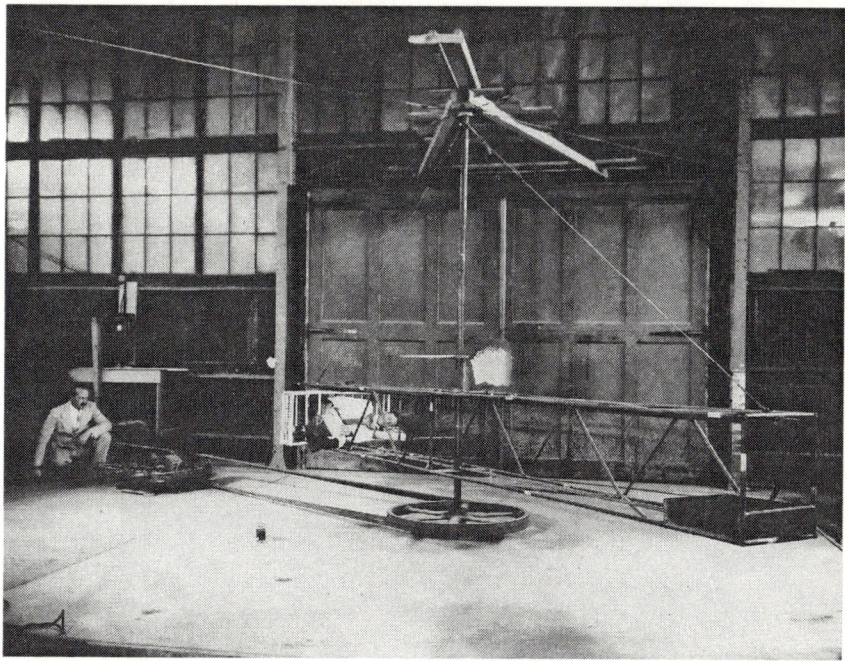

The first Wright Lab centrifuge used an electric motor to spin a test subject at one end of its twenty-foot arm, reaching as many as twenty Gs. Harry Armstrong is on the left in this 1937 photo taken in the balloon hangar that housed the device. With a cushion under his left side, Staff Sergeant Stevens is on his side on the metal frame "seat" of the device. USAF *photo.*

research facility. Laboratory investigation went by the wayside in the army.

Discovering the big tank made Armstrong think. Perhaps one way around the engineering branch's antagonism toward him would be to pick up where the docs at Mineola had left off. This might also serve as an antidote to his own feelings of boredom and inadequacy. If he focused on the pilot instead of the machine, probing the medical effects of the physical surroundings, the extreme cold, lack of oxygen, noise, acceleration, and so on, he could make a significant and independent contribution to safety, efficiency, and comfort. Armstrong wasted no time in writing up a proposal for a new medical laboratory and sending it to Maj. Oliver Echols, head of the engineering section at Wright. Echols forwarded it to Washington, D.C., where the recommendation lingered for a while and then was approved. Armstrong

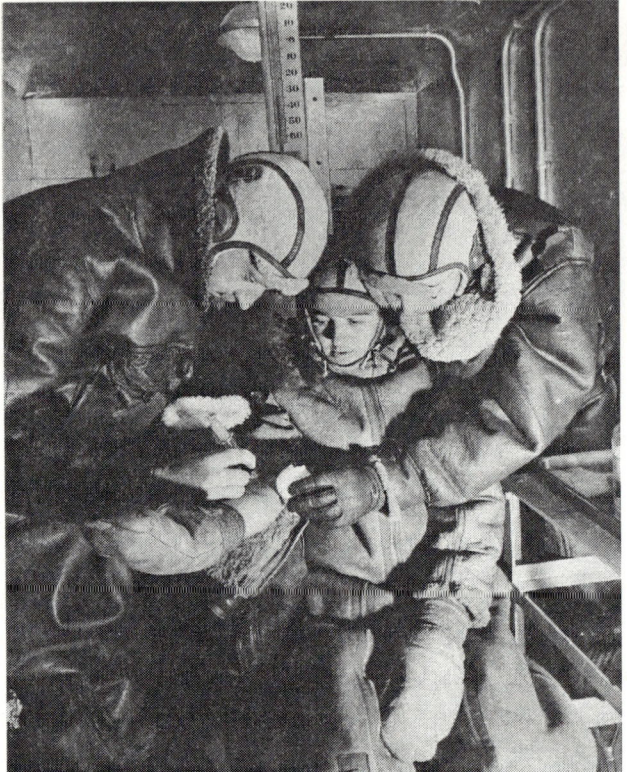

Armstrong (left) and Heim (right) draw blood from a test subject in the Wright cold chamber. USAF *photo.*

was appointed director of the new Aeromedical Research Laboratory and allowed to borrow one enlisted man from the base hospital. His budget was practically nonexistent, but it was enough to get started.[15]

BECOMING A SCIENTIST

NASA Director of Space Sciences Homer Newell, explaining to Congress in 1967 exactly what "space science" was, identified scientists by their underlying assumption that answers to questions do indeed exist and can be found in nature. Imagination is an important quality in scientists, he said, because they must be able to frame old questions in new ways or to entertain totally new questions. They have to develop novel approaches and look in out-of-the-ordinary, often unsuspected places for their answers. Practically speaking, scientists are required to measure the same phenomenon in different ways to eliminate methodological errors. They must be able to labor cooperatively with scientists from all over the world in order to develop acceptable explanations that apply anywhere in the known universe. "In this process," he added, "the scientist uses observation and measurement, imagination, induction, hypothesis, generalization and theory, deduction, test, communication, and mutual criticism in a constant assault on the unknown or poorly understood." Scientists accept results as legitimate only after open, refereed trials, meaning that scientists must present and publish papers, participate in open discussions, and if needed, publicly defend their ideas, results, and conclusions.[16]

Managing a science lab continually on the leading edge of a brand-new medical specialty could be unnerving, Armstrong discovered. He worked essentially without supervision or technical support, without a peer to talk with on a regular basis, and in an army that asked him for nothing specifically but certainly let him know if he failed to produce something they wanted. His feeling of professional solitude was intensified by having to justify both his and the lab's existence to the army at regular intervals and by the complete lack of feedback from the surgeon general's office or a corresponding facility elsewhere in the army. There simply was no one to provide guidance. In the back of his mind, too, at least for the first several years, was the knowledge that he had been trained as a practicing physician, not an administrator or a research scientist. He knew just enough about those last two jobs to get himself into a lot of trouble.

Armstrong drew inspiration from his own observations in the field and in the lab, however. As he devised the best means to define and address problems in aviation medicine, he secured the services of qualified assistants, including a Harvard-trained physiologist, and a functioning (if somewhat makeshift) laboratory. During this period Armstrong and the work he did underwent a change. He became a scientist, and the work he did became scientific research.

In 1935, Armstrong was given the go-ahead to add a physiologist to his staff. Because Harvard University owned a *high*-pressure chamber for studying the physiological effects of deep-sea diving, it seemed to Armstrong a likely place to find advice on building a bigger, better *low*-pressure device and a researcher to go along with it. He flew to Boston in the back of an open-cockpit O-25 and called on the head of the lab, Cecil K. Drinker.[17] Drinker, in turn, recommended a doctoral candidate named John W. "Bill" Heim. Armstrong interviewed Heim, who had never heard of either him or

Wright Field. The Depression was still on, however, and the work sounded interesting, so Heim decided to take the job. He reported to the lab the following summer.[18]

Heim, a thirty-two-year-old Ph.D., was just finishing up a dissertation titled "The Composition of Subcutaneous Lymph," a topic not at all related to aviation medicine.[19] He was of average height, with dark hair combed straight back and eyeglasses that sat atop a beaky nose. He always dressed for work in a suit, white shirt, and necktie, over which he donned a white lab coat, giving him an air of scholarly professionalism. In photographs from that period, Heim rarely smiles. Instead, he looks completely unperturbed, no matter what was going on with his animal or human test subjects. Entering the low-pressure chamber, Heim appears grave and confident. One of Armstrong's borrowed enlisted men is seen at the controls. In another, Heim, clad in arctic survival gear, draws blood from a test subject. In still another photo, Heim hunches over a microscope, peering at specimens taken from the brains and hearts of lab rabbits and cats.

Armstrong and Heim began to rigorously examine the physiological effects of exposure to high altitude. They made baseline runs with the centrifuge, pressure chamber, cold chamber, and acceleration devices. Then they used the mechanical exactitude of those ground devices to replicate the tests numerous times on large populations of animal subjects in ways they could not have done in an airplane. Their goal was consistency, repeatability, and total reliability of data.

Doctor and scientist devised a test for color blindness, studied altitude tolerance in animals, and examined the effects of acceleration using aircraft, the centrifuge, and an abrupt-acceleration swing they built in the balloon hangar. This device suspended human and animal subjects from the ceiling by means of four forty-foot cables, then subjected them to sixteen Gs for half a second, when a windlass brake suddenly stopped the pendulum motion. Armstrong and Heim studied the effects of repeated oxygen deprivation on the adrenal glands and metabolic processes and tested possible preventives for airsickness. After surgically inserting a viewing tube into the artery of an experimental animal and then exposing it to simulated very high altitudes in the low-pressure chamber, they were the first to observe that body fluids literally boil at sixty-three thousand feet.[20] That point became known in medicine as "the Armstrong Line."

Armstrong relied on his staff's good judgment and gave them his full support and regular feedback. As the lab grew, he allowed—within the guidelines of their military directives—his people what amounted to academic freedom to study what they wanted and to work in their own fashion. He gave himself this freedom as well. As a result, Armstrong learned much from Heim and, through his own diligence, mastered the techniques and thought processes of the research physiologist.

Before Heim arrived, Armstrong had completed a number of hands-on projects, including designing a small first-aid kit and a tool kit for extricating fliers from crashes. He had studied the conductivity of bone in flight, the effect of cold on efficiency, and the utility of gaseous vs. liquid oxygen for breathing devices. He also carried out literature studies that brought him up to speed on physiological research. He looked at data on pilot stature and performance, the physical requirements for pressure cabins, and the effect of barometric changes on the sinuses.

After Heim came to Wright, the two men undertook additional literature reviews on dental problems at high altitudes and on arctic rescue equipment. They designed an oxygen cylinder and delivery system and developed—then tested in flight—a crash helmet. Using goats in the pressure chamber, Heim studied carbon dioxide toxicity aloft and designed a new type of respiratory-gas analyzer that physicians could use aboard aircraft.[21]

Armstrong is credited with building the first human centrifuge in North America at Wright Field in 1935. The first one anywhere had been a "rotating bed" described by an English author in 1794. Although it is unclear whether that device was ever actually used, in theory patients could be strapped to it, head facing outward, and, when the bed was turned, they would fall into a restful sleep. Whirled in the feet-out position, the heartbeat supposedly slowed, and fever would be suppressed. In Berlin, a large centrifuge that early-nineteenth-century physicians thought would benefit mental patients was developed in the psychiatric ward of the Charité Hospital. It measured about thirteen feet in diameter and made some forty to fifty revolutions per minute, producing about 5 Gs at the outside edge. Fortunately for science, the physicians tested the device on themselves and noted the profound physiological changes it produced in respiration, heart function, and blood distribution. Also in the late-nineteenth century, laboratory scientists began studying centrifuges systematically, using primarily small animals. By the early 1930s, scientists in Holland and Germany were using small animals for human physiology research and publishing their findings in the open literature.[22]

Mechanics at Wright Field fabricated Armstrong's device using a salvaged electric motor and scrap-aluminum aircraft tubing. The framework had a twenty-foot diameter, with a two-and-a-half-foot seat mounted on its side at one end of the revolving arm. Adjustable, it allowed subjects to experience positive, negative, or transverse (crosswise) accelerative forces at anywhere from twenty to eighty revolutions per minute.[23] At first Armstrong and his staff gathered baseline data on how well humans and animals tolerated the stress of acceleration. Later they used it to test an inflatable belt they hoped would allow pilots to withstand additional accelerative forces. With the device, the team of Armstrong and Heim laid the scientific groundwork for modern aviation medicine. Heim stayed at the lab for thirty-two years and retired in 1968.[24]

After World War I, U.S. Army Gen. Billy Mitchell had at times made ardent calls for establishing an independent air division that could carry out offensive as well as tactical roles. Before Mitchell died in 1936, Armstrong met him and asked whether his vociferous advocacy of the airplane as a tool of war had been just a ploy to procure more government funding or whether Mitchell really had facts to support his contention. Mitchell, whose views had cost him his military career, replied that one could use history and the data at hand to project future growth. That is what he himself had done, and it had convinced him that the airplane should be used for military purposes and that the air corps must become an independent branch of the armed services.

Armstrong knew intuitively that he, too, needed to think of the future of aviation and try to deal successfully with the medical problems it would pose. At some not-too-distant point, technology would make a significant leap and put people at the controls of a machine that could reach the limits of the upper atmosphere and exceed the speed of sound. The army needed to be ready.

Armstrong got into trouble for his opinion. Speaking at a Dayton luncheon in 1935, he had been asked what speed he thought aircraft would eventually reach. He replied that certainly the speed of a .45-caliber bullet—and perhaps even greater—was likely to be reached. His remarks made headlines and drew the ire of the Wright design engineers. Armstrong was officially warned that, as a medical officer, he was not to make any more such public predictions. "Any such idea," he was told, "was pure fantasy." After hours, he was given an even more personal rebuke. At an officer's club, engineering staff who had imbibed a few too many drinks dragged Armstrong to the middle of the dance floor. There they mocked, ridiculed, and otherwise harassed the flight surgeon. Given that spouses would also have attended the base dance and that most of the attendees were in uniform, it was a humiliating experience for Armstrong. He never forgot it.[25]

FLYING WITH THE TEST PILOTS

Being able to gather data in the field whenever possible is critical to applied scientists. The army air corps did not demand that flight surgeons have a pilot's license, but the school did train them in the basics of takeoffs, landings, and maintaining level flight; it also made their flight pay contingent on accumulating a certain number of hours in the backseat of an aircraft. Armstrong chose to build up his flight time and data with a variety of pilots and in the rear of as many kinds of aircraft as Selfridge—and later Wright—could offer: some eighty-three pilots, forty aircraft, and 391 flights.

No quick, easy jaunts, these flights included a ten-day, cross-country navigational flight that took Armstrong and an O-39 observation biplane to Cheyenne, Wyoming; Salt Lake City; Seattle; Portland; Pocatello, Idaho; Cheyenne again; and then back to Wright Field. From east to west, the flying time was a grueling eight hours and five minutes without a windshield or canopy for the backseat; the return trip was only slightly shorter: six and a half hours. Armstrong flew for twelve days in an open-cockpit PB-2A pursuit bound for California. The longest leg—between March Field near Riverside, California, and Fort Leavenworth, Kansas, took seven hours and thirty-two minutes. He flew backseat on two nine-day, cross-country trips.

More often Armstrong's flights were short local hops, and he gamely went out with fledgling fliers practicing takeoffs and landings for hours on end. He flew with more than his share of beginners but also with some of the best pilots the army had. Capt. George V. Holloman took Armstrong along in his backseat for eight days of flying through the Midwest, a trip the doctor logged simply as "radio navigation." What he did not write was that these test flights were actually part of the effort to *invent* radio navigation, a means to land safely in fog, darkness, and foul weather.[26] The physician also flew often with B-17 test pilot Donald L. Putt, who would retire as an air force general a few decades later.[27]

The new Flying Fortress, an innovative type of long-range offensive bomber, was coming along rapidly by that time and needed human-factors support. Boeing's B-17 would be able to carry heavy loads of high explosives, defend itself with numerous gun positions, and stay aloft for a dozen hours or fifteen hundred miles. That meant that oxygen systems, cold-weather gear, crash safety, and other issues would have to be addressed—and soon. The bomber was test-flown in 1935, and the army air corps began receiving the first production models a year and a half later.[28] Pursuit aircraft on the drawing boards represented quantitatively similar advances in flight and combat capabilities. They, too, would benefit from the work of Armstrong and the Wright Lab personnel.

During this period Armstrong also studied cabin pressurization, which would allow passengers to travel without wearing oxygen masks or bulky arctic-weather clothing. This testing required complete and mutual trust between both flight surgeon and fliers. The test pilots would take the flight surgeon to altitude, dispense with their oxygen pipe stems, and wait for the doctor to get into a kneeling position alongside them. Then they would put the plane into a steep dive while the physician took blood samples all the way down.[29]

One observation Armstrong made while serving as his own guinea pig in the decompression chamber. He found that when he lowered the chamber pressure enough to correspond to a very high altitude, he experienced the same symptoms as a deep-sea diver with the bends. A very painful condition, the bends result when someone makes a too-rapid change from high pressure to low pressure, which causes nitrogen bubbles to form in the tissues and blood. These build up typically at the joints and cause pain and stiffness but can also produce tightness in the chest, convulsions, and even death. Armstrong's hands would begin to feel stiff and sore, and when he rubbed them together to improve the circulation, he could feel small bubbles in his tendons. Pressing his fingers on the tendons, he could move the bubbles around. Armstrong was sure they were the cause of aeroembolism—deadly blood clots in the brain and lungs.

The best test protocol for verifying this theory, he decided, would be to go into the Mineola low-pressure device with a rabbit, take it to thirty-five thousand feet, allow it to die during the ascent, and then immediately dissect it—still in the chamber—to look for nitrogen bubbles in its blood. Accordingly, he entered the chamber with an animal and the equipment, donned his oxygen mask, and signaled the private at the controls to "take him up." Glancing at the standard aircraft altimeter mounted inside the chamber, Armstrong watched the altitude climb as he waited for the rabbit to die.

He had noticed in the past that whenever they reached thirty-five thousand feet, the altimeter failed to record any further climbing. Everyone had assumed that the old Mineola chamber simply leaked air in at the same rate as the vacuum pump pulled it out. Standard procedure, therefore, was to simply let the pump keep running in order to maintain a steady altitude.

Once he and the dead rabbit had climbed to thirty-five thousand feet Armstrong began his dissection. Absorbed in the task of scrutinizing the rabbit's tiny arteries and veins for nitrogen bubbles, Armstrong was unpleasantly shocked when he glanced at the altimeter and discovered that the chamber was only at twenty thousand feet. He gestured vigorously through the porthole window for the enlisted man at the controls to take him back up. Armstrong glared, too, for effect, wanting to impress on the man that he had just ruined the experiment. The private ignored him, and the gauge continued to register a descent. At ten thousand feet Armstrong saw the post surgeon appear at the window, looking very excited. When he reached ground level, the two men outside opened the door.

Armstrong had become unconscious right in the middle of the dissection, the private told his angry boss, and had fallen off the stool and straight to the floor. The private had called for the post surgeon and then begun to take the chamber back down, watching the still form of his superior officer through the porthole the entire time. All of a sudden Armstrong had gotten up, sat back down on the stool, and gone right back to his dissection as though nothing had happened.

The lab director stared at the two men in disbelief. Not until someone noticed the enormous bump rising on Armstrong's head did he realize what had indeed happened and how close he had come to experiencing a fatal embolism right along with the rabbit. Later they determined the cause of the accident: The ancient altimeter had simply topped out at thirty-five thousand—higher than even the B-17 would fly. However, the sturdy vacuum pump had gone right on sucking the atmosphere out of the chamber. Armstrong had ascended to about forty-five thousand feet, some two miles higher than the peak of Mount Everest, where even an oxygen mask would not have been enough to maintain consciousness.[30]

The one story people always told about Harry Armstrong was about the time when he jumped out of an airplane. He told it on himself as well but fudged on the date and place. He said it had happened in 1935 at Wright Field, when the event actually took place in 1929, while he was still a student at the SAM at Brooks Field in San Antonio, Texas.

Armstrong and his classmates had watched a demonstration on proper bailout technique and the care of parachutes. After some discussion, the group dispersed, leaving Armstrong and the sergeant who had given the lecture alone for a few minutes. M.Sgt. Erwin H. Nickles had the novel idea that it would be possible to drop infantrymen from airplanes during combat, but he lamented to the flight-surgeon trainee that he was ready to give up on the whole idea because almost none of the soldiers were able to follow his instructions about proper bailout, especially the direction to count to ten before pulling the ripcord. Perhaps they briefly lost consciousness or panicked when they jumped, he speculated, or something else happened that made them forget what they had learned.

The sergeant looked at Armstrong out of the corner of his eye. "I sure wish some doctor would make a jump and try to handle it."

Harry Armstrong heard the silent plea but didn't say anything to Nickles. He went on his way, but the thought of the sergeant's dilemma—and of having an adventure himself—kept going through his mind. The next time the monthly notice went out asking for volunteers to jump, he put his name at the top of the list.

The jump plane was an open-cockpit affair based at a nearby airfield. An instructor gave Armstrong brief instructions on how to exit the craft, how to deploy his chute, and what to do when he landed. Armstrong put on two parachutes, one the standard-issue army trainer for larger-sized soldiers, the other a smaller backup parachute that was strapped to his stomach. He wore an ordinary, summertime flying uniform and a gabardine helmet but no goggles.

The plane took off and circled until it had attained an altitude of twenty-two hundred feet. Looking down, Armstrong could see the grassy landing strip and two attendants waiting to time his free fall and take photographs of his descent. The airspeed indicator showed they were moving at 119 miles per hour. At a signal from the pilot, Armstrong climbed onto the right side rim of the biplane's cockpit, grabbing the back of the copilot's seat with his left hand for stability in the hurricane-force wind. He held tight to the ripcord with his right hand, then threw himself out chest and shoulders first, pushing off against the edge of the cockpit.

He quickly shut his eyes as his body began to somersault, making one revolution every two seconds. In his written report, Armstrong remarked that he felt no nausea or vertigo at that point, "although the author is quite susceptible to both from any swinging, tumbling motion, or disorientation." After a brief period, he opened his eyes and discovered that the fear of falling that he had experienced while anticipating the jump had given way to a pleasurable experience. He likened free fall and the sensation of being held up by the air pressure to being gently lowered onto a bed of cotton. He had not blacked out or lost his awareness for even a second. Mission accomplished, the doctor pulled the cord at one thousand feet.

One school of thought is that Armstrong changed the date on the paper he wrote about his experiment to avoid getting anyone in trouble. A more likely explanation is that it did not occur to him at the time to write an article for publication. Being the first physician to jump out of an aircraft using a parachute seemed like a natural thing for a doctor to do to satisfy his own curiosity while helping out a fellow soldier.[31] His willingness to jump was the mark of a flight surgeon. Writing up his findings in 1935, however, was the action of a scientist.[32]

PROFESSIONALIZATION

By January 1937, the low-pressure chamber was operational, and, although still in the basement, it was at least in a real laboratory. The group had been allocated about 120 by 30 feet of air-conditioned space marked off by steel and glass partitions. Into this space they managed to fit a small office with three desks and a reference library, a well-lit operating room, a stock room, a dust-proof balance room with high-precision analytical scales, a physiological laboratory equipped for metabolic and blood-gas studies, and a biochemical lab with everything needed for full blood analysis and general chemical studies. A fume hood, a sink, compressed air, a device for smoking data-recording cylinders, a water still, a small centrifuge, and a refrigerator also occupied the facility.

The altitude chambers claimed the most square footage. Armstrong and Heim now had three: two with a capacity of three cubic feet, for small animals, and the Mineola device for human subjects. The small chambers were insulated and had balsa-wood cabinets for dry-ice refrigeration. The chambers could be evacuated individually or via the lab's main vacuum system. The human chamber, 31 feet long and 8 feet in diameter, was divided into three sections horizontally, with the first acting as an airlock for the next two. Those could be evacuated to simulate an altitude of 80,000 feet and cooled to sixty-five degrees below zero.[33]

Visiting scientists began to call on the lab at this point because now there was something to see and do when they got there. Well-known aviation-medicine specialists like Ross McFarland and Bruce Dill, both from the Harvard Fatigue Laboratory, came and carried out some of their experiments at the lab. McFarland, who was medical coordinator of Pan American airlines, undertook large-scale psychological and physiological studies of airline pilots in the late 1930s. Dill, the lab's informal director, was scientific leader of the International High Altitude Expedition to Chile in 1935.[34] The aviation-medicine community began to recognize that the Wright operation was no longer a one-person show but a world-class laboratory.

Although military aviation had been fairly dormant in the 1920s and early 1930s, civil aviation grew rapidly, both on the ground and in the air, flourishing even in the Depression. This can be attributed in great part to leaps in aeronautical engineering made in the United States and Europe: the cantilevered wing, metal stressed-skin construction, and streamlining from Germany and Holland; engine cowlings from NACA's new wind tunnel and laboratory at Langley, Virginia; and wing flaps, retractable landing gear, and variable-pitch propellers from American aircraft designers. A dozen colleges and universities had enrolled a total of fourteen hundred aeroengineering students, all presumably hoping for careers designing the next generation of American aircraft. Jimmy Doolittle's blind flight paved the way for instrument flying at night and on cloudy days, an indispensable capability for a viable airline system.

Better designs meant safer, smoother flights and thus contracts to carry passengers and freight. In 1928, there was already enough air traffic to generate the need for union representation in the form of the National Airline Pilots' Association (the Air Line Pilots Association after 1931). Scheduled airlines carried nearly one hundred seventy-five thousand passengers in 1929, and thousands more flew on nonscheduled carriers as well. Pan Am, the first U.S.-based international carrier, opened with government backing the same year. In 1936, the first modern-looking airliner entered service: the twenty-passenger, dual-engine DC-3. Just four years later, passengers were able to fly in a comfortable, pressurized aircraft, the Boeing 307, which could fly on top of stormy weather, thereby reducing delays and cancellations as well as the nausea caused by flying through the turbulent air of the lower atmosphere.[35]

Increasing aviation activity also brought about a need for some sort of regulation, particularly with regard to who was qualified to fly passengers. In 1926, the Department of Commerce organized an aeronautics branch and named Louis Bauer to head it. A World War I flight surgeon and commander of the school of aviation medicine at Mineola, Bauer found that his first task was to set federal standards for civilian licensing and for the physicians who would conduct the new medical-screening program. The first thirty-seven physicians he appointed as examiners included a few SAM graduates and former members of the armed forces, but otherwise none had aviation-specific training. To rectify this, Bauer called a meeting of air-minded physicians, and in December 1928 they founded the Aero Medical Association. The group held its first meeting in 1929 at the National Air Races in Detroit and began publishing the *Journal of Aviation Medicine,* which Bauer edited. As aviation grew, so did their membership.[36]

Perhaps because of the group's initial focus on civilian medical examiners, Harry Armstrong did not attend a meeting until September 1934.[37] The military sent a contingent that year because the conference was held in Washington, D.C. Armstrong listened to a paper by the SAM's head of psychology on developing an apparatus that screened out unsuitable pilot candidates on the basis of eye-hand coordination and reaction time. Two other papers dealt with equilibrium and blind flying, and a fourth with the effects of age.

Three years later, at the group's first international meeting in New York

City, Armstrong read his first paper to the Aero Medical Association. Taking advantage of the host city's prominence as a hub for transatlantic passenger ships, the organizers had invited scientists from Europe. Commercial aviation was now global in scope, airlines were opening up intercontinental routes, and European work in aviation medicine, particularly in England, Germany, Holland, the Soviet Union, and Italy, had been impressive. They hoped that some of the continent's key researchers would make the trip. Dozens did, and twenty-one were elected honorary members. It was the largest meeting in the group's nine-year history.

A cardiologist presented a controversial paper on whether it was suitable for heart patients to fly, a great concern in the days of unpressurized aircraft. Another researcher spoke on the effects of reduced oxygen pressure during altitude acclimatization. The director of air commerce for the United States described the challenges of his office. Armstrong's paper reported on the research he had been doing with Heim on short exposures in the low-pressure chamber.

It is likely that Hubertus Strughold, a physiologist who held a position in Germany comparable to Armstrong's and who was also quite involved in altitude-chamber research, attended this talk and asked a few questions, if only to show off the English he had learned during a fellowship year in the United States. Armstrong would surely have noticed him at the banquet when the "distinguished foreign guests," including Strughold, were introduced. The scheduled dinner speaker was absent, so the new honorary members were asked to say a few words about themselves. Strughold gave a short speech calling for increased cooperation in aviation among all nations.

Whether they met at Armstrong's talk or at the dinner banquet, Armstrong would have seen a man of not quite forty in a suit of European cut. He was of medium height and build, with sandy hair and vivid blue eyes. He had a pleasant face and a friendly demeanor, chatting and laughing with a group of doctors, enjoying cigarettes and cocktails, and charming their wives with his shy and somewhat awkward attention. He had a rather strong accent, all rolled *r*'s, *v*'s for *w*'s, and *ja* for *yes*, mixed together to produce a voice that sounded like movie actor Peter Lorre, only without the menace. For his part, Strughold would have met a tall, trim, dark-haired man with a high forehead, large brown eyes, a military moustache, and a ready smile. He was accompanied by a slim woman, somewhat younger, clad in a ball gown or a tailored suit with hat and gloves—in short, the gracious wife of a doctor and army officer. As both men recalled later, they hit it off immediately and had a pleasant time talking shop during the three days of the conference.[38]

ETHICS: HUMAN EXPERIMENTATION
AND SELF-EXPERIMENTATION

Discovering early on that it had the authority to speak out on issues such as physical and age standards for pilots, both civilian and military, the Aero Medical Association helped set federal policy at a time when aviation regulation was completely new. Another function of a professional organization is to establish the minimum acceptable ethical practices in its field.

The American Medical Association (AMA) had not mentioned the subject of human experimentation in its first code of ethics. Despite much public debate over what was called "human vivisection" in the early part of the twentieth century and a strong effort by the country's premier physiologist, Walter Cannon, to put the matter before the AMA in 1916, discussion of regulation had come to naught. It was not until 1940 that the association required physicians to obtain consent (but not necessarily voluntary, informed consent) and to do animal testing before beginning their research.[39]

The Aero Medical Association appears never to have established a formal code of conduct for its members. One explanation for this might be that many of its members were in the military, and their conduct was covered by army or navy regulations. They might also have assumed that since every member was a licensed physician, it would be redundant to stipulate behavior already covered by the AMA and the Hippocratic oath. The association might also have reasoned that a laissez-faire attitude was necessary to avoid discouraging research. Because some members had gone to medical school outside the United States, they might have been exposed to different philosophies and methodologies, and members who lived in foreign countries were subject to different laws anyway. In 1931, Germany, for example, had created one of the first regulations on research in the life sciences. That country allowed human testing in order to develop new therapies, provided that unambiguous, informed consent by the patient or a legal representative had been given, animal tests had been done first, and the risk-benefit ratio had been carefully calculated and considered.[40]

No one seems to have specifically addressed autoexperimentation, in which the investigator serves as the test subject. There is a long history of physicians developing vaccines or medications and testing the compounds on themselves first, family and friends second, and only then on larger test groups. Certain diagnostic procedures, including heart catheterization, were practiced on the inventor first as well. Aviation medicine was unique, though, in making self-experimentation a routine, daily occurrence. Many experiments were hazardous, including those in test chambers and field studies on high-altitude tolerances, G-force limitations, parachute deployment, and sudden aircraft-cabin depressurization. Others were dangerous because they involved actual backseat flying during test flights of new aircraft or systems. Risks in the field, which often meant the Rocky Mountains, the Himalayas, and the Andes, included avalanches, hypothermia, frostbite, pulmonary embolism, and altitude-related pneumonia. Military physicians viewed such perils as an unquestionable part of their duty as soldiers.

Taken for granted in aviation medicine, self-experimentation was rarely discussed among the physicians themselves, and it was quite uncommon for anyone to receive a medal for that sort of work. Occasionally a reporter would ask about a particularly torturous examination and be told that the flight surgeon would not ask another person to submit to a test that the physician was not willing to undergo. The doctors also felt that they were simply the best-trained people for the job. Every one of the aeromedical specialists in this book, American and German, subjected himself to thousands of experiments during the course of his career.

RECOGNITION: THE WRIGHT LAB AND THE COLLIER TROPHY

One of the lab's biggest successes was a collaboration with the Mayo Clinic in Rochester, Minnesota.[41] Former Mineola doctor Walter Boothby headed a research team there that included an army air corps reserve physician who had graduated from the School of Aviation Medicine in 1937, W. Randolph "Randy" Lovelace II, and an active-duty flight surgeon, Capt. Otis O. Benson Jr.[42] The Mayo team set out to provide fliers with an oxygen mask they could wear continuously at high altitudes and that would not inhibit their motions in the cockpit. Military, private, and commercial aviators were still "smoking" their oxygen. For his own use, Armstrong had jury-rigged a mask from a painter's respirator, placing a piece of tape over the hole where the canister went.[43] After doing the research and sketching out an idea for the mask's construction, the Mayo doctors had a clinic craftsperson fashion the apparatus and then tested it on themselves at the Minnesota lab. Lovelace also gave one to Jacqueline Cochran, who was entering the Bendix transcontinental air race.[44] Then Lovelace and Boothby carried it to Wright Field for Armstrong's expert opinion.

The military doctor pronounced it "totally inadequate." Compared to gripping a tube in one's mouth for hours on end—one that froze to your lips in the cold—the prototype must have been somewhat better, but Armstrong pointed out that a mask that covered only the nose would not work on a pilot who had a cold or simply forgot to breathe only through the nose. Besides, the connection between the mask and the "rebreather bag," the balloonlike object suspended beneath the mouth, was a series of metal valves that froze shut when Armstrong tested it in the Wright cold chamber. There was no way to incorporate a radio microphone, either.[45]

Armstrong redesigned the mask to suit air corps applications, substituting sponge rubber for the metal valves, among other things. By the end of 1938, the Mayo Clinic's new mask had been tested in flight and in the Wright low-pressure chamber several times. Boothby reported on the mask at the annual meeting of the Aero Medical Association—held for the first time at Wright Field—and his report was also published in the *Journal of Aviation Medicine*.[46]

Since this was Armstrong's first experience working with an outside contractor, he failed to realize the commercial implication of his assistance. He was chagrined to find that the army had provided his services free of charge but would now have to pay the clinic patent royalties for every mask the military eventually bought. Over the course of World War II, the invention must have made the Mayo Clinic millions.[47]

Of some consolation was the Collier Trophy for 1940, which went to Boothby, Lovelace, Arthur H. Bulbulian, and Armstrong for developing the mask. The award was usually given to aeronautical engineers, but Cochran, a member of that year's selection committee, had decided that the oxygen-mask project presented an excellent opportunity to bring Franklin Roosevelt's attention to the aeromedical field and to Germany's leadership in the area. She nominated the group and convinced the Collier committee to grant them the award.[48] The four men and Cochran flew to the White House for the presentation of the trophy by President Franklin Roosevelt.

EXPECTING WAR

By the end of the 1930s, research in aviation medicine was divided into two areas, theoretical and applied. Everyone interested in aviation medicine conducted basic research into blood oxygenation and physiological functioning, aeroembolism, conditioning and acclimatization techniques, and gravitational stress. Applications differed, however, depending on what particular operational needs, if any, a sponsoring organization might have, and resources varied as well. In the Netherlands, physiologist and pilot Jacob Jongbloed studied the effects of high altitudes on pilots while working as a military flight instructor.[49] After the UK entered the war against Germany, Canada, part of the British Commonwealth, began an aviation-medicine research program under the supervision of Frederick Grant Banting, codiscoverer of insulin. The Italians and Swiss used their Alpine facilities for basic research into high-altitude physiology. The British began a serious program to engineer a pressure suit that would keep pilots who were performing tight aerial maneuvers from blacking out. Germany had had one small aviation-medicine center near Berlin since World War I and in 1934 set up several others that tackled both theoretical and applied situations, including flying at altitudes of up to twenty thousand feet.

America saw World War II coming a long way off. There was no doubt the United States would be drawn into the fight and ally with Britain and whoever else was left standing against fascism. Between 1939, when war broke out between England and Germany, and December 1941, when Japanese actions propelled the United States into the conflict, the army's flight surgeons had opportunities to make professional connections in Allied, Axis, and neutral countries. Some of these encounters were intentional, especially those with soon-to-be-allies, but just as many were fortuitous acquaintances that came about because of the nature of the scientific profession to share, inquire, and learn from each other. Either way, these contacts would prove useful later.

In 1939, then major Armstrong forged a relationship with British Air Commodore Harold Whittingham. The pathologist and aviation consultant had arrived in Washington, D.C., for a joint meeting of the Association of Military Surgeons and the International Congress of Military Medicine and Pharmacy, and Armstrong was assigned to be his aide. Armstrong reported for duty, but the Englishman told him that he did not want an aide. He invited the American in to talk shop for a bit, however, and then stated bluntly, "You know we're going to have a war. We're in desperate circumstances. Since World War I we have not done a single bit of research on aviation. Would you consider taking me out to your laboratory at Wright Field?" He added quickly that he was not asking to be told any secrets.

Armstrong was surprised that the air commodore had ever heard of him and his laboratory. "We don't have any secrets," he replied. "There's a problem, though. I'd have to go to the State Department and get their approval. It's unfortunate, because if I were your aide I'd have to comply with all your wishes, and we could leave this afternoon."

"You're my aide," the other man replied.

The two flew right out to Dayton, and Armstrong gave Whittingham a complete tour and introduced him to the others in the lab. The commodore went home to London "with an armload of information."[50]

Another international connection required some Pentagon finagling. In early 1940, the Canadian government requested through the Banting Institute that Harry Armstrong, whose tour as head of the Wright Field lab would soon end, be detailed to the institute for a year as a consultant. The army turned down the request because the United States was still neutral in the European conflict, and such an assignment would be considered direct aid to a combatant. Armstrong was disappointed, but three weeks later he was surprised when orders arrived for him to report to the University of Toronto—as a postgraduate student in the Banting lab.

He departed in July, leaving Bill Heim as acting director until Maj. Otis Benson took over in September. Armstrong knew his government was skirting the law, but to cover its tracks and also for his own interest, he carried out some research in Toronto. He had just finished a master's degree in science at the University of Cincinnati but went through the paces again in Canada. He wrote a thesis titled "Physiologic Effects of Breathing Cold Atmospheric Air" and went home in February 1941 with a second master's degree, this one in physiology. Not coincidentally, the Canadians installed their first centrifuge in Toronto the same year.[51]

As soon as his stint in Canada was over, Armstrong was sent to London, assigned ostensibly to temporary duty at the U.S. embassy. Whittingham, by then an air marshal and a Knight of the British Empire, had written to the army asking for the loan of an air corps medical officer for three months to help them with some sticky aviation-medicine problems. "Armstrong would be acceptable," he said, with forgivable understatement. By that point, Britain had been involved in an air war with Germany for almost two years. However, Armstrong's early exposure to combat medicine with the British would give him—and American aviation medicine—a head start on preparing for the United States' imminent entry into the fray.[52]

Chapter 2

THE GERMANS

The roots of aeromedicine are in decades of theoretical and applied research carried out in well-equipped European laboratories by highly regarded life scientists of the late-nineteenth and early-twentieth centuries. German physiologists were particularly interested in questions of high-altitude respiration, partly because of the proximity of Alpine research stations and the popularity of mountaineering and also because of that nation's fascination with flight. Airplanes, zeppelins, gliders, and balloons, all of which were in vogue there after 1900, exposed pilots and passengers alike to new and deadly forces and stresses, and researchers attempted to understand these and prevent airborne calamities that occurred all too often. Even after Adolf Hitler and the Nazi Party came to power in 1933 Germany led the world in aviation physiology studies.

An early priority of the Nazi Party was Germany's rearmament as an air power. Shortly after assuming office, Hitler and the head of his new Luftwaffe, former World War I ace Hermann Göring, began pouring money into aviation-related scientific and technological research. This work included medicine, and the government established or enlarged at least half a dozen institutes of notable size and broader scope than before. Funding went into advanced studies of high-altitude respiration, decompression, and bailouts; ejection seats for jet and rocket-powered aircraft; high-speed acceleration and deceleration; radiation hazards; windblast; fuel toxicity; the effects of cold on the body; psychology; and vision.

A key figure in this work was Hubertus Strughold, a physiologist and Ph.D. A dedicated civilian scientist with a strong aversion to politics, Strughold led the Luftwaffe's premier aviation-medicine research laboratory, a counterpart to Harry Armstrong's facility at Wright Field. He had a strong interest in creating and maintaining international ties, particularly with the United States. As part of this effort, he established Germany's leading aviation-medicine journal, the *Zeitschrift für Luftfahrtmedizin,* which functioned as Europe's version of the Aero Medical Association's *Journal of Aviation Medicine.*

Strughold's story not only chronicles the rise and fall of Germany as the global authority in aviation medicine but also expresses an idea of what it must have been like to work within the Nazi regime without selling one's soul to the devil. He dealt with ethical issues under a legal system very different from the one that Harry Armstrong lived with. The open communication that was and is the hallmark of science had also become a thing of the past under Hitler. Science itself would be threatened by the pseudosciences that Hitler and many of his coterie subscribed to and by rabid anti-Semitism that decreed which areas of medical research were scientific and which were not. The Nazi regime also offered tempting enticements to favored scientists, including the opportunity to experiment on human beings—at a research facility called Dachau.

HUBERTUS STRUGHOLD AND THE NEW LUFTWAFFE

Germany's counterpart to the Wright Lab and the School of Aviation Medicine's research facilities was the Luftfahrtmedizinische Forschungsinstitut (LMFI), or Aviation Medicine Research Institute. This was a product of World War I by way of the Versailles Treaty, which had disbanded Germany's army and navy and forbidden it to have any military aircraft, even dirigibles. That action had amounted to a red flag for Germany, which already led the world in aeroengineering research and the manufacture of high-speed aircraft.

By the late 1920s, aviation leaders such as Hermann Göring and Erhard Milch, director of Lufthansa, the national airline, were not content to limit German aviation to sport gliding and soaring, nor were aircraft manufacturers like Junkers and Dornier, who had skirted the treaty by building factories abroad. With the Nazi acquisition of power in 1933, Göring and his allies established clandestine fighter-pilot schools in Germany and in Russia, which was then on good terms with the Third Reich. Similarly, they reorganized Lufthansa as a paramilitary organization with aircraft that could easily be modified for wartime service.

A physician-scientist and pilot, Heinz von Diringshofen, had been doing aviation research on his own, and, although his exact relationship with the Luftwaffe is not known, he recruited physician Theodor Hannes Benzinger in 1934 to head what would be the new Luftwaffe's aeromedical department at the Erprobungsstelle (testing center) at Rechlin, near Lake Müritz, between Berlin and the Baltic.[1] In Berlin, a Wilhelmine-era civilian research agency, the Deutsche Versuchsanstalt für Luftfahrt (German Aviation Research Facility), had been maintained throughout the Weimar years and in 1934 added a medical branch under physician Siegfried Ruff, an accomplished pilot. Erich Hippke, a physician who had no aeromedical background, went to work for the new Reich Ministry of Aviation in 1935; two years later he was made chief of medical services for the Luftwaffe.[2] He was given the green light to build up Germany's expertise in aviation-related, human-factors sciences and did so by forming new research units. One of these was the LMFI.

Von Diringshofen set up the new institute in Berlin and then tapped a thirty-seven-year-old Westphalian junior professor to lead it. Just as Harry Armstrong seemed to come from nowhere and then became the acknowledged leader in American aviation medicine, so did this researcher from Germany's hinterlands come to be the preeminent figure in aviation circles in his country. His name was Hubertus Strughold.

Strughold's father had been a science teacher and school principal, his mother a housewife, farm-reared but with some higher education and a love for poetry and classical music. The family, which included two brothers and a younger sister, lived in the small town of Westtünnen in central Westphalia, a farming area in northwest Germany. Hubertus took organ lessons as a youth and developed a liking for Mozart, Bach, and, later, popular American music. Until his father's death in 1911, when the boy was thirteen, the two would go for long walks in the woods. Otherwise parental supervision was fairly lenient for the era.[3]

As a boy Strughold had become interested in astronomy. His father had built him a treehouse, and from that lofty vantage point he viewed Halley's comet in 1910. Later he attempted to observe a solar eclipse but used a viewing glass that wasn't smoked quite enough and burned the retina of his right eye.[4] That experience did nothing to deter his enthusiasm for natural science.

Strughold did not serve in the military during WWI, perhaps because he was still in gymnasium (high school) until the last few months of the war. A teen from a family of practicing Catholics, he spent the Sundays of his war years filling in as church organist after the regular musicians were drafted.

When it came time for college, the war was still going on, and Germany had just made it through what was known as the "turnip winter" because people were reduced to drinking turnip coffee and smoking turnip cigarettes. Some three-quarters of a million German civilians died of malnutrition and hunger during the conflict. After graduating from gymnasium in the nearby town of Hamm, Strughold enrolled at the University of Münster, a cobblestoned city and largely Roman Catholic, only thirty miles northwest on the Aasee River. He could walk home in just a few days, he reasoned, if things became that dire again.[5]

Strughold knew that he wanted to study the application of the physical sciences to human physiology and biology, so he took courses in anatomy, physics, chemistry, and zoology; to satisfy his own personal interests, he also studied astronomy and logic. His chief professor was a Rudolf Rosemann, a gifted lecturer in physiology and a specialist in digestion.[6] During his five semesters in Münster, Strughold also took advantage of the many fraternity parties and other social activities at the coed school and learned all of the latest dances. After Münster, he said later, "I was always unbeatable on the dance floor."[7]

As was the custom in Germany, Strughold studied at several different universities to learn from as many experts as possible and to acquire flexibility and a broader outlook.[8] For a semester in early 1921, he moved ninety miles northeast to the University of Göttingen, then a mecca for physics, math, and aeronautics. That summer he went on to the coed University of Munich, a Jesuit school and the largest in Germany. Seventy-six-year-old Nobel prizewinner Wilhelm Konrad Röntgen, director of the Institute for Experimental Physics there, was still giving lectures, and Strughold attended these. The second instructor who drew him to Munich was Ernst Ferdinand Sauerbruch, an innovative chest surgeon and developer of prosthetic limbs. Strughold may have heard of Sauerbruch's use of the low-pressure chamber to make opening the chest during surgery a more survivable procedure.

Highly intelligent, Strughold could master difficult studies and still find time to indulge his love of history, philology, and music. Bavaria was all that he could afford in terms of going "abroad" to study, and Munich was the scene of near-constant political turmoil at the time. He took advantage of its Alpine setting and cosmopolitan atmosphere, though, spending much of his time enjoying the city's artistic and nearby wilderness resources. He visited at least one art gallery every week and took up painting himself. Standing on the bridge over the green-tinged Isar River with the other artists and painting the view, he would be rewarded now and then when a young lady would stop to chat with him about his picture. He would go dancing in the evening and occasionally be able to afford a beer or two. Every Saturday he and some friends would go hiking, leaving the rope-and-piton climbing to others but enjoying the flora and fauna, comradeship, and majestic vistas.[9]

At some point, his eclectic interests jelled well enough for the young Strughold to decide on a career in physiology, the study of the functions and processes of living organisms.[10] In Germany the field was akin to biophysics (in the United States it was allied to biochemistry), and as such it attracted those who were mechanically inclined.[11] Germany, England, and France led the world with about a hundred years of what could be called fairly modern research and instrumentation development.[12]

For his graduate work Strughold chose the University of Würzburg, known for its excellent medical and physiology programs.[13] It was the home of Max von Frey, a renowned Austrian zoologist who had studied under pioneer physiologist Carl Ludwig at the University of Leipzig. Von Frey was highly regarded for his research in blood circulation and sensory physiology, and peers and students described him as an excellent teacher, modest, and warm hearted. He also invented research tools, including the pressure pulse-recording instrument, and was the first to use an artificial lung experimentally.[14]

The practice in Germany at that time was for would-be physiologists to first obtain a medical degree for an anatomy and life-sciences grounding to their studies and then to earn a doctorate and add the research, physics, and instrumentation component. Strughold reversed the usual order of things and went straight to von Frey and told him he would like to study with him and get a Ph.D., even if he had to do the work there at Würzburg but earn the degree elsewhere. Von Frey took him on and assigned a thesis topic. The two spent a year together at Würzburg, and through his mentor Strughold came to learn about the work of August Krogh of Denmark; Joseph Barcroft of England; and Anton Carlson, Carl Wiggers, and Walter Cannon of the United States, all of them friends of the cosmopolitan von Frey. The lab, in fact, attracted many American visitors, including Wiggers, and von Frey in turn went to Scandinavia, Britain, and the United States fairly often.

Because he had already put in five semesters at the University of Münster, Strughold turned his doctoral project in to Rosemann and was granted the Ph.D. cum laude in 1922. He then went back to Würzburg and von Frey for the M.D. This time he produced a paper titled "The Distribution of Pain Spots on the Skin," which earned him a medical diploma summa cum laude in 1923. Those accolades plus the straight A's Strughold received on his oral exams won him a refund of the fifty million marks he had paid to take the state medical-licensing exam. Postwar economics, however, had reduced the value of the currency from the cost of a nice suit to the price of a pack of cigarettes in just a few weeks.

After graduating, Strughold stayed on in von Frey's lab. There he did more research on the eyes and on the physiology of touch and occasionally helped teach some of the seminars. For his work he was paid a modest salary.

To earn his *Habilitation*, a certification required to become a faculty member at German universities, Strughold took a leave from Würzburg in the winter of 1926–1927 to go to the University of Freiburg in southeast Germany. There he researched the patellar tendon reflex. With the *Habilitation*, he was able to return to Würzburg and become a *Privatdozent*, a sort of freelance lecturer.[15] Although at that grade he was not paid by the university, Strughold was allowed to develop classes he thought might be of interest, list them in the university catalog, and teach them using university facilities and resources.

Something happened in May of that year, however, that forever shaped Strughold's teaching and research: the solo transatlantic flight of Charles Lindbergh.[16]

Physiology Meets the Airplane

To say that Germany in the 1920s was obsessed with aviation would be an understatement. Civil engineer Otto Lilienthal had developed the first controllable glider in 1891 and received considerable attention for his attempts to build the first airplane. As a boy, though, Strughold—and nearly everyone else with eyes—had gazed, fascinated, at another German flying machine: the zeppelin.

In July 1900, Ferdinand Graf von Zeppelin, a count and retired military officer in his sixties, had flown a homemade, lighter-than-air vehicle for twenty minutes. After a few years of experimenting and looking for financing, von Zeppelin found his hydrogen-filled craft becoming a fixture in the German skies. Some of them more than four hundred feet long and powered by a pair of 105-hp Daimler engines, they attracted throngs who would stand and gape at these behemoths slowly gliding by. Factory workers and school children left everything to go outside when a zeppelin passed overhead. The public donated thousands of marks to the graf to keep his research going after the first few zeppelins met with disaster; a few even sent him sausages, ham, poetry, and warm socks. At public exhibitions, hawkers sold (without the graf's permission) Zeppelin cigars, Zeppelin cookies, Zeppelin shoe polish, Zeppelin perfume, as well as pencils, spoons, firecrackers, cheeses, suspenders, and cleaning agents with his bald head and moustache affixed, implying fine German craftsmanship. By 1914, his new German Airship Company had taken nearly seventeen thousand well-to-do Germans on pleasure rides. The schoolboy Strughold had likewise fallen in love with the cigar-shaped vehicles and closely followed the newspaper accounts of developments in aircraft design and flight.[17]

Consequently, Lindbergh's solo, nonstop transatlantic "hop" made aviation physiology, in Strughold's mind, the up-and-coming field.[18] He went to von Frey and said, "Here is where physiology can make a new contribution." Heretofore high-altitude field research had been done in the Alps, he continued, but an aircraft could go significantly higher and do so much faster and more efficiently. Von Frey was pleased at this kind of thinking and encouraged Strughold. That fall, the young scientist read everything the library had to offer on high-altitude physiology, then told von Frey that he thought he could create a "cocktail of lectures" that would attract students. Thus, in the winter of 1927–1928, Würzburg's new *Privatdozent* offered the world's first university course in aviation medicine: "Flight Physiology of Man." He charged no tuition and attracted fifty or sixty students.

Strughold loved everything about teaching: having an audience, mentoring young minds, drawing chuckles from students, and working hard to make his own enthusiasm for a subject contagious. The best way to spice up his lectures, he decided, was to do his own research and present the results directly to the students. The obvious platform for that sort of work was the sky above him, and who would make a better-informed and more willing test subject than himself? So, in the summer of 1928, he went to the Würzburg city airfield along the Main River. He engaged the services of a balloonist who agreed to take the new doctor and his scientific apparatus up to test the effects of altitude on the human organism.

Strughold's financial situation by then was better than it had been as a student, when he had subsisted on spinach and rolls with margarine and had lain in bed for days at a time to conserve energy. He had to budget carefully for his equipment and his trips aloft but was still a bachelor, not too far removed from the self-discipline of those college days, and he managed to set enough aside.

Reporting to the airfield, the young professor climbed into the balloon's basket with the pilot. They ascended, and Strughold used a dynamometer, a device for measuring mechanical power, to determine the strength of his muscles at higher and higher altitudes, topping out at thirteen thousand feet. Given the college weekends he had spent painting Bavarian mountainscapes, he undoubtedly took at least a little time to enjoy the view of the city below, the river valley, and the hills in the distance both north and south.

Strughold's physiology training would have told him something about what to expect at the altitudes a balloon could reach. The higher the balloon rose, for example, the colder the air would get. Ears would pop at a certain altitude, both rising and during the descent. If the balloon went *very* high, he would begin to notice the symptoms of what scientists had already identified as those accompanying a lack of oxygen: headache and shortness of breath. Accounts of balloon travelers as far back as the late 1700s warned researchers that beyond that point they would experience vomiting, unconsciousness, and death.

As a research platform, the balloon was a start, but Strughold quickly realized its shortcomings. For one thing, it did not ascend or descend as rapidly as an airplane and could not make sharp, banking turns. These maneuvers caused aircraft pilots to suffer a loss of vision and equilibrium, have difficulty breathing, or even lose consciousness, but not all of these happened to balloonists. Strughold's only mishap came as a result of the inability to steer the airship in any direction but up and down. On one flight, balloon, passenger, and pilot were blown all the way to the Czech border, over a hundred miles to the east.

Perhaps he could try simulating some of the effects of high altitude on the ground, Strughold decided. The university did not own a low-pressure chamber, but it had a device into which he could blow nitrogen, removing oxygen in the process, thereby bringing a test subject inside (himself, naturally) to the equivalent of seven thousand feet. This he did, and periodically an assistant drew blood samples that Strughold analyzed for evidence of hypoxia.

The young professor shared his balloon adventure and experimental results with his students, who were suitably impressed. This was not enough, however. Mulling over the problem of gaining access to high altitudes often enough to get good lecture data week in and week out, Strughold decided the only logical solution was to learn to fly. He went to the airfield outside of town, atop a mountain known as the Galgenberg, and approached the director of a new flying school, ace pilot Robert von Greim. Strughold found that von Greim was very interested in science and quite willing to take on a new pupil and even be a test subject himself now and then. A deal was struck; Strughold signed on for six marks per lesson.[19]

Just seven years older than Strughold, von Greim had downed an incredible twenty-eight aircraft during the war and earned accolades as a "tank buster" over France. The Bayreuth native was a big, broad-shouldered, dark-haired, blue-eyed man, friendly and likable in a fatherly sort of way. As a soldier he was loyal, steadfast, and a genuine leader of men. His awards included a Hohenzollern Hausorden with swords, the Pour le mérite ("Blue Max"), and the Knights Cross of the Bavarian Military Order of Max Joseph, which allowed him to use the title of *Ritter* (knight). After the war, von Greim was able to use his reputation and connections to earn a decent if somewhat precarious living as a pilot. He raised money for a POW charity flying mock dogfights against ace Ernst Udet, and in 1920, he took a good friend, Adolf Hitler, on a flight from Munich to Berlin after the right-wing Kapp Putsch there (Hitler was allegedly airsick the entire trip). The Allied Armistice Commission had confiscated his plane, but for a time von Greim directed a group of pilots who flew mail between Nuremberg and Munich. He got back into the aviation business full time by going to China for three years in 1924 as head of Chiang Kai-shek's Nationalist Air Force.[20]

In 1927, Ritter von Greim had just come back to Germany from China when Strughold knocked on the door of his new flying school. The ace was operating two other flying schools in Nuremberg and Munich and was busy with another postal contract while also serving as director of the Bavarian Air Sport Society. In all likelihood, he was also renewing acquaintances among German flying friends, including Udet and Göring, who were talking about resurrecting the Luftwaffe in spite of the Versailles restrictions.[21]

The two men soon struck up a friendship based on a mutual interest in the flying environment. Strughold would don his leather flying helmet and goggles and climb into the front seat of von Greim's German-built Klemm, an open-cockpit sport monoplane, and the two of them would take to the air for a combination flying lesson and science lab.[22] In between learning and practicing the basics of seat-of-the-pants flying, Strughold and von Greim took turns being the test subject.[23]

Regardless of whether they ever talked politics, von Greim must have relayed to his student a sense of the conditions under which military pilots worked. Most likely he also conveyed what it felt like to have lost a war, to have buried many friends, and to have forfeited the esteem of nearly all of the civilized world. Strughold certainly found the older man to be eager to help him and sought his advice on both flying and personal matters.

The young scientist flew as pilot five or six times and needed only to solo to get his license—when a letter arrived in the mail from New York. It was an acceptance of his application for a Rockefeller Foundation fellowship. This was an honor not only because of the high standards of scholarship required to obtain these appointments but also because of the fellowship's international significance. Since 1920, the United States had overtaken Germany in many aspects of physiological research and had fairly quickly become the best place to study. Furthermore, the program was a concerted attempt by the Notgemeinschaft der Deutschen Wissenschaft (Cooperative Aid Council of German Science) and the Americans to get around the ostracism of German science after WWI, which was Germany's punishment for using poison gas on the battlefield. Especially promising young German scientists were funded for studies in European and North American labs.[24]

Should he finish the flying lessons before he left for the United States? Strughold asked von Greim. Skip it, advised the practical-minded pilot. If Strughold did so much as break a finger, he would be ineligible to go. The flying would keep.[25]

So Hubertus Strughold, M.D., Ph.D., packed his steamer trunk in September 1928 and took the S.S. *Dresden* from Bremen to New York for a year of studying the heart under Carl Wiggers at Western Reserve University in Cleveland and sensory physiology with Anton Carlson at the University of

Chicago.[26] His pilot's license remained forever unearned, but the seeds had been planted for the work he would do for the rest of his life.

A Year in America

Letters of reference in the Rockefeller files show that the sandy-haired young man who arrived in the United States was quiet, courteous, highly intelligent, and socialized well but that his English needed a bit of work. Strughold signed up for some ten hours of tutoring to brush up on his grammar-school English and then plunged right in.[27] He knew his subject thoroughly, having learned from von Frey not only the necessary science but also the hands-on ability to design and use instrumentation.

Carl Wiggers, head of the physiology lab at Western Reserve University in Cleveland, was considered the leader in circulatory physiology. Strughold was to be part of a team studying oxygen deficiency in the heart. One of his jobs was to operate on the canine test subjects, and before long the German found that he could open a dog's chest, install manometers and electrodes in its heart, and close the chest again in only twenty minutes. This greatly reduced the anesthesia and shock risk to the animal, and it was therefore less likely to die. Also given the task of recording canine hearts in action, Strughold developed a cinematographic procedure that Wiggers used to study aortic insufficiency.[28]

The team began work on a project aimed at reviving hearts after electric shock.[29] The research was funded by the power industry, which in the late 1920s was engaged in the enormous process of electrifying the country but faced increasing costs supporting widows whose husbands had been killed on the job. During Strughold's time at the lab, they succeeded in restarting the heart of one dog.[30]

Before he left for Carlson's lab in Chicago, Wiggers did Strughold the honor of hosting an evening symposium on aviation medicine. Among those invited were Albert Wright and Edward C. Schneider, the latter a former Mineola lab scientist known for earlier high-altitude research on Pike's Peak in Colorado. Strughold gave a paper, "The Sensory Mechanisms Involved in Aircraft Control." Not only was it his first public reading, but he had also written it in English.[31] By August, his command of the language would improve enough to enable him to serve as translator for another visiting German scientist.[32]

Cleveland was a steel town, and its economy was growing rapidly, aided by the immigration of many workers from central and eastern Europe. During his evenings and on weekends there, Strughold began to indulge his love for things foreign and for the arts by plunging into the city's burgeoning social scene. He soon found the best places to dance and discovered the talking pictures and vaudeville. There were parties now and then, and it seemed as though everyone had one of those new home entertainment centers: the radio.

When he moved on to the University of Chicago for the next four months, he found the added excitement of being in a metropolis with modern art galleries and contemporary American music, which was completely unlike the Mozart and Bach he had played at the church in Westtünnen. Strughold fell completely in love with America of the Roaring Twenties. From now on, he decided, everything about him would be completely "modern."[33]

In Chicago Strughold performed experiments in the lab and gave a seminar paper on oxygen deficiency and the sensory mechanisms in flight.[34] A local reporter attended the seminar and wrote an article about the talk, extolling the medical acumen of "the German educator."[35]

Strughold attended a four-day physiology congress in Boston that August and quite likely visited the laboratories at Harvard Medical School. At various points during his year, he traveled to Johns Hopkins University in Baltimore, Columbia University in New York City, the medical schools at the universities of Wisconsin and Michigan, the Mayo Clinic, the new Woods Hole Oceanographic Institute on Cape Cod, and Philadelphia, meeting his American peers individually and in groups.[36] He was awestruck but delighted by the easy familiarity with which colleagues and even professors and students addressed one another, using first names instead of the burdensome string of titles that Germans used to keep each other in their place.[37] Even A. J. Carlson had a nickname—"Ajax"—so when his Cleveland colleagues gave *him* a new appellation, Strughold happily accepted it in his enthusiasm for this crazy modern place, America.[38] Herr Doktor Professor Strughold went to the United States, but "Struggie" came home to Würzburg.[39]

Strughold resumed his teaching and research tasks under Max von Frey in 1929. Encouraged by the response to the aviation-physiology course he had offered before going to the United States, Strughold created another class, this time charging the standard lecturer's rate. He was delighted when twice as many pupils showed up.

He linked up again with von Greim, and the two would go out and fly loops and rolls, studying their physiological reactions in flight by attempting to hit a bull's-eye on a piece of paper with a pencil. Von Greim would fly the plane in a giant loop, and Strughold, taking a paper target and a pencil with a blue point on one end and a red tip on the other, would try to hit the center with blue while going up and red on the way down. Then he would take the controls, and von Greim would have a turn. They would fly slow rolls and fast rolls and attempt the same tests again. They would write their names on a piece of paper, over and over, flying higher and higher without oxygen, to measure the degradation of their coordination as their altitude increased. They would climb as high as von Greim's new double-decker Udet Flamingo could go, then dive back down over Würzburg until one or the other of them blacked out. They would make turns and loops in the sky until one person's vision faded to the dull red that meant that three or four Gs were pushing the person's eyeballs too far outward. If they had looked up on the right day, Strughold's students would have seen their favorite teacher hanging upside down from an airplane harness for the full two minutes it took to fly across the city.[40]

HITLER COMES TO POWER

By 1931, Strughold was free to leave Germany. He thought about returning to America and staying permanently. Within a year, though, Max von Frey was dead, and, as heir apparent, Strughold decided to stay on in Würzburg.[41]

A bigger change came in January 1933, when Adolf Hitler and the National Sozialistische Deutsche Arbeiters Partei (NSDAP), already nicknamed the "Nazis," took over. One of their first actions was to place the party stamp on every aspect of university life. Students were told to attend ideology lectures, Jewish professors and those who would not join the party were in most cases fired, certain organizations were banned, and students were coerced into joining party-sponsored groups, sometimes under the threat of expulsion or of not being allowed to take their exams or obtain professional licenses. Hitler put the country under a form of martial law, suspending civil rights and rounding up political opponents of every stripe for internment at special "camps" near Berlin and a small southern city named Dachau. Newspapers, too, were replaced with party organs, making it more difficult to assess the goings-on and predict what would happen next. Strughold escaped party membership and expulsion, but Würzburg was a small city, and he wondered whether he would be able to sit tight in his laboratory and outlast this new regime.[42]

One of his old classmates from von Frey's lab took a different route. Heinz von Diringshofen had gone on to the University of Hamburg for more study with the low-pressure chamber there. Now an excellent pilot, he developed and conducted a number of in-flight physiology experiments, much as Strughold had done, and with his engineer brother Bernd invented new test instruments.[43] He also involved himself in the clandestine rearmament process in the early 1930s that had recruited pilots for a resurrected Luftwaffe.[44] Perhaps he knew Milch at Lufthansa, or Göring, or maybe the notion of participating simply appealed to von Diringshofen as a nationalist or pilot stifled by restrictions on owning and flying aircraft.

Around 1934, someone within the Luftwaffe, presumably at the very top, asked von Diringshofen to start a laboratory to carry out the sort of research he had done at Würzburg and Hamburg. He procured rooms at a military academy just west of downtown Berlin, and, again with Bernd's help, installed a low-pressure chamber and designed a ten-foot centrifuge, the only one in Germany. This apparatus could take both monkeys and humans to twenty Gs.[45] Someone, either von Diringshofen or a superior, named the facility the Luftfahrtmedizinische Forschungsinstitut (LMFI), or Aviation Medicine Research Institute.

Von Diringshofen did not stay on but left to head the Sanitätsversuchs-gruppe der Aufklärungsgruppe Jüterbog (Medical Research Group of the Jüterbog Reconnaissance Group). One reasonable supposition is that he departed because the LMFI was intended for theoretical work only. At Jüterbog he had a late-model Heinkel He-70, high-speed bomber with a modern glass canopy at his disposal.[46]

Instead, one day in 1935, the phone rang at Strughold's lab at Würzburg. Von Diringshofen was offering him the job as head of the new lab. As director, Strughold would report to Erich Hippke, chief of the Luftwaffe's medical corps. On military matters, Hippke reported to the Luftwaffe High Com-mand, that is, Hermann Göring, via Field Marshall Erhard Milch, but with regard to medicine and science, Hippke had the last word.[47] The influence and access the job would offer were obvious.

Not only was this a professional coup for Strughold, but it also offered him a chance to get out from under the local party microscope and move to a big city, where he hoped the political scrutiny would be less direct. Besides, Berlin's fast pace and modernity appealed to him. Würzburg was certainly more urban than Westtünnen, which Strughold claimed was known only for its "solid" citizens and pumpernickel bread, but it was still a small city. With just one lone airport and von Greim departing for the Luftwaffe, bucolic Würzburg was also a backwater of German aviation.

When he left for Berlin, Strughold brought with him one of his assis-tants, Hans-Georg Clamann, some four years his junior. Clamann was a native of rural Groß-Schwülper, in Braunschweig, where his father was the town's physician. Strughold and Clamann had met a few years earlier when Strughold had visited the physiology lab at Heidelberg where Clamann was working on an advanced degree, conducting research in pediatric cardiology instrumentation. Clamann seemed to be an excellent foil for the Westphalian. Both were natives of small towns far from Berlin, both had grown up in middle-class households, and both had a strong philosophical bent. Clamann, however, was media shy whereas Strughold welcomed the press. Clamann was a doer while Struggie was a theorizer and a down-to-earth man rather than a conceptualizer. Strughold's inspiration was "bringing order into diffused matter." Clamann could be counted on for the practical running of the lab.[48]

BERLIN

Germany's capital city was a great change from rural Westphalia, the smaller university cities, and even from the metropolis of Munich, where lederhosen-clad Bavarians could still be seen on the streets. Berlin was on low ground, its elevation less than two hundred feet above sea level, and most visitors described it as bland in appearance and very Prussian in character. Architecturally it was a comparatively new city since most of the main structures in the downtown and western end had been built less than a century before. Railroads, streetcar tracks, and bus lines traversed the city in all directions, giving it a much faster pace and befitting its status as the world's fifth largest city. Moreover, it was the major railway hub in central Europe and an important inland port because of its numerous shipping canals and its location at the confluence of the Spree and Havel Rivers. The population was more than eighty percent Evangelisch (Lutheran) and slightly more than ten percent Roman Catholic. The five percent that had been Jewish was already disappearing.[49]

The year 1935 was one of relative outward social calm in Berlin. Although uniformed men were everywhere and the stiff-armed Hitler *Gruß* was now more common than a handshake, it was still fairly early on in the "de-Jewification" of the country. However, Jewish physicians and lawyers were already gone, and the Jewish population was only months from losing its citizenship rights altogether. The major Jewish-owned newspapers were being "Aryanized," that is, taken over by non-Jews, with no compensation paid to their former owners. It was still several years before the Kristallnacht, however, and before the mass roundups and deportations.

Social policies were enforced through civil measures such as granting government jobs only to party members, mandating *Winterhilfe* collections for the poor, drastically curtailing the enrollment of women at the university, and seizing Jewish estates and artwork, some of it from fashionable Charlottenburg homes only blocks from the LMFI. Two years earlier, party propagandist Josef Goebbels had organized a boycott of Jewish stores, and a mob-led book burning had destroyed thousands of volumes by hundreds of authors from Germany and abroad. The burning of the Reichstag, which had prodded Hitler into declaring a state of martial law that had never been lifted, had taken place two years earlier. Also two years earlier, massive public-works projects, in particular the new autobahn, had put ten thousand unemployed adult Berliners back to work and kept teenagers occupied with city-beautification projects. Food shortages appeared to be a thing of the past, and the restaurants and hotels were doing a brisk trade.[50]

In short, 1935 was an in-between time when one might convince oneself that things were improving in Germany overall, that the future again looked bright for Germany in the world arena, and that this man Hitler really knew how to run a country. The Jews were merely being resettled. If a few individuals or small groups got hurt, that was too bad, but it would ultimately be of benefit to the people—to the *Volk*.

The building the LMFI occupied was on the grounds of an old military academy at the edge of Charlottenburg, an upper-class suburb on the west side of Berlin. An all-brick building housed the labs and offices, and the academy made a lecture room across the quadrangle available for LMFI use as well. The trees and green grass of the academy grounds were well tended. Everywhere there were cadets and older men in the dark Luftwaffe uniforms.[51]

The academy complex was bounded on the north by the city's horse track and technical college, on the west by the college of art and music, on the south by the west-end theater, and on the east by the city zoo. The zoo itself was at one end of the 630-acre Tiergarten, a combination park and wildlife sanctuary that was also home to a former royal hunting lodge. The Stadtbahn (city railway) lay between the academy and the zoo's main entrance. The area also had several pleasant hotels for visiting guests and many eateries to choose from, most of which served wine and beer, and the formal restaurant at the zoo was said to be excellent.[52]

One of the first scientists Strughold hired was Hans Hartmann, a high-altitude physiologist who had studied at the University of Göttingen under Hermann Rein, a former Würzburg classmate of Strughold.[53] Hartmann was an avid climber and had already made a name for himself in the Alps and on a Himalayan research expedition in 1931. He had brought medical equipment along and gathered physiological data on himself and his companions, then published articles on his findings in *Klinischen Wochenschrift* (Clinical Weekly) and the *Zeitschrift für Biologie* (Biology Review).[54] His exploits had also been described in newspaper accounts of the trek to Mount Kanchengjunga in Nepal and in a popular book written by the expedition's organizer.[55]

With a generous budget, Strughold was able to hire as he pleased. Before long he had added to his staff ophthalmologists Ingeborg Schmidt and Heinrich Rose to research color and night vision, depth perception, and luminance; Lothar Landschek for studies of muscle reflexes; respiratory specialists Ulrich Luft, Erich Opitz, Otto Gauer, and Hermann Becker-Freyseng for low-pressure-chamber research; and blood-pressure researchers R. Koenen and Otto F. Ranke for centrifuge work.[56]

Visiting scientists and Luftwaffe physicians detailed to the LMFI periodically made the lab a busy place.[57] Additionally, along with the directorship came an appointment as associate professor at the University of Berlin, authorizing Strughold to oversee the dissertation research of doctoral candidates.[58] Clamann, Luft, Ranke, and Becker-Freyseng received appointments there as well, with the result that students came to the capital city from other parts of Europe and Asia to research under the LMFI team.[59]

THE PROFESSIONALIZATION OF AVIATION MEDICINE IN GERMANY

Germany had no organization that paralleled the Aero Medical Association.[60] This may have been because of concerns that the party might co-opt such a group or because of laws against freedom of speech and association after 1932 or even because Germans themselves simply felt no need for such an organization. A group interested in aviation medicine founded the Wissenschaftliche Gesellschaft für Luftfahrt (Scientific Union for Aviation) in 1929, however, and held annual conferences at which papers were read and discussed. The Lilienthal Gesellschaft (Lilienthal Association), which had a broad aviation theme, was also established well before the Nazis came to power. Strughold belonged to both of these latter groups.

The head of LMFI certainly felt a call to continue mixing with his peers, both domestically and abroad. Strughold described in a 1950 book the significance of such get-togethers during the Hitler years:

Considerable importance was attached to personal contact between scientists. For this purpose medical scientific discussions were held, in which for one or two days a large complex of problems was treated before a forum of experts. . . . [O]nly one topic was discussed . . . and an especially long time was devoted to discussions. . . . [C]are was taken that the attendance did not become too large (about forty to seventy people).

These discussions offered . . . the possibility of getting thoroughly

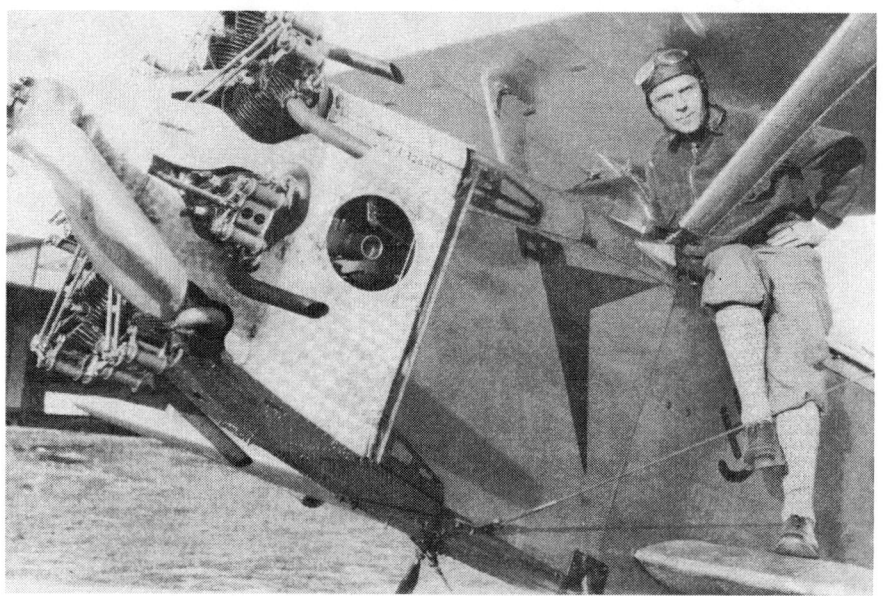

Strughold and his flying instructor, ace and future Luftwaffe general Robert von Greim, practiced aerobatic stunts in this Udet U-12 Flamingo over Würzburg. They gathered physiological data for the young professor's lectures, often flying until one or the other blacked out. Photo courtesy of Roland Dornes.

acquainted with the latest status of a certain field of research. . . . The scientists could exchange their opinions and experiences; they could make and hear suggestions. Moreover, they could make new scientific associations which, in the long run, are indispensable for any productive research. Since during the War, the usual large conventions were not held, such special discussions in a smaller circle were of the utmost importance.[61]

Although Strughold does not say so directly, another function of these meetings that would become increasingly important was the ability to speak face-to-face with like-minded people, to size them up, and to communicate without fear of Gestapo phone taps.[62]

Germany already had one medical journal that focused on high-altitude and aviation medicine, a hallmark of the professionalization of the specialty. Journal publishing, too, was affected by the politics of the 1930s. Ludolph Brauer, then at the University of Hamburg, had in 1933 founded the first aeromedical journal in Europe, *Acta Aerophysiologica*.[63] Up to that time, re-

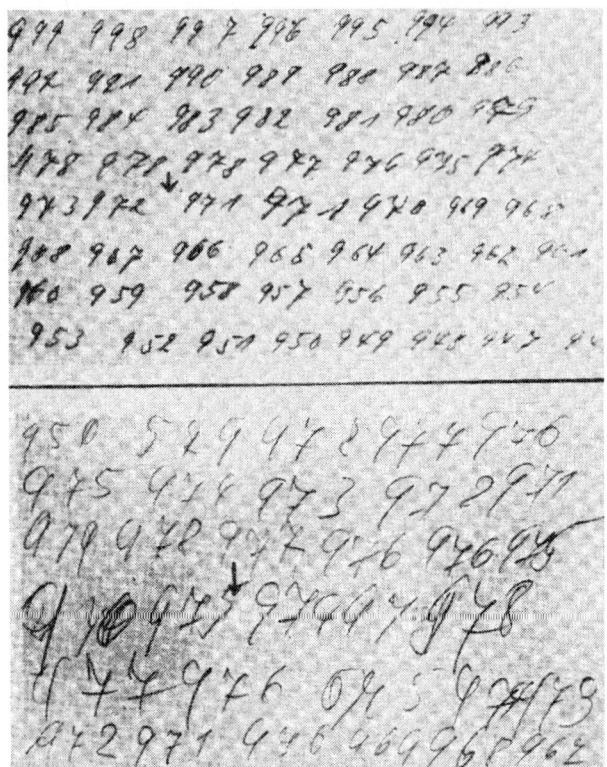

Handwriting samples show the effects of oxygen deprivation. The figures on the bottom represent altitudes simulated in a high-altitude chamber. Reprinted from Sicherheit und Rettung in der Luftfahrt *with permission of the Deutsches Museum.*

search had been published in biology journals or technical periodicals such as the *Zeitschrift für Flugtechnik und Motorluftschiffahrt* (Journal for Aviation Technology and Motorized Flight). After only one year, however, publication of *Acta* ceased. Brauer had a reputation for supporting academic freedom and the participation of Jews in science, so it is likely that he or his publication met with party disapproval.[64]

In 1936, Strughold, Rein (now director of the Department of Physiology at the University of Göttingen), and the seventy-one-year-old Brauer established the *Zeitschrift für Luftfahrtmedizin* (Journal of Aviation Medicine). Who suggested the alliance and whether it was a way for Strughold and/or Rein to help Brauer in some fashion or just a fortuitous combination of talent is difficult to say. However, Strughold used his position during the Nazi years to help others who were not in good standing with the party, and this may have been one such case.

The periodical was modeled after the well-regarded scientific and medical journals of the day, with papers based on original research, book excerpts, foreign news, reviews, and special bibliographic issues, and illustrations accompanied the articles. The LMFI did most of the editorial and publishing work, probably because of its larger staff size, central location, and access to resources. It is not clear whether the journal was peer reviewed.

Three journals sponsored by the Nazi party premiered shortly after *Luftfahrtmedizin*. These were the *Luftfahrtmedizinische Abhandlung* (Essays in Aviation Medicine), a bulletin for university lecturers edited by Werner Knothe, Artur Pickhan, and Georg Weltz of the University of Munich; *Mitteilungen aus dem Gebiete der Luftfahrtmedizin* (Reports from the Field of Aviation Medicine), descriptions of practical applications sent to field medical officers by the head of the Sanitation (medical) division; and *Schriften* (or *Berichte*) *der Deutschen Akademie der Luftfahrtforschung* (Reports of the German Academy of Aeronautical Research).[65] This last periodical would have covered a variety of aviation topics.

Because of the difficulty of obtaining copies of these journals, it is impos-

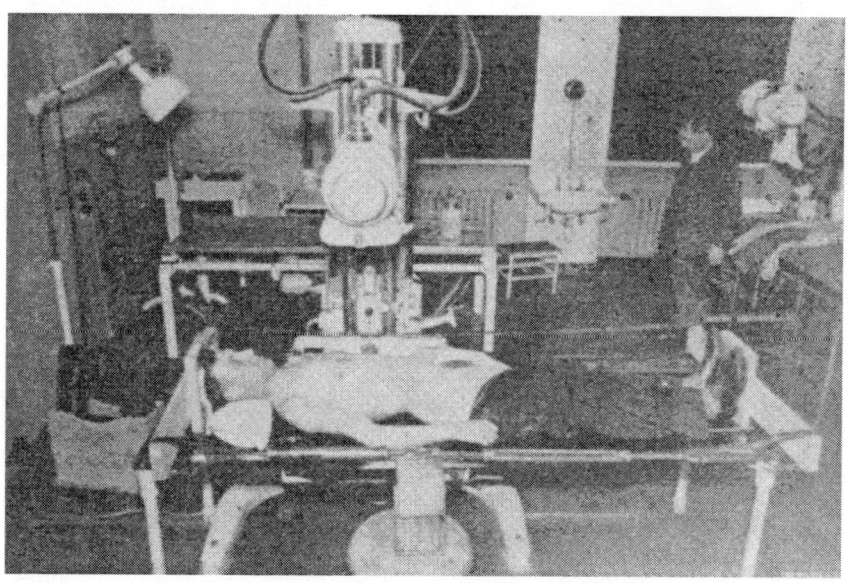

Research at the DVL's aviation-medicine facility in Berlin, under the supervision of Director Siegfried Ruff, at right. Reprinted from Sicherheit und Rettung in der Luftfahrt *with permission of the Deutsches Museum.*

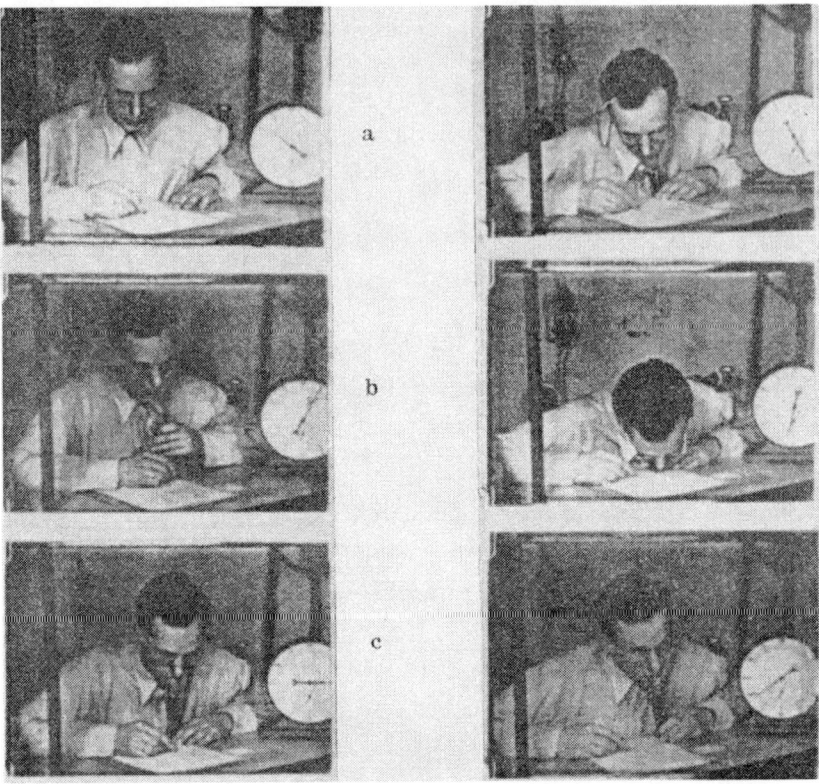

One of the medical phenomena researched at the LMFI was the rare "paradox effect," in which subjects who had first been deprived of oxygen, then were given an ample supply, suddenly experienced a seizure or catatonic reaction, as in the top two photos on the right. German researchers first observed this in 1938. Reprinted from German Aviation Medicine: World War II.

sible to know with certainty how much crossover there was among authors who submitted to these publications. Clamann and Strughold had one article each in *Luftfahrtmedizinische Abhandlung* during the mid-1930s.[66] They may have submitted them to help get the other publication off the ground, to placate authorities who might want to know why these two respected scientists did not publish in party-affiliated journals, or simply to inject some variety into their résumés. An examination of the citations in *Luftfahrtmedizin* does not show any other LMFI researchers publishing in party-supported, aviation-medicine journals, which may reflect their political beliefs or direction from Strughold. It is perhaps telling that the fascist-government-sponsored journal for Italian aviation-medicine researchers, *Rivista di Medicina Aeronautica*

(Journal of Aeronautical Aviation), reprinted only articles from the *Zeitschrift für Luftfahrtmedizin* and none from the overtly Nazi-sponsored publications. Perhaps the science was better, or the Italians were subtly protesting government control.

The increasing number of journals reflected the large number of research organizations studying aviation medicine in Germany compared with the United States, whose only military-sponsored research facilities were then at Wright Field. The Institute for Flight Medicine at the Deutsche Versuchsanstalt für Luftfahrt (DVL) under Ruff and the Luftwaffe test facility in Rechlin under Benzinger were joined by a pathology unit supported with Luftwaffe money at the University of Freiburg.[67] Weltz organized a research group at the University of Munich around the same time, but it was taken over by the Luftwaffe in 1941.[68] In addition, the Reich Research Council awarded contracts to other academic labs and to private industry.

Inevitably, there was some duplication of effort and rivalry, but most of the time these institutions interacted smoothly. They functioned independently of one another, assigning themselves projects on the basis of the scientific

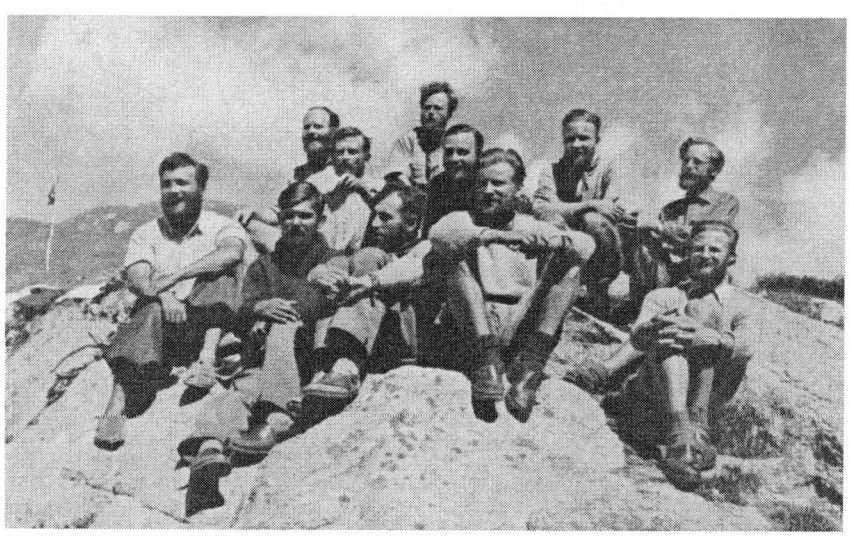

The 1938 German Himalayan expedition failed to reach the top of Nanga Parbat, but everyone returned home safely. From left to right, front: Alfred Ebermann, Herbert Ruths, Fritz Bechtold, Bruno Balke. From left to right, second row: Maj. Kenneth Hadow, Mathias Rebitsch, Ulrich Luft, Paul Bauer. Top row: Flight Captain McKenna and Rolf von Chlingensperg. Hadow and McKenna were from Great Britain. Not shown: Ludwig Schmaderer. Reprinted from Nanga Parbat: Berg der Kameraden, *with permission of the Deutsche Alpenverein.*

interests of the leaders and key researchers. On occasion they collaborated on a single project, or one group would lend equipment to another. From time to time the LMFI would also work with one of the Kaiser Wilhelm Institutes on a project. According to Strughold, that atmosphere of casualness and independence was exactly the way the researchers wanted it and, to him, was the hallmark of scientific independence and creativity. Erich Hippke seldom interfered, considering it his duty only to evaluate the researchers' results and pass them on to aircraft designers and Luftwaffe leaders as needed.[69]

RESEARCH

In 1936, the most formidable problems German aviation medicine faced were those that challenged researchers everywhere: aeroembolism and oxygen deprivation at high altitudes. The LMFI focused on determining the limitations of the human body with regard to differing levels of oxygen and atmospheric pressure. How long could someone go without oxygen—or without *enough* oxygen? How high could one fly before bottled oxygen was a requirement? What other factors determined these boundaries? Could anything be done to acclimate a pilot to high altitude or to lessen the injury to the pilot?

The effects of acceleration also posed a significant problem. Dogfighting required fast turns, dives, steep climbs, and other quick maneuvers. With those moves came blackouts, grayouts, or redouts, the different types of visual reactions fliers had to such maneuvers. With jet aircraft capable of speeds that exceeded five hundred miles per hour already on German drawing boards, keeping the pilot alert, conscious, and able to see clearly during all of these activities would only become more critical.

Strughold thought that his own best technical contribution to these problems was in classifying the atmosphere itself from a medical point of view. He also came up with the concept of *Zeitreserv* (time reserve), known in the United States as the "time of useful consciousness."[70] In the opinion of others, his greatest feat during the LMFI years was bringing together the talented scientists who accomplished important research at the institute.[71] An enormous amount of leading-edge medical research was going on, and, regardless of whether it actually took place at the LMFI or was only published in its journal, nearly all of the work that occurred in Germany can be linked to Hubertus Strughold.

As one example, in 1938, Hans-Georg Clamann began working on the problem of oxygen poisoning, first alone and then with Hermann Becker-Freyseng, a twenty-eight-year-old physician who had graduated from the University of Berlin three years before. Oxygen poisoning—breathing difficulties and even death—had been observed in pure-oxygen environments many times, but scientists debated whether the cause was a lack of the nitrogen found in the atmosphere, a poisonous effect of oxygen itself, the pressure of the carbon dioxide in the blood, or something else altogether. Using pure oxygen during flight had great advantages. It was much more efficient in terms of size and weight to take a small bottle of pure oxygen aloft than to use the bulkier mix of ordinary atmospheric gases. However, if it killed the user, that was small consolation.

Clamann and Becker-Freyseng used themselves as subjects in a test of the toxicity of the pure-oxygen environment. They set up air-conditioning inside one of the decompression chambers and raised the oxygen content inside to ninety percent, well above the atmospheric level of twenty-one percent. Then they went inside and waited.

Nothing unusual happened during the first twenty-four hours, but on the second day Clamann experienced prickling and a numb sensation in his fingertips, while Becker-Freyseng had an elevated pulse rate and body temperature and experienced some difficulty in breathing. On the third day, Becker-Freyseng also began to feel numbness and prickling in his fingers, and in both men these sensations spread to all of their fingers and toes. Becker-Freyseng's temperature and pulse rose again, and he experienced transitory pains in his knee joints. At night, Clamann was awakened by strong heart palpitations, and his pulse rose to one hundred ten beats per minute. Becker-Freyseng, meanwhile, began to experience painful breathing, and his rate of respiration increased greatly. On the morning of the fourth day the experiment was halted when Becker-Freyseng experienced sudden nausea and began vomiting. His temperature was 100.5°F. He was sent to the hospital, where the diagnosis was pneumonia caused by the pressurized, high-oxygen environment. In about a week his pulmonary symptoms disappeared, and in another week the numbness and tingling in his extremities also went away. Blood tests on both men showed that they experienced a temporary dip in red-blood-cell counts and that the carbon-dioxide pressure in the alveoli was as much as twenty-five percent below normal.

The two repeated the experiment, remaining in the chamber another four days but with the atmospheric pressure reduced, as it would be in actual high-altitude conditions. This time there were no problems, only one annoyance that both observed and wrote up in the official account of the experiment: flatulence. X rays showed that their intestinal gases had expanded, pushing up on the diaphragm and leading to abdominal pain and some reduction in their ability to breathe.[72]

Another example of leading-edge work is that of Hartmann and Luft.

Friends in the Deutsche Alpenverein (German Alpine Club) offered Hartmann an opportunity to attempt to climb a second Himalayan peak, the daunting Nanga Parbat, where four Germans had died from effects of the high altitude and the elements in 1934. He accepted enthusiastically in spite of having lost the front of both feet to frostbite on an Alpine expedition.[73]

Hartmann invited his medical-school friend and climbing buddy Uli Luft, now also a physiologist and an LMFI colleague, to come along. In the spring of 1937, a team of eight Germans (including three scientists from other disciplines) made the slow sea voyage to India. With gear plus food and pay for native workers, they undertook an arduous, three-week overland journey across India to the foot of Nanga Parbat, a twenty-six-thousand-foot peak in what is now Pakistan. They were accompanied to the base camp by a few British military officers and dozens of native porters, a few of whom would help them ascend the peak. The group also kept diaries and took still and moving pictures for the books, talks, and documentary film that would help cover their expenses. Using lab equipment they had hauled from Berlin, Luft and Hartmann did blood and respiratory experiments to determine the effects of altitude and physical conditioning.

Then, on June 18, expecting to catch up with the rest of the team and the nine porters at encampment V, just above twenty thousand feet, the tall, red-bearded Luft set out from base camp with three porters. However, no one was at the encampment. In the worst mountaineering accident in history, all seven of his European companions, including Hans Hartmann, plus nine porters had been wiped out by a monstrous avalanche. Luft spent the next few weeks running the effort to search for their remains.[74]

A year later Luft returned to Nanga Parbat and resumed the work Hartmann had begun. He took along another mountaineer friend from medical school, exercise physiologist Bruno Balke, whose father, a physical-education instructor, had from a very early age instilled in Bruno a near-fanatical belief in sports as a way to maintain physical and mental health.[75] Balke had begun helping his father coach younger pupils when he was only six and had supported himself through college (his bachelor's degree was in physical education) and then medical school as an instructor of gymnastics, fencing, skiing, handball, and other sports.[76]

In addition to paying their respects to the many German dead on Nanga Parbat, the two carried out additional blood and pulmonary studies to determine high-altitude acclimation, one of Balke's special interests. Data on the eight mountaineers in the 1938 party, who had spent three months above 14,000 feet and seven days at 23,000 feet, preceded by many ascents in the altitude chamber in Berlin, showed that highly acclimatized people could survive and work at surprisingly high elevations. At a simulated 32,800 feet, more than 20,000 feet higher than the point at which military aviators are told to put on their oxygen masks, Luft noted that most were still lucid enough to complete an assigned writing task. Overall, highly acclimatized people gained at least 3,000 feet in altitude tolerance.

By the time war was declared against Britain, Luft had gained an international reputation for his work on high-altitude acclimatization and respiration. The application was, of course, pilots who went from sea level to 30,000 feet or so in just minutes. The mountaintop fieldwork of Luft, Hartmann, Balke, and another LMFI researcher, Erich Opitz, showed that acclimatized aviators could ascend to 28,000 feet without oxygen masks.[77]

Such research was typical of the work done in the German labs in the 1930s. In the United States, scant mountaintop high-altitude work was being carried out, and the sole low-pressure chamber devoted to aviation medicine was at Wright Field. The Luftwaffe's other labs, in particular those under Benzinger and Ruff, also undertook research using airplanes. Benzinger, Ruff, and von Diringshofen were all licensed fliers and had dedicated aircraft at their disposal. Wright Field again was the only place in the United States where research in the air was taking place and then only when Armstrong could get a pilot and a plane. Germany had a huge advantage over the United States in personnel, equipment, facilities, money, and brainpower.

From the beginning, Nazi-party affiliation was an issue for Strughold and others at the institute.[78] Nearly all of Strughold's peers at other labs had been party members since the mid-1930s. Siegfried Ruff of the DVL joined in 1938.[79] The head of the aeromedical institute at the Luftwaffe's Rechlin proving ground, Theodor Benzinger, had been a party member since 1933.[80] Georg Weltz at the University of Munich became one in 1937.[81] Heinz von Diringshofen, who emigrated to Argentina after the war, was likely a party member, too. Hartmann and Luft had seen local climbing clubs and the sixty-four-year-old Deutsche Alpenverein forced to become part of the Reich's new division of sports in 1934, as had Bruno Balke's motorcycle club. Göring personally usurped Strughold's Lilienthal Society.[82]

At the university research centers, Nazi-party membership was also the norm for the professors in charge. All were government-sponsored institutions that received their funding from both Berlin and their home state or province. Party members controlled the purse strings and put the Nazi imprint on curriculum, hiring, and extracurricular activities by mandating courses in National Socialist ideology and membership in Nazi student organizations. Furthermore, the party controlled students' access to licensing exams; thus medical students could graduate with a medical degree but be unable to practice if they did not show proper enthusiasm for the Nazi state. The 1933 purge of the professoriat had also served as a warning to any academics who might have been thinking of going their own ideological way.[83]

There were exceptions. Nobel physicist Werner Heisenberg was able to say "no" to party recruiters, and his international reputation made it difficult to replace or punish him. He sought out the patronage of Heinrich Himmler as political protection, a genuine deal with the devil, telling himself that he could thus protect German physics from ruination under the Nazi system. Biographer David Cassidy explains this reasoning as emblematic of German intellectualism that was held over from an earlier era. "German academics shunned overt involvement in political intrigue as antithetical and detrimental to scholarly objectivity," he notes. "Politics were beneath the dignity of an academic aristocrat. [O]penly opposing the new regime meant descending into the dirty world of politics, while openly supporting or even tacitly acquiescing to one-party rule was seen as somehow apolitical and objective."[84]

Ironically, for a scientist who did not want to join the party or any of the Nazi-sponsored professional societies, the military could be a good place to hide. The army had weighed in on Hitler's side very early in his regime because of his pledge to restore Germany's military power. However, career officers in monarchical Prussia had traditionally avoided joining any political party so as not to give the appearance of unwillingness to defend the emperor. This provided a useful excuse for Strughold, a civil servant and (because of his job) a lieutenant in the Luftwaffe medical corps reserve, to turn down recruitment offers from party officers.[85] Because of his refusal, those of his staff who wished, Luft and Clamann among them, were likewise able to remain off the party rolls.[86]

It is not quite true, as Strughold claimed later, that no one on his permanent staff had been a Nazi—"only the janitor and the man who took care of the animals," he said.[87] Hans Hartmann may have become a member prior to the LMFI's founding, although he had died well before the war began. Likewise, Hermann Becker-Freyseng, who worked only part-time for the LMFI during the war, was also a party member.[88]

Hans-Georg Clamann had managed to avoid party membership with casual rebuffs: "I don't have my wallet," or "I don't have a pen with me," or "I'll get back to you."[89] Having a sister and mother in Great Britain may have given Luft some respite from the pressure. He never joined the party either, although his friend Balke, as an ethnic German living in the Sudetenland, had become a member of the Ausland Organization der NSDAP (Foreign Branch of the NSDAP) in 1939.[90] Balke did not work for the LMFI, however.

It may be that one story Strughold told about his close call with party recruiters is true. It fits a pattern that other historians have described, namely, that German fascism so strongly supported scientific research that it sometimes overlooked a lack of party credentials, chalking it up to the typical scientist's aversion to politics.[91] It also just sounds true because it has often happened that the scientifically literate have been able to use the ignorance of others to their advantage by means of bedazzlement, fear, or both.

Two officials from the air ministry came to Strughold's office at the LMFI one day, ostensibly on business. They talked with him long enough to establish that they were aware of and impressed by the contributions of the LMFI to the up-and-coming field of aviation medicine. Strughold knew that their real mission, though, was to enlist him in the party because of his standing within this new medical specialty.

"Let me give you a tour of the lab," Strughold suggested, showing the two officials out the office door. He brought them past offices where his physiologists engaged in all kinds of mystifying technical work involving sophisticated X-ray, optical, filtration, respiration, and electrical devices. He explained the studies that were under way to test for color vision and depth perception in pilots, to remove the salt from small amounts of seawater in the event of a ditching, or to aid the heart and lungs in adapting to higher altitudes. His researchers did not have time to involve themselves in politics, Strughold stressed, and their scientific knowledge was too precious and their work too demanding to ask such involvement of them. The officials nodded and looked impressed—but not *too* impressed.

The LMFI director then took the men down to the basement. "Let me demonstrate an experiment," he said, escorting his unwanted guests over to the low-pressure chamber. The device looked something like a very wide hot-water heater made of thick steel and with various pipes and valves projecting from its top and sides. A small window mounted on a door that resembled that of a bank vault gave visual access to researchers observing the reactions of subjects undergoing tests inside.

There was an experiment in progress. Two of Strughold's assistants were inside the chamber at a simulated altitude of twenty-three thousand feet, well above the altitude at which supplemental oxygen was considered necessary for flying. One man had a mask on, the other did not, and, as the three observers watched, the one without oxygen lost consciousness. The pen with which he had been writing slipped from his hand; his eyes closed, and his head hung as his whole body began to slide forward in his seat. The other assistant in the chamber gave the unconscious man oxygen, and immediately he recovered.

Strughold could see that his guests were impressed but not awed. Casually he added, "Our studies are all very risky. They require great ability on the part of the assistants and great responsibility. If the man did not get oxygen now, he might be dead in five minutes."

There was room for three inside, Strughold added, and he would be happy to take the others up to the same altitude. Of course there would be side effects; one person might become very depressed, whereas another might feel very cheerful and intoxicated. The reactions were not entirely predictable. The offer provoked an immediate and, to Strughold, nervous "no," with the visitors claiming they had another appointment in an hour's time.

Strughold expressed his regret and led them on to the centrifuge, which he explained exposed subjects to various degrees of gravitational pull. The person riding the fragile-looking, open-sided device could either rotate in a forward or backward seated position or lie down and be spun in either direction. One of his assistants had ridden the centrifuge for two minutes and experienced fifteen times the force of gravity. Strughold had done so himself, as a matter of fact. Would the visitors like to have a turn?

"That did it," Strughold said. "The older one said to the younger one, 'Herr Oberregierungsrat, we must go in five minutes. We cannot stay.' So they were very eager to quit the conversation; they did not even start their actual topic and they left as quick as possible. They never came again."[92]

Nazi Germany and the Rest of the Aeromedical World

From the beginning, Strughold made it a point to foster a cosmopolitan atmosphere at the LMFI, just as Max von Frey had treated his Würzburg laboratory as a salon where foreign guests were always welcome. He maintained contact with and welcomed visits from Swedish and Norwegian researchers and responded to scientists who requested reprints of various *Luftfahrtmedizin* articles.[93] The lab maintained a subscription to the *American Journal of Physiology* and the *Journal of Physiology*, a British publication, and occasionally copies of the *Journal of the American Medical Association* found their way to Berlin.[94] Every three months, *Luftfahrtmedizin* excerpted articles from foreign journals and reviewed books published in the United States, Italy, France, and elsewhere. Once the war began, visitors from Sweden were occasionally able to bring copies of Allied journals they could still obtain due to their nation's neutrality. The *Journal of Aviation Medicine* was not among them, however.[95]

Besides the Himalayan expeditions in 1937 and 1938, Strughold also financed trips for Luft and Erich Opitz to mountaintop research stations in Switzerland, Italy, and Austria.[96] The Himalayan work would have meant considerable interaction with the British government in India. The Jungfraujoch station, founded with funds from the Rockefeller Institute's International Education Board, was chartered by the Swiss government but supported by stipends from other nations. The Capanna Regina Margherita, a more primitive station in the Italian Alps, had hosted especially hardy and intrepid physiologists since the 1890s.

The work at the LMFI and Strughold's reputation brought at least one American to his Berlin doorstep. Randy Lovelace was touring Europe on a Mayo Clinic fellowship, learning new surgical techniques, observing facilities and equipment, and generally making himself better acquainted with aviation medicine's leading edge.[97] His stay in the German capital coincided with the return in 1939 of German troops from Spain, where they had been supporting Generalissimo Francisco Franco. Lovelace saw those troops march in and others headed for the invasion of Poland march out.

Lovelace had heard of Ulrich Luft, too, because of his work both in the mountains and at the LMFI, but the two men were unable to meet. When Lovelace arrived in Berlin, Luft was high atop the Jungfraujoch, eating quite well, he recalled later, because, with war imminent, all the other guests had abandoned the station. When they attempted to return home, however, the military had commandeered the roads, vehicles, and gasoline, and it was a long and uncertain week before scientists and gear arrived back in Berlin.[98]

Strughold did not get to spend much time with Lovelace. They arranged to meet one evening for discussion, but Lovelace was called away to a medical emergency in England that required his expertise: the salvaging of the British submarine *Thetis,* which had sunk in Liverpool Bay, killing ninety-nine people. However, Lovelace went home and prepared a report on the Luftwaffe low-pressure chambers that went to the desk of Franklin D. Roosevelt.[99] The Americans and Germans would not meet again for nearly another decade.

After his success at the Aero Medical Association event in New York, where he had met Armstrong and introduced himself to the American aviation-medicine community, Strughold appealed to Luftwaffe medical corps chief Erich Hippke to have a similar international convention on German soil. Hippke agreed. Strughold and his staff organized the conference, which was held at the Ministerium in Berlin in late October 1938. Attendees came from several European countries, including Denmark, Holland, Austria, Switzerland, Romania, Yugoslavia, and even China.

Hippke himself gave the opening address, using it as a platform from which to publicize German aviation's return from the dead. He thanked the heads of other Luftwaffe departments, the aviation-medicine specialists, the many medical students who acted as test subjects, Hermann Göring, Erhard Milch, and, finally, "the man, who no less than anyone else we must thank for Germany's resurrection, our Führer, Adolf Hitler." Guests then heard aviation medicine touted as a profession that represented the acme of German science and culture, as Hippke declared that German medicine was truly *völkisch*—reflective of the soul of the people. He emphasized that his country's advances were solid evidence that German science had risen from the nadir of the last two decades. "[I]t is the most brilliant evidence of the inner health and fitness of German spiritual life that German science has arisen like a phoenix from the ashes," he declared, "clear and pure and ready for action as never before, in spite of hindrances on so many sides. So, too, in aviation medicine, in which for us everything is new, scientists go forward to do their work with joyful hearts and light in their eyes."

He closed on a topic close to the NSDAP's heart. The relationship between people and machines, he implied, needed to become completely symbiotic in order to benefit the German state. So, too, science, the universities, and the state must become as one, with teacher becoming pupil and vice versa. Aviation medicine should be a "little sister" to the science and technology of flight, so that, as humans stand "with astounded eyes before a new world, and step by step have to recognize that its size had become ever more immense, they will not go astray."[100]

The leaders of German medical science had thrown a ball and invited the world (or at least Europe) to witness the debut of its offspring. Without a doubt it was a proud day for Hippke, Strughold, and the directors of the other German aviation-medicine institutes. They were far ahead of any other nation on the continent and had a comfortable lead against the United States in pressure-cabin research, mountaintop-acclimatization studies, and work with human centrifuges. By 1939, Germany would have many times the number of aviation-medicine research centers as any other nation and be on the leading edge of ejection-seat acceleration, wind-blast research, and even weightlessness studies. It seemed as though there was no area of aviation medicine in which the Germans would not excel.

Chapter 3

WORLD WAR II

World War II, particularly the war in Europe, marked a watershed period for aviation medicine. Overnight, the U.S. Army had to turn a sleepy medical school into an institution that could crank out physicians, nurses, and technical specialists who were able to work in combat conditions, train other field personnel, and labor in the cold of northern Europe or the heat of the malarial Pacific islands. The war also forced the Wright Lab and the new research arm of the school to attain levels of technical and organizational sophistication needed to serve a postwar jet-and-missile military. Harry Armstrong established a hybrid medical unit in England that functioned as both a training center and a field research facility. All of these actions ultimately redefined the relationship between the school and the lab at Wright Field in a way that would continue through to the flight of the first Americans in space.

In contrast, for Germany's medical teams the global conflict marked a heady time for aviation medicine followed by a precipitous decline in fortunes as the nation descended from world supremacy to dissolution in the face of Allied victory. A few scientists took advantage of the wartime environment to do research on human subjects that went far beyond the boundaries of science and into sadism. Most, however, could do nothing more than hunker down and work as best they could.

ORGANIZING FOR WAR IN THE UNITED STATES

The scale of the job facing American aviation medicine during World War II is nearly impossible to comprehend today. After 1919, demobilization had reduced the army to near skeletal proportions. Increasing it to a force equipped to wage a massive war around most of the globe required an infusion of colossal amounts of money and personnel. Adding those troops was the greatest immediate challenge to aviation medicine.

A few statistics help convey the scale of growth at that time. Over a three-and-a-half-year span during wartime, the army medical corps would have to care for twelve hundred times the number of personnel it had tended in the twenty-four years since 1918, amounting to nearly 2.4 million officers and enlisted men by January 1944 alone. It had to screen thousands of would-be pilots and airmen, then train them to deal with the medical problems of high-altitude flight, primarily hypoxia, which could be fatal to an entire crew. Seven thousand Americans earned pilot's wings in the nineteen years before the war; some seventy-five thousand went through military pilot training each year after WWII began. Using knowledge gained while caring for a relative handful of army aviators, balloonists, and dirigible pilots flying in unpressurized, often open cockpits a few thousand feet above the ground, flight surgeons were now supposed to deal with the bends, aeroembolism, frostbite, deafness, and battle wounds. Moreover, they would have to do so while at very high altitudes during long flights and while fighting a more intense, sustained, and deadly air war.

In anticipation of the airplane's expanded fighting role, the War Department established the U.S. Army Air Forces (AAF) on June 20, 1941. As for the School of Aviation Medicine, the Aero Medical Laboratory at Wright, and the flight surgeons serving in AAF squadrons, the army tried various organizational systems and then finally decided in February 1942 to make them a separate group within the air surgeon general's office, reporting to the chief of the AAF. Following Armstrong's own example, during the 1940s and into the 1950s, personnel from the lab at Wright Field would work there and then move on to the school, leading to a blurring of affiliations, experiments, and functions during WWII and the early Cold War years. Overall, however, the lab continued to emphasize the interface of people and machines, while the school kept its focus on education, theory, and research of a broader nature. While the school was extremely busy training huge numbers of personnel and evaluating new student pilots, the people at Wright tested devices and systems in specific wartime applications.

The total number of AAF casualties in Europe and around the Mediterranean exceeded 94,000, and nearly 30,000 were deaths. Thus four-fifths of the total AAF casualties worldwide were a result of the war against a single nation: Germany. Asian warfare accounted for only twenty-two percent, and stateside deaths less than one percent.

THE SCHOOL OF AVIATION MEDICINE: TRAINING AND CURRICULUM

In October 1931, Armstrong's army alma mater, the School of Aviation Medicine, had moved from Brooks Field, south of San Antonio, where it had been for five years, to Randolph Field, northeast of the city. Randolph was a new base, built in response to overcrowding at both Brooks and nearby Kelly Field.

World War II changed the SAM curriculum drastically. The school added courses on arctic survival and tropical diseases and increased class size while cutting the training period from three months to nine weeks. Physiology training for flight surgeons had been didactic until the school added a low-pressure chamber and six hours of practical work in December 1941. Student doctors stayed in the chambers for three hours at thirty-five thousand feet, a requirement for graduation. After March 1944, they had to take a flight in the cold chamber at forty below zero.

The school also brought in a complete B-17 fuselage as a training prop. Between November 1942 and February 1944, the school held field bivouacs of up to six days, giving doctors hands-on practice in different working environments. It dropped flight training from the required curriculum and instead offered it as an optional two-week course. Other changes provided training specific to combat medicine or to the geographic areas where the AAF was operating. The school added a course on army paperwork in 1941, then pistol and machine-gun training. In late 1942, it gave tropical medicine department status, a nod to the war in the Pacific, and added field sanitation, first aid, and shock treatment to the curriculum.

The school's other function was to instruct and indoctrinate student pilots and aircrews. This meant giving a thorough flight physical to pilot candidates when they arrived at Randolph, Kelly, or other preflight schools, screening them for any of the many defects that would make them ineffective military pilots, and demonstrating to troops the hazards of oxygen deprivation. At flight school proper, the school trained aircrews—navigators, bombardiers, radio operators, and gunners—in the use and care of their oxygen equipment.

The army had to hire a great many aviation physiologists for this last task. It also wanted them young so they would be able to withstand the stresses of repeated simulation flights with the cadets.[1] The physiologist's job was to brief the cadets on what to expect, seat them inside the chamber, check that each soldier's mask was on tight and had oxygen flowing, then slowly take them up to altitude, remain with them at thirty thousand feet for twenty minutes or so, and finally bring the group back to normal altitude. The whole session lasted about two hours.[2] The air surgeon's office set the qualifications for physiologists as a Ph.D. in biology with an emphasis on human physiology "or equivalent training," perhaps certification as a medical doctor. It sought one hundred fifty such people but, given the scarcity of such credentials, never achieved its recruiting goal.[3]

RESEARCH RETURNS TO THE SCHOOL

A surprising amount of research went on at the school during the war years, given the workload. Scientists carried out studies during screening or by compiling and interpreting data already obtained during the intake process. The research centered primarily on sensory physiology, developing vision standards, tests, and requirements for each occupational classification; studying night vision and finding better ways to treat aviation-related eye diseases and injuries; and examining the effects of altitude, drugs, and fatigue on vision and efficiency. The school also investigated causes of ear infections and the effects of altitude, cold, and oxygen on pain and on the development of tooth decay.

The school had studied air sickness for fifteen years. Between 11 and 19 percent of combat crews in training became airsick, with figures varying by crew task. Among navigators, 65 percent became sick, but navigator-bombardiers and radio gunners fell ill at even higher rates. Among paratroopers, 25 percent got sick, some 15 percent to the point of incapacitation. School researchers concentrated on better screening methods and secondarily investigated drugs as possible preventives.

Two groups that focused nearly exclusively on screening were the psychology and neuropsychiatry departments at the school. The former operated primarily from the medical point of view, and the latter from a behavioral perspective, but there was enough overlap in testing methodology and goals to view them as a unit. The neuropsychiatrists used electroencephalographs, photoelectric plethysmographs (measurements of the reaction of the pulse to being startled), somatotyping (profiling body build), Rorschach ink blot tests, and standardized pencil-and-paper tests to predict emotional stability under stress. They obtained interesting medical data but overall ruled the tests inconclusive as predictors of the ability of a candidate to make it through pilot training and combat. The tests disproved some assumptions that had kept certain people from being accepted into flight training, however. Cadets from broken homes flew as well as those from intact families, for example, and candidates who fainted during the exam were not necessarily neurologically impaired.

In March 1942, the psychology section was given the assignment of developing or obtaining tests and testing equipment. They came up with a battery of exams that measured coordination as well as steadiness, finger dexterity, and visual discrimination, including the Multidimensional Pursuit Test, which duplicated simultaneous stick, rudder, and throttle operation. In early 1944, the physiologists began testing the Link Trainer, a small simulator that employed a photoelectric beam to measure one's ability to keep on course. Visual- and physical-coordination screening of bombardiers proved no more successful than pilot screening, but researchers never lost interest and kept trying new means of selecting the best candidates for the job.

The school and lab both investigated the actual causes of death from airplane crashes. Using postmortem exams and interviews with survivors, they determined which portions of the body were typically injured severely enough to cause death and which parts of an airplane (shattered Plexiglas, for example), did more superficial, albeit often gory, harm. The results of their work led to the use of shoulder harnesses instead of lap belts alone, different procedures for crash landings, strengthening of the parts of the fuselage likely to impact the pilot during a crash, easier safety releases on canopies, and, by June 1944, calls for an ejection seat. Both groups also did comparative studies of animals and humans and learned that the shifting of internal organs during abrupt deceleration caused most of the internal injuries.[4]

The Wright Lab and the War Effort

The lab's emphasis was on the integration of people and machines; problems in human-factors engineering, biophysics, and physics; field tests of safety, rescue, and medical equipment; and cooperation with other departments to standardize cockpits and flight gear. The creation and deployment of so many new aircraft in such a short time, compounded by the need to properly equip great numbers of personnel globally for conditions the air corps had never before experienced, made this a time of explosive growth, immense complexity, and great technical challenge.

The research and accompanying buildup was done under the supervision of Armstrong's successor, Capt. Otis O. Benson Jr. A flight surgeon from Minnesota, Benson had served in Hawaii and California, then done graduate research at the Mayo Clinic in the late 1930s, working on the Boothby-Lovelace-Bulbulian (BLB) oxygen mask and more recently at the Harvard Fatigue Laboratory.[5] Benson was three years younger than Armstrong, of average height and slim build, with the Clark Gable mustache favored by many army officers. He was a quick-witted man who kidded colleagues, occasionally with pointed humor. Like Armstrong, Benson had come to aviation medicine from another specialty, but his training and personal inclination were for sophisticated research and administration rather than his predecessor's hands-on, trial-and-error, baling-wire-and-string approach. Under Benson's command, the lab studied tolerance to prolonged cold in high-altitude flight; created an anthropological database to standardize clothing, equipment, and aircraft interiors; and improved oxygen equipment for long-range and multicrew high-altitude flights.

By the time of Benson's arrival in 1941, the lab had picked up four enlisted men, a stenographer, and two Princeton scientists, John F. Hall and Ernest A. Pinson. Two years later, the staff had grown to forty-six officers, eighty-two enlisted men, and seventy-three civilian employees. Earlier in 1941, the lab had moved into newly constructed buildings at Wright Field and acquired a new library, cold chamber, mannequin test room, and a vivarium (quarters for lab animals).[6]

The biophysics unit of the lab concentrated on cold protection. It tested thermal protective gear, primarily clothing, beginning in early 1942. By October 1943, an improved, electrically heated suit was in production after extensive testing at the lab's refrigerated altitude chamber and all-weather chamber.

The physics unit provided technical assistance with issues of light, heat, sound, electricity, and mechanical forces such as acceleration and deceleration, in particular developing instruments and recording devices to carry out and quantify research. Two examples are the remote-indicating electric thermometer and watch-sized recording thermometer-hygrometer (moisture indicator), created in the course of research into crew clothing. Lab personnel also designed a new type of bicycle ergometer for use while breathing pure oxygen to speed up blood denitrogenation before ascent. While designing effective anti-G force suits, the physics unit enhanced the centrifuges, augmenting them with an auditory and visual signal-and-response system for recording reactions of test subjects to high acceleration. It also came up with a thermal-insulation meter and a control panel for regulating the heat supply to various parts of the electrically warmed suits. They improved airspeed indicators, built a wind machine and wind tunnel, and created a freezing-effect meter for frostbite studies that measured the combined effect of low air temperature and wind. They designed and built a pneumatic recorder for explosive decompression, an oxygen-moisture tester, an oxygen-tank temperature indicator, an electric pneumograph for respiration studies, and a "copper man" dummy for the thermal research team. The unit also made theoretical assessments of the optical properties of windshields and bubble canopies and methods of adding nitrogen to the carbon dioxide in life-raft inflation devices so that they would operate at very cold temperatures.

The ophthalmology section worked on matters pertaining to fields of vision, goggles and sunglasses, contact lenses, and night vision. These were tied primarily to aircraft and instrument-panel design issues. They studied the optical qualities of Plexiglas, the degree of curvature of the IBM canopy, and advantages of the new "bubble" type versus the older ribbed and reinforced variety with its more restricted field of vision. The section also studied goggle design and construction, instrument luminescence, and ways to compensate for the high nose angle of fighter aircraft so that the pilot could shoot accurately.

Oxygen-mask redesign was ongoing because so many things could go wrong and so many possible weight-and-supply issues had to be addressed and readdressed. In 1941, during the Battle of Britain, Benson visited England, where he obtained and sent back to the lab a few of the Auer demand-type oxygen regulators captured from German soldiers. These were heavily modified by two civilian contractors working with the Mayo Clinic and Harvard, and their modifications resulted in the A-12 oxygen regulator.[7]

Wartime also brought new organization and funding to aviation medicine as a whole. Franklin Roosevelt established the Office of Scientific Research and Development (OSRD), which included among its eight committees one on aviation medicine. Director Vannevar Bush knew that scientific research was no cookie-cutter operation; consequently, he encouraged initiative and creativity and backed up that verbal support with money. The committee toured the lab in Dayton and wrote a check for $2.4 million to place the facility at the cutting edge. Because of this, the lab wound up administering twenty-eight research projects at universities around the country.

While at Harvard, Benson had learned about anthropometric (body measurement) research from the school's physical anthropology specialists. By 1942, it was apparent that the AAF needed to solve various problems of hatch and clothing sizes, parachute and helmet design, and gun-turret sizing. As a result, the lab made a comprehensive physical survey of aircrews and incoming personnel with guidance from Harvard.[8] Interestingly, the team first collected sociological data on incoming cadets to see whether region, occupation, or ethnicity reflected a difference in body sizes. They combined those results with others they already had, such as skin pigmentation and photosensitivity. Finally, four Harvard-trained observers took body measurements at AAF stations where student pilots were sent after passing their physicals.

The observers sent their data to Harvard daily, and workers at the Peabody Museum there encoded it and keypunched IBM cards for tabulation in what was a groundbreaking use of computing technology. Data pertinent to gun-turret construction were immediately sent back to Wright as soon as the first thousand cards were in. Special needs that came up later, in particular for the next generation of oxygen masks, required that the basic data be supplemented with additional measurements, and for this the lab drew on pilots who were already on flying duty, medical students from the University of Cincinnati, women in the AAF Nursing Division and the Women's Air Force Service Pilots, black Reserve Officer Training Corps (ROTC) students nearby, and members of the lab itself.[9]

U.S. Army Reserve Col. Randy Lovelace had been called up in February 1942 and was already working at the lab under his former Mayo colleague. Raised on a New Mexico cattle ranch, Lovelace had learned to fly as a naval cadet.[10] He was tall and dark haired and described by Jacqueline Cochran as resembling the actor Cary Grant. It was a flatteringly accurate physical comparison, although test pilot Scott Crossfield, who met Lovelace some ten years later, described his demeanor as one of "cordial aloofness."[11] The army sent Otis Benson overseas as surgeon for the Ninth Air Force in early 1943, supporting the Royal Air Force (RAF) in North Africa. He ultimately became surgeon for the AAF's entire Mediterranean theater, and Lovelace took over the lab in Benson's absence.[12]

In November 1942, Lovelace and two Boeing pilots made the first aircraft flight with pressurized breathing equipment, flying to 42,000 feet in a Boeing B-17E. With a Lockheed pilot and wearing a second mask design, Lovelace made another flight to nearly 45,000 feet in a P-38. These two flights proved that pressurized breathing equipment could work effectively above 40,000 feet, but one problem still remained: bailout. If a pilot or crew jumped and then pulled their rip cords early, they could freeze, be shot, or simply run out of air before reaching a breathable altitude. If they went into free fall instead, they might spin out of control and lose consciousness. To resolve the question of whether to pull early or late, the New Mexico physician personally undertook the Wright group's most attention-grabbing experiment during the war years, winning for himself the Distinguished Flying Cross. It was a parachute jump, designed to test a small portable cylinder that contained about twelve minutes of oxygen, enough for a high-altitude emergency bailout.

Even though Lovelace had never parachuted from an aircraft before, it was not something the newest lab director would delegate to a subordinate simply because it was risky. So, in June 1943, a B-17 with novice jumper Randy Lovelace aboard took off, followed by an observation aircraft that would monitor his progress and take pictures of the descent. Lovelace wore cold-weather aircrew garments developed at the Wright Lab, a back-type parachute connected to a static line that would open automatically, and a chest-type parachute as a backup.

As the plane approached the jump altitude of 40,200 feet, Lovelace climbed into the bomb bay, faced the rear of the aircraft, and surveyed the terrain below. The B-17 was nearly eight miles above Euphrata, Washington, and he could see the Columbia River and green farmland. The Flying Fortress flew at a steady speed of two hundred miles per hour, and when the flight surgeon stepped off, he was hit by a blast of air that, at that altitude, was fifty degrees below zero. The parachute opened nearly instantly. The combination of the wind blast and arctic air knocked Lovelace unconscious. His thick outer gloves were torn off, and a thin inner glove on his left hand peeled off as well. Fortunately, the breathing apparatus remained strapped to his face and continued to work.

Observers on the ground and in the aircraft could only watch as the limp form of the thirty-five-year-old physician dangled in the air for twelve long minutes, then hit the ground hard, and lay motionless. Miraculously, Lovelace's injuries were minor. His unprotected hand had frozen, however, and required six months to get back into usable condition.

The army learned a great deal from Lovelace's experience, including some things they had not been testing and that would not have been discovered in an altitude-chamber simulation or with an anesthetized animal or manikin. The biggest revelation was the initial shock at jump altitude. Everyone had assumed the jolt would be less severe at high altitudes due to the thinner atmosphere, but the reverse proved true. When the researchers later did the math, they learned that when Lovelace stepped off the back of the plane, he had sustained about forty Gs. The army immediately changed its procedures and warned jumpers to remain in free fall until they reached an altitude at which it was safe to open their parachutes. Descending from such a height—Lovelace had set a new world altitude record for parachuting—was also safer than dangling in the cold, unbreathable air for ten minutes or more. Lovelace had his Wright crew design better ways to keep gloves and other clothes on the jumper, and they also went over the parachute and discovered points at which it needed strengthening. The chute itself had barely survived Lovelace's fall, proving that nylon fabric was superior to silk.[13]

To follow up on the test bailout, the lab and the Mayo Clinic did further work at Muroc Dry Lake in California, where they looked for ways to measure the forces a jumper sustained when a parachute opened. The device they developed was called a recording tensiometer. The lab also used Muroc to develop an automatic opening device and an aneroid-controlled microswitch for parachutists.[14] Given the incessantly warm, sunny weather at Muroc and the isolation of the site, it is no surprise that the Wright Lab would set up a field station there for both human-factors research and the test flights of jet aircraft right after the war.

Beginning in the mid-1930s, Harry Armstrong had led the research into explosive decompression and searched for answers to the question of what might happen if a pressurized cabin suddenly depressurized due to an enemy bullet or other rupture. His technique had been to drill different sized holes in the low-atmosphere chamber and to fit each one with a correspondingly sized cork. He would climb inside, have a technician take him to altitude, and then pull out the smallest cork. The atmosphere rushed out, but he experienced no discomfort at all, let alone injury or death. Repeated tests with larger and larger holes led to the same result, which was a great relief to the army and aircraft manufacturers, who no longer worried that a single bullet hole might cause instant hypoxia and kill an entire crew.[15]

Then, toward the end of the war, the army brought into operation the B-29 Superfortress, which had started out as the Very Long Range Bomber. Pressurized, it could reach 42,000 feet. Under Lovelace, the lab examined the effects of rapid decompression more carefully. More than one hundred subjects, including flight surgeons and other officers, simulated going from 8,000 feet to 30,000 feet in less than a second. No ill effects or incapacities were noted. Thus the notion that explosive decompression would be fatal to everyone inside an aircraft was proven to be incorrect.[16]

Before Lovelace transferred out of the lab in September 1945, he established a new psychology branch and supervised the building of a second centrifuge, a machine shop, and a wood shop.[17] He also put in some time at the front, flying a mission over Czechoslovakia in a B-17 to test a new pressure-breathing mask under combat conditions and surviving an air attack by German fighters. Lovelace also played a role in the air evacuation of the wounded from Normandy to England during the first few days after the invasion. That same year, he made two trips aboard B-17s from Foggia, Italy, to Bucharest to evacuate American fliers. He received the Air Medal for his role in several missions flown by the Fifteenth Air Force.[18]

Immediately after VE Day, Lovelace and two lab associates went on a secret mission to Sweden, England, and Germany and brought back information on the Swedish Saab corporation's successful ejection-seat design. In Sweden he also obtained a German ejection seat for the Wright aeronautical experts to reverse-engineer. By July 1945, the lab had begun its own ejection-seat research, mounting a telescoping catapult atop a new thirty-foot tower to test the explosively charged device on a willing test subject.[19]

RESEARCH GOES TO ENGLAND: ARMSTRONG AND THE CENTRAL MEDICAL ESTABLISHMENT

A combination of distance, numerous aircrews, and the urgency of combat led a significant number of both school and lab functions to be carried out in the field. This was particularly true in the Eighth Air Force, which was based in England and charged with air support and the bombing of northern and central Europe. The "Mighty Eighth" was organized in January 1942, and by May, its first combat personnel were in England. One of its missions was to validate the belief of the commanding general of the army air corps, Hap Arnold, that the air forces could perform missions of their own and not simply provide air support to ground forces. Proving this required the Americans to push for a new bombing strategy. Rather than drop their explosives at nighttime as the British did, they would carry out high-altitude precision raids and do it in the daytime.[20]

Most of the heavy bombardment in Europe was carried out by Boeing B-17 bombers, four-engine aircraft with gun turrets mounted in various locations on the fuselage and in the tail section and a Plexiglas nose occupied by the bombardier, who also had several guns. The B-17s carried a crew of ten and a widely varying number of bombs, depending on their size. Fully loaded with bombs and gasoline, they struggled to attain the 145 miles per hour needed to lift off of the marshy grass runways that were typical of the rainy British Midlands. Returning on fumes with just the crew, the plane might be flying at 195 mph. They flew eight- or nine-hundred-mile missions, some as long as thirteen hours and nearly all on oxygen and in extreme cold. Without bombs, the aircraft could reach an altitude of about thirty thousand feet. Thus, early in the war, at least, they were able to return to bases in England at an altitude higher than some of Germany's fighter aircraft could reach.

Protection for the daylight bombers—as well as insurance that the target would be effectively hit—included fighter escorts and enormous flight formations. In a typical mission, three squadrons of B-17s might take off from England and meet at a prearranged spot over the water as a bomb group of 51 airplanes. Bigger missions could involve an entire air division of three such bomb groups flying in tiered formation. On very large raids, multiple divisions, three or four such 153-aircraft units, would group together, flying an aerial "train" that stretched for miles and dropping their deadly cargo for what must have seemed to those on the ground like eternity.[21]

One aeromedical field contribution was made by the flight surgeon who had preceded Armstrong at Wright Field, Brig. Gen. Malcolm Grow. By October 1942, seventy percent of Eighth Air Force wounds were due to low-velocity German missiles, *fliegerabwehrkanone*, or flak. Consequently, Grow, then surgeon of the Eighth Air Force, personally took on a project to design body armor for use in the air. When complete, his flak suit weighed more than twenty pounds: seven pounds for the front vest only (worn by the pilots), sixteen for the full vest (worn by the bombardiers, navigators, and gunners), and five or six for the sporran (worn by the standing crew). A sort of ripcord allowed the crew to take off the vests before bailout. Later Grow's team developed armpit and neck guards and the quick-release "Grow helmet," which weighed half as much as an infantry soldier's helmet and had cutaways around the ears.

The flak gear was not universally popular. Ball-turret gunners, for example, were short men whose station was a hydraulically lowered cylinder that hung beneath the fuselage and behind the bomb bay. The occupant fired a machine gun, half-sitting, half-reclining and with his knees up around his ears. His station offered no room for a parachute and scant space for flak garments. Similarly, the bombardier in the clear nose of the plane was also in a tight space and exposed to sunlight. To drop bombs, he had to clamber up and over the bombsight, lying flat on his stomach with his head against the Plexiglas. The added warmth of the flak gear was not always welcome, and the bulk made it nearly impossible to do his job. Once the aircraft entered the airspace over a heavily defended German industrial center, though, a bombardier might take the components of a flak suit or two and use them to line his station, reserving one to sit on. Between the helmets and the armor, Grow's gear cut the death rate from flak or shrapnel from 35 to 21 percent.[22]

Another more formal operation was the Eighth Air Force's Provisional Medical Field Service School, later renamed the Central Medical Establishment (CME), which opened on August 10, 1942. It was the brainchild of Harry Armstrong, who had observed that many early casualties were the result of insufficient medical and safety training among the aircrews. An onsite education facility might reduce this, Armstrong reasoned. The CME was divided into five units: altitude training, psychiatry, research and development, instruction, and the Central Medical Board.[23]

The first challenge was to instruct the AAF personnel, especially the medical staff, in aviation physiology and the use of life-saving gear. This was practically all the CME did in 1942. In 1943, the bases in England began to get more graduates from the SAM, so the CME began to include recent medical discoveries, problems specific to the Eighth Air Force, and administrative work. It trained 438 medical people in the next nineteen months and another 640 people to be "unit equipment officers" to reduce casualties caused by failures in protective gear. The equipment-officer program expanded to include officers from the Ninth Air Force and a few from the Twelfth and Fifteenth Air Forces, who were fighting in the Mediterranean theater.

The CME also gave classes in psychiatry to a medical representative from every combat group. It used mobile altitude chambers to train medical personnel, both commissioned and noncom, in diagnosing and treating medical problems in aircrews. Seemingly small and unrelated things such as creating detailed diagrams of ditching procedures saved approximately 650 lives.

Another scheme established mobile medical units at Royal Air Force stations to which returning American crews might be taken after ditching in the North Sea or English Channel. Jurisdictional disputes between the RAF and AAF had resulted in costly delays in treatment. This move raised the survival rate from an incredibly low 1 ½ percent in early 1943 to a much more robust 43 percent in 1944.

A leading cause of death remained anoxia—lack of oxygen. About twenty percent of these deaths occurred among men who were on their first high-altitude mission and who had insufficient training in the proper use of oxygen gear. Some of them were holding their masks on with their hands, others did not understand the mask's components, some plugged them into the wrong outlet, and many used borrowed, ill-fitting masks. In February 1943, the CME began putting crew members in the new low-pressure chambers, and by the end of the year the CME had trained more than a thousand soldiers. Anoxia due to poor indoctrination practically disappeared from the casualty list.

Maintenance of the breathing devices in flight was the second component of the antianoxia efforts. During their six-to-eight-hour missions—ten, eleven, or more if the target was Danzig or Vienna—crew members were ordered to constantly check each other and avoid isolation. They frequently had to wring out the sponge-rubber portions of the older models of oxygen masks to avoid freezing, and many soldiers simply modified them on their own, so the army finally issued everyone two masks. The CME designed a special baffle for later-model masks that worked significantly better in extreme cold. By November 1943, the number of anoxia deaths had plummeted from 27 to just 7 per 100,000, a reduction of sixty-eight percent.

Early on, half of the injuries were the result of frostbite, mostly to the hands or feet, but the face, neck, and ears of crew members exposed to wind blast were also "bitten." The chief culprit was, again, altitude. The average temperature inside a B-17 at bombing altitude ranged from a low of forty-five

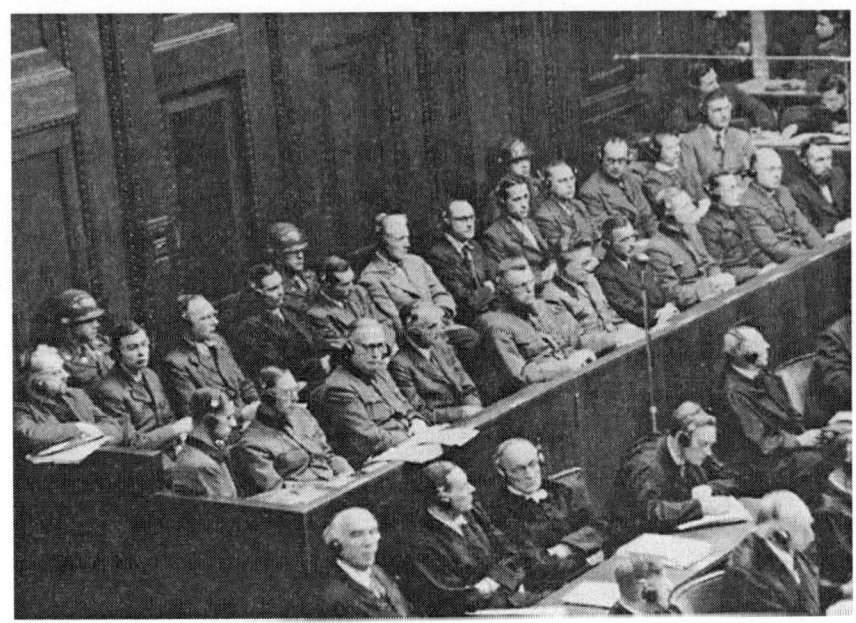

In the dock at Nuremberg, U.S. v. Karl Brandt et al., *Ruff is second from left in the top row. To his left are another defendant, then Romberg, another defendant, Weltz, Schäfer, and Becker-Freyseng. Oskar Schröder is in the front row, fourth from left. U.S. National Holocaust Museum photo.*

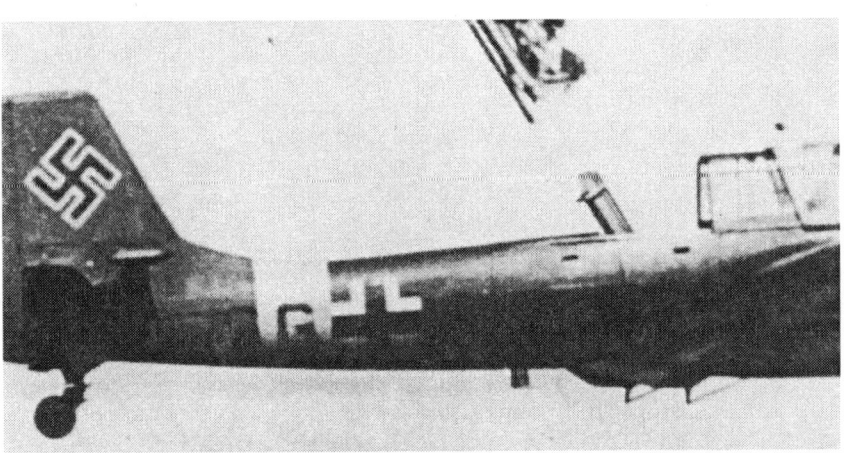

The first human tests of an ejection seat were carried out at the Rechlin test station in 1941. Reprinted from Sicherheit und Rettung in der Luftfahrt, *with permission of the Deutsches Museum.*

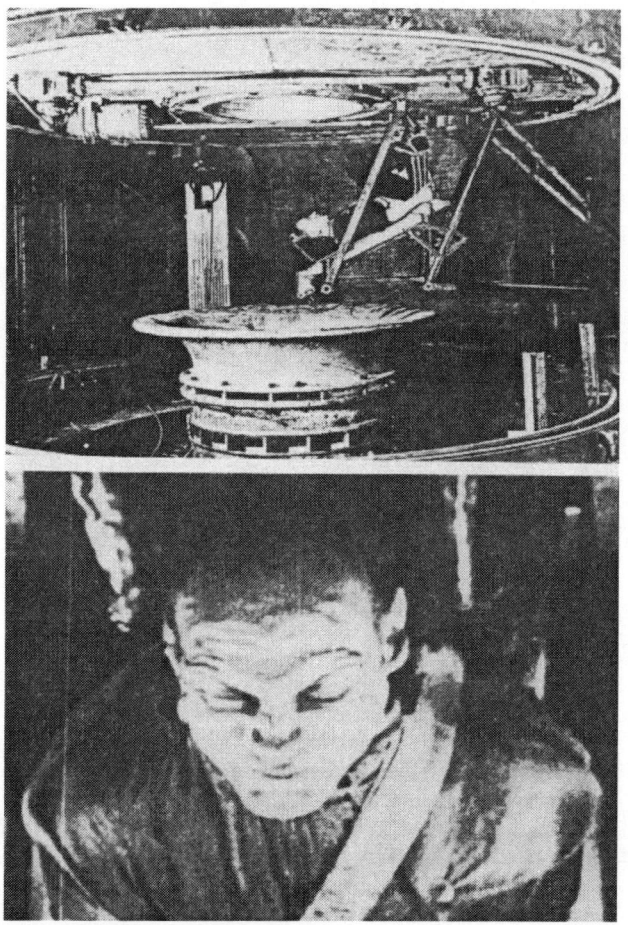

Ruff used an aircraft manufacturer's wind tunnel to examine the facial effects of high-speed, high-altitude bailouts. The volunteer test subject here is one of his lab employees. Reprinted from Sicherheit und Rettung in der Luftfahrt, *with permission of the Deutsches Museum.*

degrees below zero (Fahrenheit) during the winter to a "high" of six above in summer. Between November 1942 and December 1943, more than sixteen hundred crew members were removed from duty because of frostbite, and the following year the number continued to rise, albeit slightly. The injured missed ten and a half days on average, and seven percent never returned to combat.

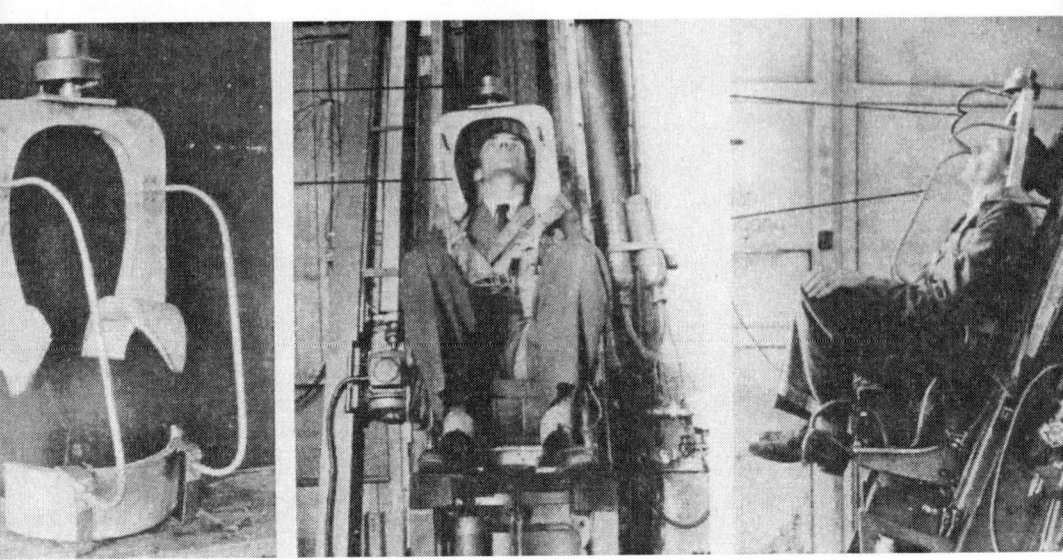

Another research tool was this vertical accelerator outfitted with an oscilloscope. It was used at the Heinkel aircraft manufacturing plant to test the effects of abrupt acceleration and deceleration on the human frame. Reprinted from Sicherheit und Rettung in der Luftfahrt, *with permission of the Deutsches Museum.*

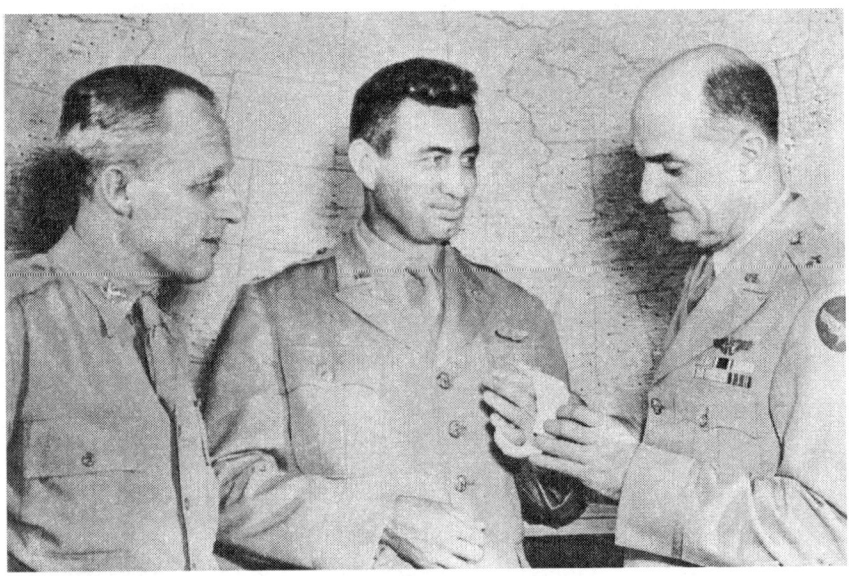

Randy Lovelace displays his frostbitten hand. He received the wound—and the Distinguished Flying Cross—for a daring high-altitude parachute jump (his first) to test an oxygen bailout system. National Library of Medicine photo.

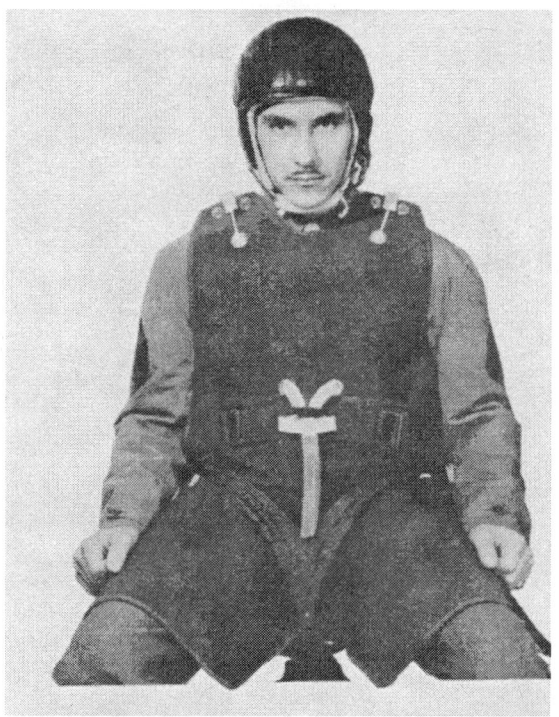

The flak suit and helmet worn by American air crews during WWII were the creation of Malcolm Grow, later the first surgeon general of the U.S. Air Force. U.S. Army photo, reprinted from Medical Support of the Army Air Force in World War II.

The CME focused on developing better protective gear, including electrically heated clothes, shoes, and rescue blankets. Tail and ball-turret gunners usually wore heated suits later in the war, as did waist gunners if enough electricity was available. The suits were known to catch fire, though, if misused. A few of the men wore them in the rain or during preflight warm-up exercises. Others donned them (improperly) over the uniform or with too many pairs of socks. Sometimes the wearers simply didn't maintain their suits.

Modifying the aircraft was a second means of preventing frostbite. Wind blast was a major issue for gunners because they had to remove Plexiglas windows over their guns, creating large openings in the fuselage, in order to pivot their weapons. The CME worked with engineering and bombardment groups to develop an insert to reduce wind blast in the B-17's tail. It recommended other modifications to deflect the wind at the waist and increase the electrical current available for heated suits.

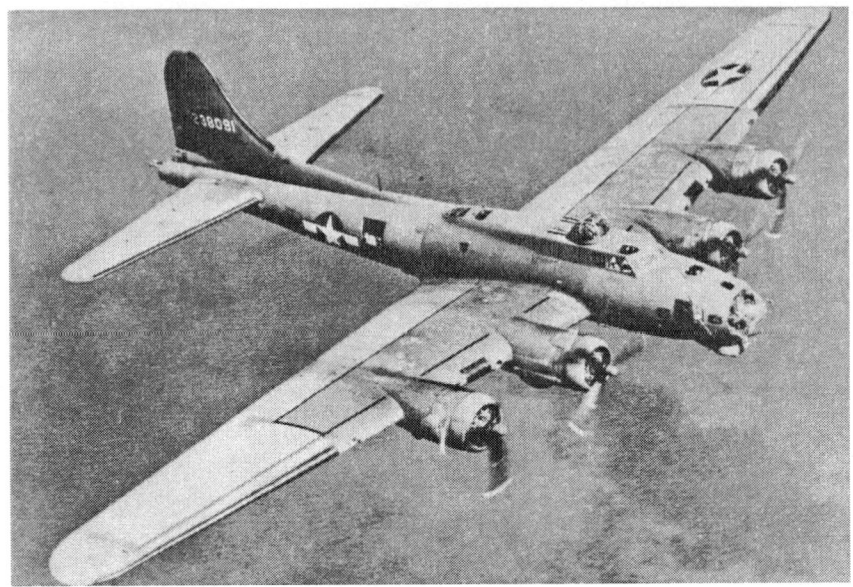

B-17 "Flying Fortress." USAF photo.

Armstrong became chief surgeon of the Eighth Air Force in March 1944, still a year before the victory in Europe. By then the Mighty Eighth had a combined strength of nearly 190,000 men and women, including 300 flight surgeons. Total medical personnel numbered almost 4,000. The strategic goal they were supporting was round-the-clock bombing of Germany.[24] The end of Hitler's Third Reich was approaching.

GERMAN LABORATORIES AND THE WAR

During the war, things were very different for aviation medicine in Germany. The Luftwaffe fought primarily a defensive war after 1942 and did not, as a rule, carry out long-range bombing sorties. It also did not engage in extended high-altitude flying early on but preferred strafing tactics and dive-bombing using smaller aircraft. German airplane designers sought to give their pilots an edge by making their vehicles more maneuverable, faster, or able to carry more armament. High-speed turns, climbs, and dives exposed their pilots to great accelerative and decelerative forces and the accompanying problem of blackout.

Once the Allies moved to higher altitudes of operation, the engineers at Junkers, Messerschmitt, Fokker, Dornier, Heinkel, and other companies responded with pressurized cabins, higher-altitude capability, and faster speeds for their own pursuit aircraft. Germany developed and deployed the first jet to fly in air-to-air combat and the first rocket-powered airplane. In 1938, German aircraft designers started working on ejection seats and entire ejectable cockpits for their new high-speed aircraft.[25] Consequently, around 1940, German labs began to test human performance, including bailout, at altitudes above thirty-five thousand feet. They also looked at the effects of extreme cold and reaction to speeds exceeding five hundred miles per hour and G forces of twenty times the normal force of gravity. Late in the war,

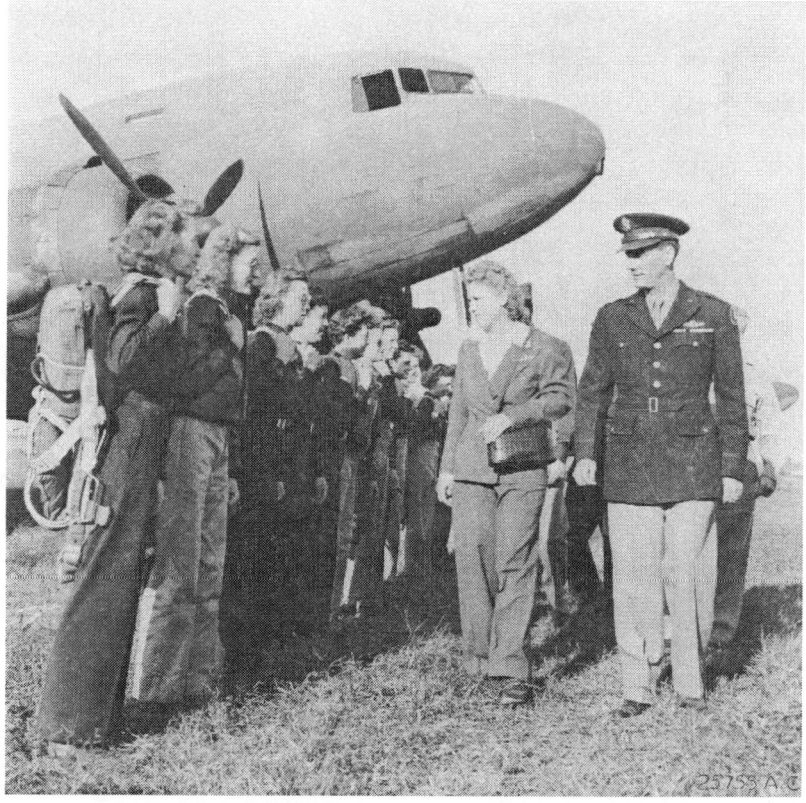

WASP director Jacqueline Cochran inspecting a group of women pilots who were responsible for towing airborne targets to provide novice gunners with practice before heading off to war. Photo courtesy of the Texas Women's University WASP Collection.

they began working on issues raised by the V-1 buzz bombs that had been modified to hold suicide pilots. With jet and missile research, any parity that American medicine had achieved early in the war was shifting again to favor the Germans.

Postwar records, particularly transcripts of the war-crimes trials of the Luftwaffe leaders, give the impression that infighting was rampant within the German air force and that few actually subscribed to Hitler's vision of racist, genocidal expansionism. Much of such testimony remains suspect as the self-serving rationalizations of those charged with capital offenses. On the other hand, it has also been demonstrated that Heinrich Himmler's Schutzstaffel (SS) was a rival for Luftwaffe power and authority and that Hitler was a very capricious leader. Adept political maneuvering and extreme adaptability were required to stay in Hitler's good graces. Because of this, people farther down the chain of command wound up working on projects that started and stopped or achieved "wonder-weapon" status overnight; they might also find that their funding had suddenly been cut off. Scientists were subject to serving time as ordinary field physicians on some far-away front. Technical designs, particularly building construction, were subject to the Führer's artistic whims, and even the highest-placed people were constantly on guard lest someone find—or even suspect—a Jew in their family tree. Hermann Göring's own second-in-command, Erhard Milch, had to "prove" his own illegitimacy in order to avoid the taint of his father's alleged Jewish ancestry. The Nazi regime brought chaos, deceit, destruction, and immorality to its military, and as a consequence, many of the actions, projects, decisions, and behaviors make little sense to us today. That, however, does not make them any less true.

THE WEAPONS AND THE RESEARCH

In 1933, Hitler established the Luftwaffe and Reichsluftfahrtministerium (Air Ministry) under Hermann Göring. From their inception, research was to be a critical function because Nazi leaders had plans that required a superior military. Engineering-oriented human-factors studies similar to those at Wright Field went on under the auspices of the Technisches Amt (Technical Office) at the Deutsche Versuchsanstalt für Luftfahrt (German Aviation Test Facility; DVL) in Berlin and at the Luftwaffe test station in Rechlin. In this manner, research was supervised by the same center that monitored the design and testing of new military aircraft. Theoretical work and studies somewhat removed from immediate applications to the military were under the supervision of the Chef des Sanitätswesens (chief of medical services). These included Strughold's LMFI, the institutes for aviation medicine at the universities of Hamburg and Munich, von Diringshofen's Sanitätsversuchs- und Lehranstalt (Medical Research and Teaching Institute) at Jüterbog, and the Institut für Luftpathologie (Institute for Aviation Pathology) at the University of Freiburg.[26]

The Technical Office had to deal with a proportionately larger number of aircraft makers than the Allies since German firms produced a great array of designs rather than banding together to build just a few models in large numbers. Each manufacturer also had a favorite design or application for its aircraft, and political conditions favored some companies over others. Junkers and Messerschmitt, for example, were allowed to use conscript labor in their manufacturing plants. In contrast, Klemm, a family-owned firm that had specialized in sport aircraft, saw its operation taken over by the Nazi govern- ment after turning down the "opportunity" to build military aircraft.[27]

Most of the leading-edge designs were technical successes but the problems of maintaining production while under bombardment, the scarcity of raw materials, and the caprices of those at the top of the party or the Luftwaffe hierarchy meant that most were never mass produced. One example was the Henschel Hs-130, a bomber that could go higher than forty thousand feet. Technically that was quite an accomplishment, but the Luftwaffe had no real reason to fly bombing missions at that altitude, so the design languished. The Heinkel He-178 was the first jet aircraft developed and actually flown. It was tested very early in the war, in 1939, but never mass produced—the prototype was already on display in the Berlin Air Museum in 1943, when it was destroyed by an Allied bomb.

Another early jet aircraft, the Messerschmitt Me-163 Komet, could fly at 600 miles per hour. Streaking past Allied pursuit aircraft, it was nearly unbeatable, but it used highly volatile and toxic propellants that made ground operations ungainly and very dangerous. It went into production near the end of the war, and some 370 were used, but they were too late to turn the tide. Similarly, the Messerschmitt Me-262, a single-seat, jet fighter-bomber, flew first in April 1941, going 540 miles per hour. Nearly 1,300 were produced, but it was September 1944, seven months before the war's end, before they finally reached the Luftwaffe squadrons. Only a hundred flew in combat.[28]

These new designs raised questions of physiological adaptation to high altitude, both in flight and during bailout and descent. One aircraft, for example, was known for its ability to climb to altitude very quickly, reaching fifty thousand feet in under three minutes. The pilot would need an ejection mechanism, a bailout bottle containing oxygen, and a protocol for how and when to eject in an emergency. High-speed, high-altitude bailouts exposed pilots to conditions of low pressure, thin atmosphere, and severe wind blast.

Siegfried Ruff and Hans Romberg at the DVL and Ulrich Luft and Erich Opitz of the LMFI researched the physiological responses to rapid ascent using low-pressure chambers in their labs or hauled into the Austrian Alps. Their work showed that pilots without oxygen felt fine while going up because three minutes was usually within their *Zeitreserv*. However, if they went past that reserve, they developed hypoxia. Moreover, the time needed to recover consciousness after a blackout depended not on the altitude itself but on the time previously spent at similar altitudes, that is, it depended on a pilot's conditioning. An additional danger was that pilots who were aware of oncoming sickness might immediately descend to a more manageable altitude but still pass out since the effects of oxygen deficiency are not quickly reversible.

With high-speed aircraft, a mastery of linear acceleration was important for evaluating the forces involved in crash landings, parachute openings, ejection-seat use, and any future manned missile flights. Ruff and Otto Gauer of the LMFI were the main investigators in acceleration forces. In one instance they evaluated captured anti-G suits from American P-51 Mustang aircraft. In another experiment Siegfried Ruff, who believed it would be possible to send a human being up inside a missile, shot off an unmanned V-1 using a catapult and captured the launch on film.[29]

When aircraft makers introduced new jet- and rocket-propulsion units, pilots blamed them for a variety of real and anticipated disorders, such as impotence, upper-respiratory ailments, and deafness. Scientists had to study and either prove or disprove such connections, sometimes examining the complainant to determine what other factors in the pilot's life might account for the symptoms. One pilot who claimed to have a nervous disorder actually turned out to have multiple sclerosis. Other pilots were simply overworked and likely undernourished. Reports of hearing impairment seemed more reasonable, and one researcher developed a new audiometer to precisely evaluate hearing impairment among fliers and test-stand workers.

A complete list of research projects would show many that were set aside due to the war before any useful conclusions could be reached or mass manufacture begun. One example is body armor. The von Diringshofen brothers and the team at Jüterbog studied captured American flak suits and found their resistance to gunfire to be very high. However, a lack of materials sidelined the Germans' plans to make suits for their fliers, and time ran out before an alternate plan to weave synthetic fibers into a bulletproof vest could be carried out. Similarly, the University of Berlin began, but did not finish, a study of the toxicological problems associated with rocket-propelled fighter aircraft. Ruff did not complete his V-1 launch studies, and the universities of Heidelberg and Strassburg could not complete their work on the use of drugs to improve altitude tolerance. The DVL obtained data on dental problems among fliers but never tabulated them. Researchers created and tested heat-radiation-reflecting suits, but a shortage of aluminum prevented their manufacture and distribution to rescue personnel in cities under bombardment. An electric blanket for use by water-rescue teams did not even reach the testing stage.

A major part of Germany's aviation-medicine research was abandoned solely for political reasons. In January 1942, the Luftwaffe abolished the use of psychological screening among pilot candidates on the grounds that it gave only a "snapshot of the personality, but it would not provide a motion picture which gives a true reproduction of the actual psychic processes; likewise it would not permit prediction as to the future fitness of the flier."[30] Perhaps not, but this policy prevented medical personnel from accumulating a large body of data that could have served as a point of reference in future research.[31]

The order came from the office of the chief of the medical service, Erich Hippke. It may have been personal preference, a lack of useful data on the validity of psychological evaluations, or a dearth of personnel and resources. Another likely reason is Nazi prejudice against psychiatry as a "Jewish" science: invalid, *unvölkisch*, and likely to corrupt the German people. Tellingly, an American who met one such psychologist who had emigrated to the States after the war remarked several years later that the German was "bitter toward the Nazis, having stated that his career had been threatened by the . . . regime back in 1942 when [they] had reduced psychology to a second-rate science."[32] In his postwar writing, Strughold did not explain the thinking behind the decision but stated "Some psychologists, however, stayed with their units giving advice on purely military questions," indicating that this had been a top-down decision and that unit commanders still wanted advice. Whatever the reason that psychiatry and psychology fell out of favor, subsequent research in the Luftwaffe was officially limited to attempts to improve efficiency by means of caffeine tablets, cola beverages, and benzedrine.[33]

THE DACHAU EXPERIMENTS

German aeromedical researchers believed that humans made the best test subjects despite the fact that injuries and even one death were known to have occurred due to the low-pressure chamber.[34] When subjects fainted inside the device, they later did not recall even feeling ill, let alone losing consciousness; they simply resumed working as though nothing had happened, much like Armstrong had done in Dayton.[35] Working on oneself, like-minded coworkers, and the occasional flying cadet from the academy next door was more efficient than recruiting and training outsiders, too. Furthermore, medical journals would have reinforced the belief that this practice was the norm in the rest of Europe and North America.[36] Because the Nazi regime devalued individuals and saw human worth only in the capacity to produce for the state, keeping this sort of experimentation within a small, closed community of trusted colleagues must have strengthened the professional bond and thus been emotionally and spiritually valuable.

Autoexperimentation also tended to separate practitioners from accusations of conducting "Jewish science." Hitler had already applied that label to psychiatry and theoretical physics because the seminal work there had been done by Sigmund Freud, Albert Einstein, Niels Bohr, and others with Jewish ancestry. The label "Jewish" sentenced adherents to professional ostracism, isolation, and ridicule from the Nazi government, which controlled university appointments and funding. Self-experimentation was Aryan, the thinking went, since the Talmud prohibited endangering one's life. Experimenting on someone else was a "Jewish" (and by implication, cowardly) thing to do.[37]

There was no such thing as staying too far away from embroilment in the party and its pursuits. In an affidavit for the Nuremberg court after the war, when several colleagues were tried for their role in experiments at Dachau, Strughold stated that the Gestapo "took measures against" dissident doctors and labeled them saboteurs. He cited two of his researchers who had been threatened after stating that they were unable to corroborate someone else's research findings. Those physicians, he revealed after the war, were ophthalmologists Heinrich Rose and Ingeborg Schmidt. During the hearings, it also came out that Heinrich Himmler had personally uttered threats against aviation-medicine researchers who shied away from using human subjects or who preferred to use Luftwaffe pilots instead of condemned criminals. The party supported the research of its loyal members, regardless of the quality of their work, and truth was not always welcome in the Nazi Party.[38]

A few aviation-medicine researchers placed themselves in even worse positions than Rose and Schmidt. They became involved in deadly SS-sponsored work and were unable to extricate themselves without exacting the punishment Himmler had promised for "weak" doctors who were "traitors" to the Reich for their views on human experimentation. That penalty was death.[39] In 1941, Siegfried Ruff and Hans Romberg of the DVL and Georg Weltz of the University of Munich made the mistake of agreeing to work with an unscrupulous would-be researcher, medical doctor Sigmund Rascher. He was a personal acquaintance of Himmler via his wife, reportedly one of the SS leader's former lovers. Rascher did not possess the academic credentials to merit the title of scientist and was conducting research in pursuit of his Ph.D. and *Habilitation*.[40]

Rascher, who later told Ruff that he had had his own father sent to a prison camp, used his Himmler connection to gain access to human subjects at Dachau. He then exploited the expertise, staff, and specialized equipment of first Weltz and then the DVL to conduct experiments in killing by means of the low-pressure chamber.

Thinking Rascher's request for Ruff to supervise his doctoral research legitimate, Hans Romberg agreed to monitor Rascher's actual fieldwork at Dachau while he himself took advantage of the offer of test subjects to carry out studies involving response time during emergency high-altitude bailouts. In wartime it was extremely difficult to find young men in Berlin who were available as volunteers, and the researchers at the DVL had been up in the altitude chamber so often they were too acclimated to be of use.

To Romberg's shock, Rascher calmly asphyxiated an inmate in the chamber one day even as Romberg was telling him to bring the victim down to a lower altitude because the inmate's EKG was showing evidence of heart distress. Instead, Rascher announced that he was going to do an autopsy on the man inside the chamber, looking for aeroembolism in the heart, and needed Romberg's help. Romberg entered the chamber, and Rascher sent the altitude so high that Romberg blacked out.

Himmler had extremely strict secrecy rules that made it illegal for Romberg to tell even Ruff anything that went on in the prison camp. Still, Romberg headed for Berlin to report the killing to his boss. He did not trust the telephone. Coming back to Dachau, he found the barometer on the altitude chamber broken. Repair meant a trip back to Berlin and a two-week wait. When Romberg got back to Dachau again, he found that Rascher had killed a second inmate. A few days later he killed a third. This time Romberg confronted Rascher, and the two argued violently. It ended when Rascher waved a letter under Romberg's nose and told him Himmler had ordered the work and Romberg was not to interfere.

As soon as he could, Romberg found a phone, called Ruff in Berlin, and conveyed the news of the two new deaths without giving the secret away to SS eavesdroppers. Ruff had already gone to Erich Hippke and gotten him to order the equipment returned for "urgent use at the front," a ruse to avoid charges of treason for interfering with SS work. He had also informed Hermann Becker-Freyseng, who was then detailed to the Luftwaffe as an assistant medical advisor, and the latter had contacted the chamber manufacturer and told the company to deliver nothing else to the SS; only Luftwaffe orders were to be filled. Everyone sweated out the return of the chamber, which took several slow weeks due to wartime logistics problems, then prayed that no one would notice that the "urgently needed" chamber was sitting in the DVL parking lot. Rascher's intent to test subjects literally to death became even clearer in the last few days, when a large electrocardiograph device arrived at Dachau. Romberg spun a lie for Rascher, telling him there was too much electrical interference at the camp for it to work there.[41]

To complete his accreditation, Rascher launched a series of infamous experiments in which he slowly froze Dachau inmates to death. Hans Romberg refused an invitation to take part, but Himmler ordered him to participate in the project, where he tried his best to be invisible when it came time to do the work.[42] The SS physician froze Jews, Soviet prisoners, and Catholic priests in cold-water tanks or in the open air until they lost consciousness or, in many cases, died. He filmed and photographed several of the "experiments," ostensibly designed to determine the best method of reviving pilots downed in cold seas. Himmler came to watch some of the tests. A proponent of *völkisch* "science," he told Rascher to go to the North Sea and find out what the common folk used to warm victims of extreme cold. Romberg was there that day and reported that Himmler said he thought "that a fisherwoman could well take her half-frozen husband into her bed and revive him in that manner. Everyone said that animal warmth had a different effect than artificial warmth." Romberg objected and was met with a painful silence. Himmler had his way, so for his next bizarre test Rascher used naked female prisoners to warm the nearly dead male inmates.[43]

Konrad Schäfer, who was on the LMFI payroll but working in a position Strughold had arranged for him at an industrial lab, found himself in a similar nightmare, although not of his own making. On his own, he had developed Wolfatit, a legitimate chemical means of purifying sea water, and tested it on animals and on four or five human subjects, including himself. An engineer from a technical college in Vienna, a man named Berka, had meanwhile concocted a yellowish tomato-based recipe he called Berkatit to disguise the taste of seawater. It was patently impossible to make seawater potable this way, but since it was much less expensive than Wolfatit, which required silver, someone high up decided to test the recipe. According to Schäfer, Berka had already tried it on several soldiers in Vienna, who reported that it had made them thirsty and given them diarrhea. Someone coerced them into changing their report and threatened Schäfer with a visit to the Luftwaffe's Erhard Milch if he did not agree to the test. The proposal to evaluate the two methods side by side came across Becker-Freyseng's desk, but against his advice a group of doctors tried it out on two dozen hapless Gypsy inmates at Dachau. The "tests" involved undergoing six to twelve days of water deprivation, drinking saltwater, and having painful lumbar and liver punctures to judge the effect of the Berkatit. Some expected it to make the kidneys more efficient. Instead, it proved to be torture for the inmates and may have caused one death.[44]

Ruff, Romberg, Schäfer, and Weltz wound up in the docket at the Nuremberg war-crimes trials and were acquitted, but their reputations were damaged, and the U.S. Army canceled their contracts to come and work in America after the war. Becker-Freyseng was found guilty of complicity for his advisory role and sentenced to twenty years in prison (later reduced to ten). He died in jail. Neither Becker-Freyseng's supervisor, a doctor with the surname of Anthony, nor Erich Hippke were ever charged with a crime, but interestingly Hippke's successor, Oskar Schröder, who took over on May 15, 1944, long after the Dachau experiments, was charged. Berka seems to have vanished. Sigmund Rascher and his wife were reportedly ordered shot by Himmler late in the war for reasons unrelated to the medical experiments.

For the rest of his life, Strughold was periodically accused of involvement in the perversity at Dachau or at least of having known about it and failing to act. The Nuremberg testimony makes it clear that he was not on hand for the experiments or directly involved in them. However, his claims that he knew nothing before his colleagues' arrests in 1946 simply are not plausible given the personal and professional closeness of the German aeromedical community. Furthermore, Strughold, Clamann, Benzinger, Rein, Ruff, Schäfer, Konrad Büttner, Balke, and some ninety other medical experts were reportedly present at meetings in the fall of 1942 in Nuremberg and Berlin at which Rascher and his collaborators presented the results of the Dachau experiments. Schäfer admitted giving one of the papers.[45]

Strughold's former superior, Erich Hippke, also made a remark at the Milch trial that shows that he knew that Rascher was planning to conduct some sort of cold tests. The former chief of the Luftwaffe's medical branch testified that his researchers had been testing small lab animals to find a means of warming pilots who had been shot down over cold waters and, in spite of being rescued, had died from hypothermia. Experimenting on a primate would more closely mimic human surface area and volume, Hippke had reasoned. He testified that he talked with Strughold about "this question regarding the use of monkeys," but the LMFI director said that "He assured me that it was impossible at that time in Germany to get hold of apes for this experiment."[46] Whether the two talked about using human subjects is not known, and Hippke did not say that he brought up the subject with Strughold again when the lethal cold experiments at Dachau actually began. The Allies located Hippke in time to obtain his brief Milch testimony, but he disappeared again, and thus little information was obtained from him. However, it is possible that he mentioned the altitude-chamber deaths to Strughold. It is also likely that Ruff would have told his friend Strughold something of what Hans Romberg had witnessed.

Strughold always denied that he had known about and assisted in the experiments. He stated that he had been on the side of those who were opposed to the Hitler regime and that he had Jewish friends. He claimed his life had been at risk due to a close friendship in Würzburg with Friederich von Stauffenberg, cousin of Count Claus von Stauffenberg. Friederich had introduced the two in 1939, and when Claus nearly killed Adolf Hitler with a bomb, Strughold had to go into hiding for two weeks. Since he was on a list of enemies, he went from farmhouse to farmhouse, he said, until it seemed safe enough to return to Berlin.[47]

This story might have some truth to it. Some five thousand of Claus von Stauffenberg's acquaintances were arrested in the days following the assassination attempt. Strughold fell into the same socioeconomic class as that of the best-known anti-Nazi resistors in Germany: middle- or upper-class, university-educated urbanites. He lived alone and socialized only with his lab colleagues and other professionals. He was very interested in the United States and things American and was known at the time to have avoided joining the party. Perhaps he was also known to have been opposed to the regime and acquainted with intellectuals who were willing to express negative feelings about it in private.[48] He aided individual researchers who wanted to avoid military service or feared losing their employees to conscription or simply were in trouble and needed a cover and an income.[49] Thanks to the occasional Swedish visitor, the LMFI had access to a few English and American medical journals, which was probably a crime after 1939—and certainly risky. Strughold also conspired to keep private property out of party hands. Whether he might have had the courage to do more is hard to say.

After Strughold's death in 1986, charges against him intimidated the air force into taking his name off of the Hubertus Strughold Aeromedical Library at Brooks AFB, which had been dedicated after his retirement. For the same reason, the Medical School at Ohio State University erased Strughold's likeness from a stained-glass mural depicting key people in the history of medicine. The Strughold name was reportedly removed from a facility in Germany as well.[50] The holes where the library sign was still remain, and employees and retirees at Brooks still resent what they see as an unfounded slander campaign.

WAR COMES TO THE LMFI

With regard to day-to-day research, at the LMFI things moved along "surprisingly unmolestedly" early in the war, as Strughold recalled later. The only physical change at first was in the teaching duties. Because of RAF air raids, lectures were moved next door to the basement of the military academy.

Strughold was even able to get away to Austria on working vacations, sometimes to Vienna, where he would sit in a café and write scientific papers to the accompaniment of music. In Berlin he sometimes went into a beer cellar and wrote after imbibing an ale or two. Now and then he would visit the rural town in south Westphalia where his sister lived; there he was able to write, undisturbed by lab business or phone. "Those were my best papers," he recalled after the war. His intellectual pursuits and city life in Berlin needed an antidote, and roughing it in Westphalia helped him keep his "horse sense."[51]

Ulrich Cameron Luft felt safe with his wife, Alice, and son, Friederich, in their apartment in Berlin-Friedenau, a southwestern suburb just two or three miles from the LMFI. He worried more about his mother and sister, who had gone to Great Britain at the outset of the war. He had had almost no contact with them since then. He knew that his Scotland-born mother, Mary Muir Wilson Luft, had hired an attorney to try to win back her British citizenship. While she awaited the outcome with her family in Edinburgh, his younger sister, Hildegard, was incarcerated with other German nationals on the Isle of Man in the Irish Sea.[52]

Most of the researchers appear to have been exempt from actual battlefield service. All or nearly all of them apparently held a low-ranking, medical corps reserve commission in the Luftwaffe and from time to time had to take additional classroom training but were not ordered to the front. A few, including Siegfried Ruff and Hans Romberg of the DVL, did some research on troops stationed in France, and Hermann Becker-Freyseng occasionally had to travel within German-held areas as part of his Luftwaffe work.[53]

There were, of course, exceptions. In 1939, Luft's climbing friend Bruno Balke had been drafted into the army. He griped enough about the office jobs he was assigned to that he was sent to the Russian front with a fighting battalion in 1941; there, however, he contracted hepatitis and was sent back to recover. Luft heard about his condition and contacted the ailing physician through Balke's wife, Annemarie, saying that there was a job in the scientific department of the Heeres-Gebirgs-Sanitäts-Schule (Army School of Mountain Rescue) at St. Johann in the Tyrol. Did he want it? Balke wavered; he had promised his soldiers that he would return, but it was obvious that he was not fit for frontline duty. Maybe he would be of greater use in the mountains. He signed himself out of the hospital, jaundice and all, and packed for Austria.

Balke was able to use his Alpine hiatus to study the benefits of physical training at high altitudes in gaining tolerance for the thin low-pressure atmosphere. Acclimatization appeared to be a promising strategy, and Luft planned to conduct tests there in 1945 to see whether the benefits of such conditioning could be preserved at lower altitudes via daily running or similarly strenuous cardiovascular exercise. Events interfered, and Luft did not see his friend again until 1950, when Hubertus Strughold nudged Balke toward another job—with the USAF School of Aviation Medicine in San Antonio, Texas.[54]

At least three aviation-medicine specialists volunteered for short tours in battle zones. One of them, Theo Benzinger, took advantage of his Luftwaffe employment and learned to fly, then qualified further as a test pilot. He used his training and access to aircraft to personally research the toxicity of aviation-fuel fumes at high altitude, cockpit fogging and icing, and the effectiveness of air brakes in dive-bombing maneuvers. In November 1940, he requested permission from Gen. Ernst Udet of the Luftwaffe to fly ten reconnaissance and research missions over England. According to Benzinger's postwar memoirs, avoiding what seemed like the entire British air defense required skillful flying. "Diving to [the] ground perpendicularly without air brakes, pulling out on time, and riding the hedges of the British countryside were the only sensible approach to getting home after the reconnaissance mission was accomplished," he wrote. On one occasion, his tail gunner was wounded, and the radio operator was killed in a crash landing in France when a British Spitfire destroyed the landing gear on his Junkers 88 twin-engine dive bomber.[55]

Both Konrad Büttner, a physicist who did meteorological research for Benzinger, and Ulrich Luft were sent to North Africa to support the Luftwaffe's efforts in matters related to heat stress.[56] Presumably because of his native fluency in English, Luft was also sent for a short period to an evaluation station at the western front to interrogate new prisoners of war. Captives on either side were required to divulge only name, rank, and serial number, but for whatever reason—fear, despair, exhaustion, inexperience, confusion, or just plain skillful interrogation—some Allied crew members gave out information about their aircraft, troop strength, base locations, training, onboard equipment, and targets.[57] These statements were relayed to the Luftwaffe High Command in Berlin. Most of the prisoners gave only the required information, however, and some intentionally misled their interrogators. Luft, for example, passed along misinformation about venereal disease and reported incorrectly that the Americans had tablets that made seawater potable.[58]

BOMBS OVER BERLIN

In November 1943, the RAF stepped up the bombing of Berlin and made some sixteen raids on the city over the next four months. Working and living conditions became considerably worse.[59] When bombs destroyed LMFI researcher Konrad Schäfer's apartment, he and his wife moved in with the family of a lab assistant.[60] The others wondered whether their homes would be next.

The next month Strughold accepted an offer from a countess to shift part of his lab to her castle, Schloß Welkersdorf in Polish Silesia, nearly 175 miles southeast of Berlin. She hoped that making the property available to the Luftwaffe would keep it out of party hands, where it would be gone for good. Strughold relocated equipment and a half dozen employees there to work on color vision, night vision, and electroencephalograms. He shuttled back and forth, taking the new autobahn or the longer way due east and then south through Frankfurt-an-der-Oder, depending on road conditions, the availability of gasoline, and troop movements. He tried to be in Berlin at least once a week to answer correspondence. Clamann and Luft acted as deputy directors when the boss was away.[61]

The German government tightened restrictions on food and fuel and diverted nearly all resources to the front. For civilians, that meant rationing far beyond the limits set in Allied nations. Caloric consumption overall was cut and sometimes provided with no attention whatsoever to nutritional balance. A family might be given bread, turnips, and glucose, for example. Butter, meat, fresh fruit, eggs, sugar, and coffee were only memories.

Rationing laws were strictly enforced. One child of an LMFI researcher recalls looking from his living-room window at the building across the street, where a kindergarten friend lived. A car pulled up in front of the house, and three men in dark suits, hats, and overcoats got out. They did not look like the type of people who usually visited the home, and that caught his attention. One man rang the doorbell, and after a second the classmate's father answered the door. As the boy watched, the man in front pulled out a gun and without explanation shot the father point-blank in the chest. Just as quickly and silently, the three turned away, got back into the car, and drove off.

The boy knew instinctively what the visit had been about. That morning his friend had told the class that his parents had slaughtered a pig and they had enjoyed a fine meal of pork. No one but the military was allowed to keep the meat from privately owned animals; the owner was required to "donate" it to the troops at the front. The boy knew that his own father sometimes brought meat home from the lab when one of the experimental pigs "fell down the stairs," as reported on the required government form. Who else knew about the pigs? Would a man come to the door for his own Papi?[62]

Berliners had experienced air raids as early as 1940, but when the British began the heavy bombing in late 1943, they had to accustom themselves to crowding into bomb shelters in the middle of the night. Some of the shelters made the effects of the bombardment worse. People smothered in the plaster dust that was shaken lose; they baked in the heat of incendiaries or were simply crushed amid the rubble. When the bombers appeared over his own house, Strughold hid in a hole he had dug in his yard, which he felt was much safer than a bomb shelter.[63] Years later, it seemed to Hans-Georg Clamann that the group had spent most of their days rebuilding what had been destroyed overnight.[64]

With the advent of round-the-clock bombing by the Americans in 1944, air raids became a twenty-four-hour interruption. Research was disrupted by power outages and trips next door to the shelter in the basement of the academy. On several occasions, LMFI scientists met with visiting researchers across the street and inside the enormous flak tower built at the zoo. The five-story turreted structure, its concrete walls several meters thick, offered better protection and also held offices where they could confer in safety.[65]

The period after a raid could be just as dangerous as the bombardment itself. Burning debris fell from upper stories and set the clothing of pedestrians on fire. People would grab strangers and beat out the flames on the unsuspecting victim's coat. Fire storms, which superheated the air and caused tornado-like winds, sucked people right out of buildings.[66] In some places, water and utilities were interrupted or cut off completely. When the taps were running, citizens would store water, usually untreated, in their bathtubs. Some got intestinal worms as a result, and poor hygiene and even worse nutrition led to rampant gum disease.[67]

When the Americans' daylight carpet bombing of Berlin began in the spring of 1944, Hans-Georg Clamann sent his family to Groß-Schwülper in north central Germany to live with his parents. The village was 130 miles west of Berlin and not in a prime target area. Clamann's father still had a medical practice, and as one of the perquisites of his profession he was allowed to keep a supply of rabbits. As often as not, one of the bunnies was diverted to the hasenpfeffer pot. Marie Clamann, also a medical doctor, worked in the practice, and the two boys would play and hunt for dandelion greens for the family to eat.

In the last few months of the war, there was little resemblance to normality in Berlin. The three-story Clamann home in an eastern suburb took a direct hit down the chimney from an Allied bomb. Transportation, public or private, was extremely difficult, and Clamann resorted to trading pickling alcohol liter for liter for gasoline or stretching his fuel by adding hexane and alcohol from the LMFI stores.[68] Strughold's former apartment on the west side of the city was destroyed a week after he moved out.[69] Luft lost his car to a bomb and took to bicycling to work.[70] Respiratory physiologist Joseph Pichotka managed to get to work at the LMFI but one day found himself on a Berlin street where an enraged crowd was threatening an Allied airman unfortunate enough to have bailed out over the city he had just carpet bombed. Somehow Pichotka got his hands on a gun, wrested the man away, and turned him over to the Luftwaffe authorities.[71]

In desperation, Hitler promoted Strughold and other scientists and doctors. Strughold thus became a full colonel in the regular German Air Force's medical corps just two months before the collapse of the regime. Photos show him in full uniform and looking not unhappy. Perhaps it was because the promotion meant more pay or the chance to wear an impressive uniform, or his sense of irony simply made him aware of how ludicrous the new rank was. Obviously Germany was not going to win; furthermore, a uniform displaying high rank would implicate one as a Nazi when the Allies arrived in Berlin.[72]

As the Soviets prepared to move into the city, Strughold directed those at Welkersdorf castle and the LMFI to seek shelter with his old classmate, Hermann Rein, at the University of Göttingen. It was two hundred miles west and therefore less of a target than Berlin and likely to remain out of Communist control.[73] Clamann opted to go to Groß-Schwülper and rejoin his wife and two sons.[74] Luft, a native Berliner with a brother and other family members there, decided to stay in the city with his wife and son and see what opportunities remained when the dust settled. Before he left the LMFI for good, he attached his mountaineering rucksack to his bicycle and shuttled back and forth with books and records he knew would some day be collectors' items. Along with Erich Opitz, he was the last to leave the lab.[75]

PART II

Space Medicine

Chapter 4

THE PAPERCLIPS

The immediate postwar years were marked by upheaval in aviation medicine as well as unmatched opportunity. Harry Armstrong and other air corps medical officers recognized that Germany's defeat was their first chance to get ahead of the engineers. German jets and V-2 missiles were vehicles of the future that existed in the here and now, and they were bound to end up in the American arsenal. If the United States acted quickly, the experts at the Wright Lab and the School of Aviation Medicine could begin doing whatever was needed to make flight aboard such machines survivable.

With this in mind, the American physicians began recruiting their German counterparts—when they could find them. They first offered them contracts to work in Heidelberg, then asked their former enemies to come to the United States for six months and later bring their families with an eye to staying. Several dozen accepted the offer, hesitantly at first. Hubertus Strughold and many of his team recognized that this would be their only opportunity, perhaps for a very long time, to find any employment at all in aviation-medicine research. The United States, which was already shipping Nazi aircraft and missiles back for scrutiny in its own labs, was sure to be the next great power in aviation.

Neither the American nor German life scientists had ever been particularly interested in space exploration. If they even thought about life beyond Earth, it was in terms of making such a place or the vehicle required to get there safe and habitable. A few may have had thoughts of scouring the moon or planets for biochemical signs of life, but primitive plant forms were all they expected to find. Dreams of finding evidence of even extinct human life within the solar system or of colonizing space were strictly fantasy, and visions of conquering the planets and the moon belonged to German rocket designer Wernher von Braun. Still, scientific curiosity drove some to pursue research far beyond that undertaken in either the United States or Germany, and from this grew a new discipline: space medicine.

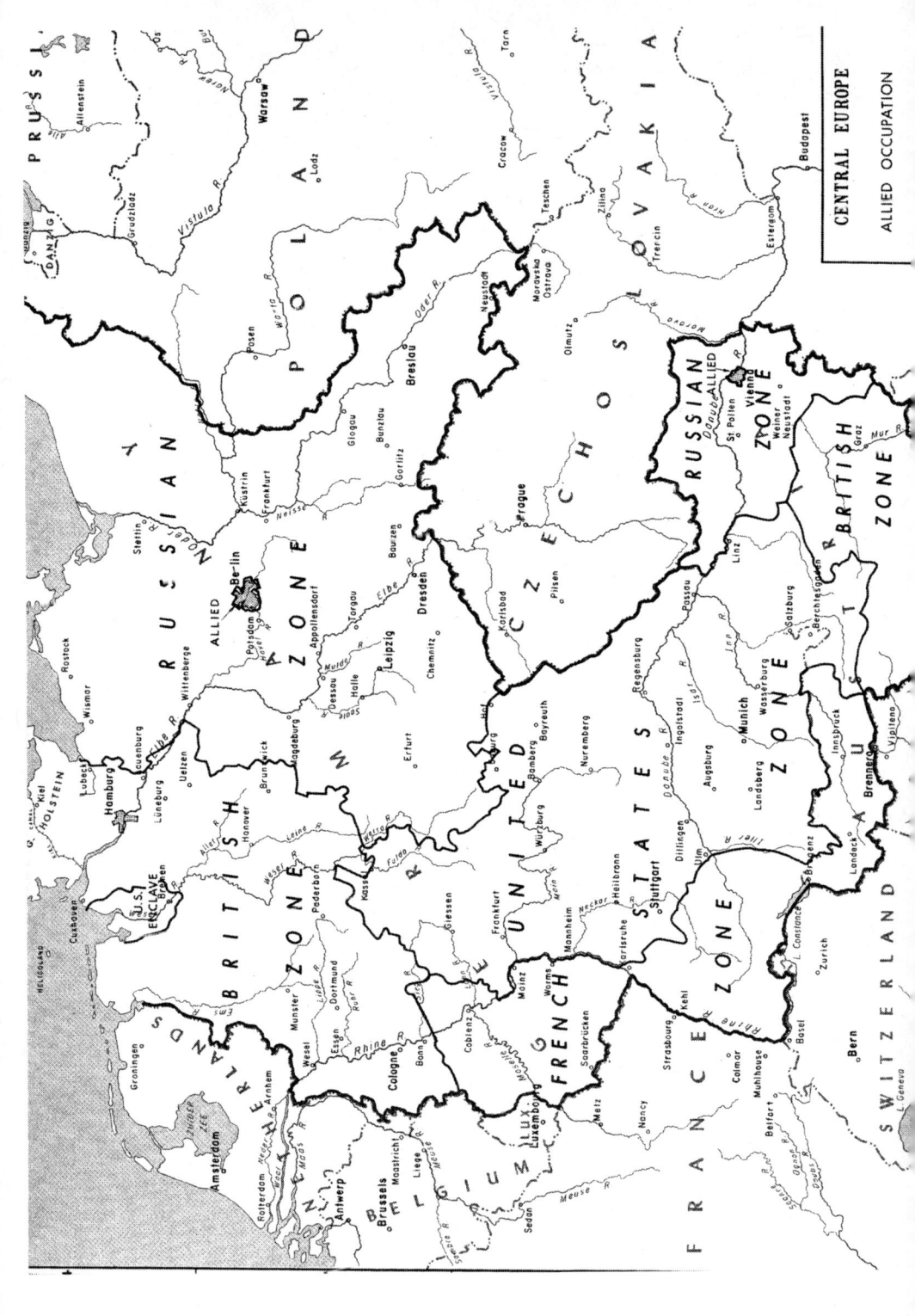

CENTRAL EUROPE

ALLIED OCCUPATION

THE SPOILS OF WAR

In 1944, three years into his tour in England, Harry Armstrong came out of his London hotel room and was walking by Hyde Park when he heard an explosion half a mile away. Seconds later, strangely, he heard the scream of the bomb *arriving*. He had witnessed German buzz bombs several times since their initial deployment that June, but what on Earth was this?

He soon found out that this "backward" bomb was another *wunderwaffen* the Germans were throwing at the Allies at the end of the war. Called the A-4 or V-2, for Vergeltungswaffe-2 (Vengeance Weapon 2), it had probably been launched from western Holland, about 160 miles away. Unlike the V-1, the V-2 was steerable, and its trajectory had taken it nearly 50 miles up. On the way back down, it built up tremendous momentum as it roared toward its target. Upon impact, it had been going about fifteen hundred miles per hour, more than twice the speed of sound, and had arrived at the target before the noise of its engine could alert people to take cover. The Germans built nearly 6,000 V-2s in the last fifteen months of the war and ultimately used 3,200 of them by April 1945. More bombs were aimed at Belgium than at England, but in all they took five thousand Allied civilian lives. Armstrong had heard the first V-2 to hit London, on September 8, 1944.[1]

The experience made Armstrong think about what an engineering feat like that could mean for aviation medicine. If one could send a projectile of that weight from Germany to London, surely the future would see such missiles hurtling along with people inside. It would certainly be a quick way to travel, he thought, but how would the occupants get down safely?

If anyone knew how to accomplish that objective, it would be the scientists involved in making the things. Although he was scheduled to go home and hadn't seen his wife and children since 1942, Armstrong volunteered to go on to Berlin with the occupation forces and try to find out what Germany's aviation-medicine specialists knew about this new form of flight. The best person to help find them, he thought, would be the man he had met at that Aero Medical Association meeting in 1937, the German who had run a lab much like his: Hubertus Strughold.[2]

LEFT: Map of Occupied Germany. After the defeat of the Third Reich, administrative and military control of Germany and Austria was divided among four of the Allied nations: the United States, Britain, France, and the Soviet Union. The capitol, Berlin, was likewise divided among the four. Map courtesy of the U.S. Military Academy.

Although it was too late to turn the tide of the war in Europe, Hitler's scientists and engineers had made good on the Führer's promises of wonder weapons. They had deployed the Me-168 Komet rocket plane, the V-1 buzz bombs, and the V-2 missile. Those who were privy to the secrets of the Manhattan Project even feared (wrongly, it turned out) that, with such expertise, Germany must be close to putting an atomic bomb at Hitler's disposal.[3] Late in the war, others in the U.S. military had begun to think along the same lines as Armstrong about the V-2 and other advanced weapons of the German military.

For many, this display of technological ingenuity brought back disturbing memories of the chief horror of World War I: poison gas. It had injured, crippled, and killed thousands, a perverse display of Germany's supremacy in chemistry. Allied nations had responded after that war by boycotting German science and culture. The Boy Scouts had even excluded German youngsters from the international jamboree in London in 1920.[4] Now, thanks to accounts of the unbelievable capabilities of German jets and missiles, some Americans decided that someone should simply lock up Germany's brightest people and throw away the key. Maj. George Fielding Eliot, news analyst for CBS and military correspondent for the New York *Herald Tribune*, wrote in the scholarly publication *Foreign Affairs* that the scientists of Germany and Japan ought to be sent to the remote South Georgia Island in the Atlantic, a bleak way station for Antarctic whaling vessels. Many in Washington wanted at least to see military research prohibited in Germany. No one really desired to repeat the mistakes of Versailles and castrate the nation, the thinking went, but hadn't the Germans shown they could not be trusted with their own genius? Wouldn't just a little humiliation be good for the proud Prussian soul?

Some felt that a relatively weak Germany would prevent a third world war, reasoning that since Germany had started the first two, it would likely be the nation that set off a third conflagration at some future point. Others, though, saw a prostrate Germany as an open invitation for Communism to spread throughout Central Europe. Franklin Roosevelt wanted the Germans to remain dependent on the United States for the time being, until they could earn their way back into the good graces of "peace-loving and law-abiding nations." He planned to eliminate Germany's military capability, punish the Nazi leadership, and eradicate any opportunities for citizens to demonstrate military fervor, even parades. The State Department wanted to both demilitarize and denazify Germany, punish its war criminals, and democratize the nation, but it also knew that, for Germany to set aside once and for all its grandiose plans for conquest beyond its geographic borders, it would have to be self-supporting and a full member of Western society.

The United States never developed a coordinated policy for Germany's rehabilitation, however. Roosevelt died, Secretary of State Cordell Hull retired, and others in FDR's cabinet saw their power diminish, leaving a policy vacuum. The only cohesiveness seemed to be in the military, which was following established guidelines as to how the Allies would administer the zone of occupation. An interim directive put forth only a week after the German surrender stipulated that laboratories and related facilities should be abolished but that scientific research would be allowed in areas that constituted no threat; these areas would, of course, be subject to constant scrutiny. All scientific findings would be published in the open press. Key scientists who were linked to wartime research would not be allowed to participate.[5]

Leaders in the military and aviation industry had been rankled by the failure of overcautious engineers at the National Advisory Committee for Aeronautics (NACA) to latch on to advances made by Germany and Britain in the 1930s, in particular jet propulsion, and were determined not to remain in third place.[6] Thinking ahead, they realized that breaking the German monopoly on such technologies could mean revolutionary advances for the nations that obtained that know-how. Some observers had already seen the advantages of such technology transfer before 1945 with the emigration of physicists Albert Einstein, Leo Szilard, Enrico Fermi, Niels Bohr, Emilio Segré, John von Neumann, Hans Bethe, Lise Meitner, Otto Hahn, Eugene Wigner, Edward Teller, Stanislaw Ulam, George Kistiakowski, Otto Frisch, and so many others out of German territory. The world's most destructive device, the atomic bomb, was taking shape in an *American* lab. These groups wanted to obtain Germany's remaining talents and technologies for the United States.

Consequently, following the Normandy invasion in June 1944, the army began deploying squads of ordnance, chemical warfare, and communications specialists to evaluate the equipment, laboratories, prisoners, and documents left behind as the Germans retreated from the French coast. These teams were quickly overwhelmed by the amount and type of materials left behind, so the Supreme Headquarters of the Allied Expeditionary Forces (SHAEF)—primarily the United States and Great Britain—set up special units called T-Forces a month later to help sort things out. As the Allies moved east, these forward scouts would locate and seize targets of interest to the military effort the instant the firing ceased.

These efforts, however, were not enough to exploit the technology they were finding. By the end of August, the Combined Chiefs of Staff responded by creating the joint U.S.-British Combined Intelligence Objectives Subcommittee (CIOS), which could compile lists of targets and provide the experts necessary to evaluate them. By the end of 1944, nearly two hundred CIOS investigators had been dispatched to France.

They had competition, though. Some of it came from the U.S. Navy, which felt the CIOS teams were too unwieldy, too army oriented, and too likely to give what they found to the British, who were not fighting a war in the Pacific. The navy also thought the atomic scientists had defined the targets too narrowly, searching for scientific expertise at the expense of technological capability. Consequently, it created the Naval Technical Mission in November 1944 to obtain equipment and personnel useful against Japan. Another rival was the Technical Industrial Intelligence Commission (TIIC), a civilian group formed by the Foreign Economic Administration, created by FDR in September 1943, in part to oversee activities in captured zones. By January 1945, the TIIC had commissioned nearly three hundred civilians as army officers and dispatched them to seek useful finds in mining, chemicals, railroads, lumber, machinery, textiles, medicine, aeronautics, and communications. A third contender was the U.S. Army Air Forces, the slowest to join. In April 1945, the AAF began compiling several hundred mobile teams as part of what was then called "Operation Lusty." Within six weeks, it had assembled military and civilian experts who were knowledgeable in medicine, law, history, industry, and the sciences to evaluate the enemy's capabilities in aviation manufacturing, radar, aerial photography, ordnance, communications, and aviation medicine.[7]

While the war in Europe was still underway, the first concern was in fact atomic weaponry the Nazis might launch against the invading Allies. The response in the United States was the creation of the Alsos unit, a joint operation of the army, navy, and Office of Scientific Research and Development (OSRD). Deployed immediately after the takeover of Paris, Alsos was charged with finding out exactly how far the Germans had progressed in harnessing the atom for military purposes. Planners took the British into their confidence to some extent but completely excluded their erstwhile ally in the East, the Soviet Union. Many historians believe President Truman's decision to drop the atomic bomb on Japan was made to warn the Soviets that the United States had the greater military might. Some mark this as the start of the Cold War, while others point to earlier decisions to exclude the USSR from key decisions, such as the one to build the bomb in the first place. It seems likely that a desire to keep Moscow from Germany's aviation and missile technology was a factor in the way the United States developed and executed its plan to grab whatever and whomever it could.[8]

The Soviet Union also had plans for obtaining German technology and talent. Stalin ordered the military to confiscate anything that seemed worth having. As the Red Army moved into eastern Germany and Berlin, troops disassembled entire factories and began taking what they needed to replace what their war with Germany had destroyed—or what the USSR did not yet have the technical prowess or capital to build itself. They loaded machine tools, printing presses, electrical devices, cameras, radios, office machines, and furniture onto trains bound for the East. They cleaned out motion-picture companies, car manufacturers, mining concerns, and manufacturers of everything from radiators to safety razors. One American observer called it "organized vandalism." They even took basic fittings and fixtures. Ulrich Luft found that the sinks in the physiology lab at the University of Berlin had been sledge-hammered from the wall, presumably to be put on a truck headed east.[9] Light bulbs and doorknobs met a similar fate.

The Soviets also laid their hands on technologies that worried them as Germany's nearby neighbor. Theirs was a geographically large but politically new nation with a very small base in high-tech things, but they had a solid tradition in aviation and rocketry. This chance to position themselves as the postwar leader in these fields was not to be missed. Thus, shortly after rocket designer Wernher von Braun and most of his team surrendered to the United States (rather than fall into Soviet hands), the USSR sent its own rocketry wizards to the northern island of Peenemünde, now in the Soviet zone, to scavenge for parts, drawings, and engineers.[10] The venture proved to be quite an effective strategy.

AVIATION MEDICINE AND PROJECT PAPERCLIP

The medical corps's scavenging effort had a rather fragmentary, albeit ambitious, start. At a July 1945 meeting at the field office of Malcolm Grow (then surgeon of the U.S. Strategic Air Forces in Europe) in St. Germain, France, a group of AAF flight surgeons, including Armstrong, conceived a plan that would set up the Aero Medical Center under the Ninth Air Force's Central Medical Establishment. It was physically created a month later at the Kaiser Wilhelm Institute at the University of Heidelberg and also pulled into its sphere the Helmholtz Institute group located in Nussdorf, about forty miles south of Munich. Official credit for the plan was given to Grow, but Harry Armstrong led one of the two four-man committees that directed the program, specifically the one charged with selecting the locations in Germany to use and the native personnel to recruit. The army outfitted the Heidelberg institute with a high-altitude chamber and allowed the German scientists free rein to research and write as they wished.[11] Immediately after VE Day, Randy Lovelace went into Germany and traveled from Lübeck to Oberammergau collecting interesting aeromedical equipment and data and interrogating more than one hundred aviation-medicine specialists.[12]

For Armstrong, Lovelace, and others, wrapped up in this project was also a simple desire to know what researchers on the other side had been working on, what discoveries they had made, and what challenges they had met during the war. It was an opportunity to meet and share experiences with their counterparts, whom circumstances had kept out of circulation for nearly six years. One scientist, an expert in ordnance, pointed out that for the Americans, the chance to discover how science and technology had functioned under the Hitler regime was like finding a unique and completed experiment, available now for analysis as to its successes and failures in goals, planning, and methodology.[13] There can be no doubt, too, that the feeling was mutual among the German scientists.

One of the first names mentioned for recruitment was Hubertus Strughold. Paul Campbell, who would become director of space medicine at the School of Aviation Medicine in 1958 and then SAM commander in 1962, had, like Armstrong and Lovelace, encountered Strughold earlier, during the German's fellowship at the University of Chicago. Campbell considered him to be an excellent teacher as well as a first-rate scientist. Early in 1945, Campbell was called in as part of "Operation Lusty" and sent to Greenville, North Carolina, where he was told only that he was part of an air staff intelligence team, a top-secret operation with four members from each of the air force's major disciplines. Rank did not necessarily matter when it came to expertise, either. There were fifty participants in his group, Campbell recalled later, ranging from full colonels down to junior officers and some civilians, including physicist Detlev Bronk, then a consultant to the air force surgeon general. They were all going into Germany the day the war was over, he was told, by parachute if they had to.

The group was privy to what was then top-secret information, including the lines of demarcation of the various occupation zones in Germany, so they were always kept under guard. They had to mark time for a while in Greenville and then were taken by train to a port and sent to England aboard the *Île de France*. Still too early for their intended purpose, the group was again maintained under guard in England until Germany's expected capitulation. Harry Armstrong, by then a colonel, took on the job of telling the four medical experts where they might best spend their time once they got to Germany. One very useful thing Armstrong had them do while they waited was interview surviving members of the German general staff (including Oskar Schröder, head of the Luftwaffe medical corps in 1944 and 1945), who had been captured and placed under arrest at a compound north of London.

The general staff turned out to be "quite cooperative," Campbell recalled, and very interested in getting things back to a state of normalcy. When the Americans asked where they might find records of German research, one of the German generals mentioned that they ought to look for two file cases that had been in his desk. He told them that he had ordered a particular German major to take the file cases to the "national redoubt" in Berchtesgaden, Bavaria, but suspected that the man had run into trouble along the way and had probably headed for the Harz Mountains, northeast of Göttingen. The most likely place to look for him there would be the one Luftwaffe hospital that was still in operation, as the accommodations were free. The Americans went there and indeed found the major. The files they wanted had already been torn up and scattered everywhere, the German stated, by Polish conscript laborers who had been freed just the day before. He took them to the spot, only to find that one of his countrymen had carefully picked everything up and put the files back together. Finding papers and publications would remain a problem for a while; Armstrong had to requisition gasoline for one German's car so that he could drive out to the countryside and retrieve his papers from the convent where he had hidden them.[14]

Because he had volunteered to stay on in Europe after VE Day, Armstrong was assigned as surgeon of the air contingent for the occupation forces in Berlin. When he arrived there, he headed for the LMFI and Strughold, but the building had been abandoned. No one whose name Armstrong knew could be found, and for months his inquiries in Berlin proved fruitless. Anyone in an American uniform who asked the whereabouts of a specific German was regarded with the greatest suspicion, he discovered; consequently the locals would either lie outright or feign ignorance in an attempt to protect a countryman. Eventually Armstrong stumbled onto Ulrich Luft, who was teaching amid the rubble that was the University of Berlin's physiology department and had a busy medical practice treating the stream of refugees coming through the capital city, many of whom had typhoid fever and other virulent and communicable diseases.[15]

Luft recognized Armstrong's name and listened as he stated his reasons for coming to Berlin and asked where everyone at the LMFI had gone. Luft decided to trust him. Except for the uniform, the man seemed to have nothing in common with the soldiers who were arresting and taking away Germans who had maintained a higher political profile than Luft and his coworkers. He seemed to genuinely want to talk to Strughold about the medical work they had done and not ask a lot of questions about anyone's political beliefs. Luft confided to him that his boss had dismissed everyone back in April, telling them essentially that they were on their own. He believed that Strughold had gone to the University of Göttingen and was working in a research lab there.[16]

Armstrong headed west to Göttingen and found his former counterpart there. The area was then under the control of the British, who were trying to restore the university to its earlier status as a center of scientific research. Strughold was not unhappy there. He much preferred the attention and personal contact of teaching to the solitude and, for him, the relative tedium of lab work.[17] The two men spoke for quite a while, Armstrong recalled later, and Strughold willingly told him as much as he knew about where his people had gone. It still took some doing to locate them. Armstrong found two of them in the Bavarian Alps, designing artificial limbs in a chicken coop.[18]

As soon as the plans to establish the new CME at Heidelberg were finalized, Armstrong went back to Göttingen and asked Strughold whether he would be willing to head the new group. He would function as a sort of senior scientist working under an American director. Because the University of Göttingen was in the British zone, Strughold's assent entailed some negotiating on Armstrong's part in London. He got his way, however, and, in November, Strughold was transferred to Heidelberg, where he spent a day as an American POW before being released to work as a civilian at the new lab.[19]

Armstrong approached Hans-Georg Clamann personally at his family home in Groß-Schwülper. Although the town's citizens were fortunate to have three physicians available, the only means they had to pay was by barter, and by this time no one had much that they could part with or that anyone would want. Armstrong came to the house one day and asked Clamann to come to Heidelberg, but the scientist declined the invitation. Armstrong left. Not long afterward, however, Clamann heard that a German colleague had been forcibly taken to Russia, so he got in touch with the American. "I've had a change of heart," Clamann said. "I knew you would," Armstrong replied.[20]

Ultimately, neither the British nor the Soviets secured any aviation-medicine researchers of note. Most of them either stayed in Germany or came to the United States, permanently or for ten years or so. At least two, Heinz von Diringshofen and an Austrian named Harald von Beckh, went to Argentina.[21]

THE ARMY AIR FORCES AEROMEDICAL CENTER AT HEIDELBERG

Even as civilians, the Germans at Heidelberg found that their movements were restricted under the terms of their six-month contract. They had to live in the building where they worked rather than with their families. They were paid food and one hundred dollars per month, but with starvation and disease rampant in the bombed-out cities, that still was enough to tempt almost everyone who had children.[22] Strughold, a childless bachelor, used his confinement to pursue his interest in history and read several volumes on the history of medicine.[23]

The army gave the Germans one directive: to reconstruct from memory, notes, and wartime journal articles the research they had done for the Luftwaffe and to present it in publishable form in English. By November 1946, the Germans at Heidelberg had finished around thirty-five studies. Fifty-nine scientists in all contributed eighty articles and three hundred illustrations, totaling nearly thirteen hundred published pages. Strughold was given the task of coordinating their efforts and of writing the introductory pieces on the history of German aviation medicine. An American, Maj. William F. Sheeley, oversaw the team of editors and translators in Heidelberg until March 1947 and then at the School of Aviation Medicine for another two years. Army medical artists helped recreate lost drawings, and the editorial staff and authors mailed their manuscripts back and forth until all were satisfied that both English and German versions were in good order. The work was time consuming and detailed, but the result was an impressive, two-volume illustrated work, *German Aviation Medicine, World War II,* that reveals in understated fashion the extent to which Germany experimented with rockets and studied problems directly related to high-speed flight.[24]

Meanwhile, the University of Heidelberg had offered Strughold the chair of the Helmholtz Institute, a very prominent position. Its previous holder had been a staunch party member, and that was now a liability. He had to go.[25] So, during the summer of 1946 and the 1946–1947 academic year, Strughold also taught physiology at the university. Once again rooms overflowed with young students who wanted to hear the lectures by "Struggie," his "official name" at the school.[26]

The army deactivated the Heidelberg center on March 1, 1947, but Armstrong had already approached Strughold, Clamann, Luft, Schmidt, Rose, Benzinger, Otto Gauer, and others about coming to the United States on short-term contracts under Project Paperclip. More than thirty Germans accepted.[27] In a 1961 interview Strughold claimed that when the offer to go to Texas came, he had not wanted to leave his teaching post but felt that he owed it to the others to see the book project through to the end. He also claimed that Heidelberg urged him to go because they wanted to make connections again with other universities. This actually seems either unlikely or a task that Strughold mysteriously neglected. He was not going to any American university in the traditional sense, although the school was part of the U.S. Army War College, a postgraduate institution, and he never became a faculty member at any other university or developed close ties with any other teaching institution.[28] Whatever his reasons for accepting, though, he happily set sail for New York.

Coming to America

In the camp at Landshut, Germany, where the Clamann family was living, Hans-Georg and Marie talked over the offer to work in America. Neither one wanted to go, but the alternative seemed to be short-term starvation and long-term unemployment for Hans-Georg as a researcher. America meant a job, but it also meant going to a land about which they had heard so many evil things over the past fourteen years. Religion was important to the Clamanns, who had a mixed Lutheran-Catholic marriage, and they knew that Americans were not religious at all. There was no music, art, or literature in America, either. The Americans still treated blacks like slaves, and worst of all, they were known to actually eat human flesh when the mood suited them. Hans-Georg was willing to go on ahead of the family, but what if something happened to him? How could he warn them if things were as bad as they had heard? Father and mother decided on a secret code: If things were so horrible that Marie ought to take the children and flee the camp, Hans-Georg would use a certain phrase in his letters home. If things were all right, he would leave it out. That made things a bit better, and the family settled down uneasily to await the day of Hans-Georg's departure.[29]

The German scientists went to the States in batches. Ulrich Luft's travel orders, dated May 15, 1947, show him going from Landshut to Bremerhaven to take the first available ship to the United States. He recalled later going next by military bus to a military airport in New York, then on to Alabama and finally to San Antonio. A total of eleven Paperclips in the group, including Luft and meteorologist Konrad Büttner, were bound for the school, and another four went to the air materiel command at Wright Field. One rocket specialist went to von Braun's group at Fort Bliss, near El Paso. Eight others went to five different naval centers in various states. Luft's orders also show him traveling with a family of 6 dependents to meet a spouse who had already been sent to Wright Field, a group of 25 dependents (spouses and children) heading to Fort Bliss, and another 20 dependents rejoining loved ones under contract to the navy. The civilians received six dollars per day as a subsistence allowance, except for the period on board ship, because the cost of the ticket included their meals. Dependents were allowed to purchase army rations at the same price as their officer escorts.[30]

When Harry Armstrong had visited the Clamann home, he had been accompanied by his driver, the first black man the family had ever seen. When Clamann arrived in the United States, he and the other Paperclips were placed on a train bound for El Paso, Texas, and were guarded by black MPs. At mealtimes, the Germans were escorted off the train and into a restaurant, where they were fed, but their guards were not allowed inside. This happened at every meal stop. They really do treat the blacks like slaves, Clamann thought. That was something he would have to consider when he decided what to tell Marie and the boys.

Clamann's train arrived in Texas, but instead of stopping in San Antonio it kept going west. The worried Germans found themselves in El Paso at a jail for POWs. This is not what we were told would happen, they said to each other. In horror, Clamann realized that what he had feared was true; they were going to be jailed forever or executed or tortured—or something. It would be foolish to wait for evidence of cannibalism. He would write to his wife right away and use the secret message to tell her that she and the boys must not come to America. He quickly wrote the letter and sent it by military post.

In Germany, mother and children waited for word from Texas. Finally a letter arrived. Marie opened it while the boys watched. She unfolded the letter and stared at it in disbelief: It looked like a paper doily. Army censorship had come down so heavily on the Paperclips that almost nothing was left of her husband's letter. Marie wept with disappointment and fear. Her one consolation was that the warning sentence was not in the remaining shreds of the letter, so it must be all right to come. Even if it was not, she decided, it was better for the family to be together. So the Clamanns packed their belongings and took the boat—in error—to the United States.[31]

Many of the Germans kept in touch with former colleagues who had stayed behind, including those who went on trial in Nuremberg. Before they left, Strughold, Clamann, Luft, and others wrote testimonial letters for the defendants and gave affidavits concerning the nature of their research. Anything declaring that these men were of good character as scientists might be useful in their defense, they thought.[32] Ulrich Luft kept up at least a thready correspondence from the United States with Hermann Becker-Freyseng's wife and in return heard from her about the situation in Germany and her husband's condition at the Landsberg prison. He also negotiated with expedition organizer Paul Bauer over the making and distribution of a film about their Himalayan experiences. Throughout the rest of his career, Luft would continue to correspond with scientists in the United States and Germany about research in high-altitude physiology.[33]

Hans-Georg, out of jail and reassured as to the safety of life in the United States, met Marie and the boys at the Randolph airfield. He would take them to their house a little later, he said. First, they had somewhere else to go. Hans-Georg drove them over to a hangar that was full of people, most of them in uniform, and long tables were set with food for everyone to eat. There was more food than the boys had ever seen, and some things were items they had never tasted in Germany. That didn't matter; it all looked good.

"We can't afford this!" Mrs. Clamann said to her husband, shocked, embarrassed, and a little bit angry that he had brought them to such a feast when they could not pay for any of it.

"We don't have to pay," he explained. "We are guests. It is Thanksgiving, an American holiday."

The children did not need such reassurance. America was suddenly looking like a great place. They ate and ate, got sick, and ate some more.[34]

ADJUSTING

By the end of 1947, not everyone on the base had welcomed the German nationals into their community. Many of the people living there had fought in Europe or lost family and friends in the conflict, and the war had not been over long enough to allow warm feelings to grow. Some of the bitterness and hostility had been directed at the scientists at the school, and Armstrong was concerned that one or more of the Texans might actually assault a German. Consequently, he cautioned the Paperclips to keep to themselves and avoid confrontations.

For the most part, that was not a significant problem because few spoke English well, if at all. Ulrich Luft spoke English with native fluency, although with a Scottish accent. Besides him, only Kurt Kramer, who had attended Cambridge University, could converse well in English. Luft acted as an ad hoc translator in various transactions and was given power of attorney by some of the Paperclips, which authorized him to act in their stead on financial and legal matters.[35]

After six months, when the families of those Paperclips who decided to stay on in the United States came over, the situation was still very tense. A number of families, including the Clamanns, Lufts, and Roses, had young children between the ages of four and eight. Harry Armstrong had met some of the youngsters in Germany and saw them as pink-cheeked little cherubs, possibly as future Americans. Something had to be done to defuse the situation, he knew, and maybe these kids were the key. So he went to the wives' club with his wife, Mary, one afternoon and stood up and asked for a moment of the women's time.

"I know that you don't care much about these Germans that are over here or about their families," he began, "but they have got a lot of children—little tots three, four, or five years old—and they are in a strange country, and the people are not very friendly to them, and this is their first Christmas away from home."

The women, all officers' wives, were for the most part looking at him with polite enough gazes that Armstrong thought his idea might be worth a try. He went on.

"Now, for the children's sake, would you consider buying a twenty-five- or fifty-cent gift for each one or some of them? We will have a Christmas party for the children. We will have one of the Germans—because the children can't speak English in most cases—we'll get him a costume, dress him up as Santa Claus, and all those that give a gift can come to this party, and we'll give the gifts to the children."

Hearteningly, the women seemed to take to the idea right away. When he left, they were talking about decorations and refreshments and what sorts of toys the children might like. All he had to do was find the Santa suit.

A few weeks later, the women held the party, and as Armstrong had hoped, it was an enormous success. The Americans fell in love with the German children and then discovered that their mothers were very nice women. Before the afternoon's festivities were over, the scientists were pretty good people, too. There was not a Hitler in the bunch. The ice was broken at Randolph, and the problem quickly came to an end.[36]

In another incident, the military police confiscated a cache of sugar—because the whole lot was infested with bugs—that one scientist had secretly been hoarding since his arrival in America. The man screamed, cried, and begged them to leave it alone. It was for his family back in Germany, he shouted, because they were starving. Two guards pinned him, struggling and kicking, while another quickly destroyed the contaminated stash. The man collapsed, sobbing and nearly out of his mind with the thought of his family perishing from famine when he had food to spare. Moved by pity, the guards took up a collection so the man could send sugar and other essentials to his family. From that day on, one of the Germans recalled, the Paperclips and their families were "Americans through and through."[37]

In 1947, American news sources were indeed reporting critical shortages of food, fuel, clothing, and housing in Germany. The Randolph commissary sold the ready-made CARE packages that the Paperclips could buy and send to friends, relatives, and colleagues still living in the grim postwar conditions. These contained measured amounts of meat, sugar, fat, cocoa, and coffee and came in small boxes for those with many people on their mailing list or large containers for those with bigger families or fatter wallets. In spite of their meager salaries—less than what base secretaries earned—the Germans sent what they could to loved ones back home.[38]

Uli and Alice Luft had a long list of people they knew would appreciate a package, so they saved enough to augment the rations with a few other items such as tobacco and even old clothes, knowing these would be welcome, too. Friends in Germany kept them informed of the situation there, and they knew it to be grave since many civilians and displaced persons, "DPs," had died right after the war due to exposure and disease. Some were bombed-out city dwellers and foreigners who had been liberated from their prison camps; they had neither a home to return to nor a desire to live in the Soviet zone. Letters from coworkers, friends, and climbing comrades told the couple that ordinary Germans, too, were in nearly as bad a shape. One mountaineer wrote to thank the Lufts for the food, sweaters, socks, and an old pipe they had put inside a package. He mentioned that his son was being sent to a special camp because he was malnourished and underweight.[39] Nearly everyone told them about mutual acquaintances left homeless by the war. Knowing that finding an intact apartment would be extremely difficult, Luft offered the use of his Berlin dwelling and all of its contents to a colleague at the university.[40]

By 1950, the Paperclips were able to start retrieving belongings they had left behind in Germany, though it would take several years for items the army believed nonessential to find their way to Texas. Sometimes creative labeling was necessary to convince Uncle Sam that doing without certain items would impair the Paperclips' ability to serve their new country. Military shipping manifests show Ulrich Luft receiving a case of "scientific equipment" that included "one tent bag . . . climbing ropes . . . one mandolin, one pair of India slippers . . . two pairs of iron climbing shoes, one hammock, one sword, one tropic helmet . . . one sleeping bag, [and] two violins with cases."[41]

THE LIFE SCIENTISTS AND THE ROCKETEERS

Securing Germany's aviation-medicine experts can be compared to recruiting the von Braun rocketry team, and certainly both proved critical to the development of the U.S. manned space program. However, the two events differ in key ways. The disparities may explain why Wernher von Braun's name is still synonymous with space exploration while the contributions of the "other Germans" are largely forgotten.

As a group, von Braun and his companions were unknowns in the United States while Strughold, Ruff, Clamann, Luft, von Diringshofen, Benzinger, and so on were personal acquaintances of the aeromedical experts or could at least be found in the scientific literature or on a bookshelf. Unlike the rocketeers, the German physicians had peers in the United States, who were already organized along similar although not identical lines. The United States had no rocket-manufacturing capability, but it had the School of Aviation Medicine, the Wright Lab, and contract researchers at the Mayo Clinic, Harvard, Yale, and two dozen other universities. It had the Aero Medical Association and people like Armstrong, Benson, and Lovelace, who knew which areas of research would be of use to the postwar U.S. military and which Germans to "acquire." Although the rocket designers had worked in secret, throughout the war the German doctors had continued to act like scientists, although they were largely isolated by politics. They published their results in appropriate scientific and medical journals, organized and attended conferences, wrote textbooks, gave talks, supervised the doctoral work of students in their field, traveled abroad, hosted guests at their institutions, and reviewed books submitted by foreign authors to the journals.[42] In this sense, the Americans got a proven product in the medical group, whereas the army took an enormous gamble on von Braun. A roll of the dice, when it pays off, is much more exciting and attention-grabbing than a sure thing.

There were also deeper personal differences between von Braun and the one German physician who headed a program in the United States, Hubertus Strughold. Although the latter was brilliant, von Braun had been a wunderkind in rocket design before such a discipline even existed. He had earned a degree in mechanical engineering and a Ph.D. in physics when he was twenty-two. He came from a wealthy and well-connected Prussian family, and his father, Baron Magnus von Braun, was secretary of agriculture in the Weimar cabinet.

During the 1950s, Wernher von Braun became a household name in the United States when he popularized the notion of space colonization via the television sets that were popping up in every American living room. Walt

Disney built several episodes of his TV show around von Braun's ideas and had the German design a portion of the new theme park he was constructing in the orange groves of southern California. Disney called the segment "Tomorrowland."

Strughold led from behind, enjoying the attention he received in the lecture hall but giving full academic freedom to subordinates and acting as mentor to numerous scientists. He made no attempt to forge a permanent team and hold it together in America. Von Braun put himself and his rockets front and center, and he promoted his group and his technology within the German Army, the U.S. military, and later the National Aeronautics and Space Administration. Amid all the attention, no one thought to ask the charismatic creator of the V-2 any hard questions about his connection with the Nazi regime.

Some people question how Strughold, a Catholic and a man of medicine, could have known about Dachau and not have publicly protested or somehow even prevented it. This is a legitimate and useful query. Strughold's failure to act on any knowledge of events that had already transpired, however, pales in comparison with the decision of von Braun and his colleague Walter Dornberger to work—to death—thousands of slave laborers in underground rocket factories. Perhaps the explanation is that the life scientists' primary interest was always the human subject, frailties and all, while the engineers' main concern was the machine and the places it could take those who controlled its power.

For the life scientists, space exploration was a natural expression of scientific inquisitiveness, but it was not the driving force behind their search for knowledge. Voyaging to the moon or planets on behalf of a specific nation or putting a human being into space to accomplish a technological coup or make a political point was never on their agenda. Von Braun and his associates, however, used their speaking engagements, Disney ventures, film collaborations, and writings to call often and loudly for American military supremacy in space, pushing the Cold War button with summonses to "conquer" space, the moon, and Mars.

Another telling difference between doctors and engineers was group cohesion and self-promotion. Strughold, Clamann, Luft, and colleagues had to be ferreted out and begged to come to the United States, while von Braun marched his people and their blueprints into the arms of the Americans, having decided that the Soviets were too incompatible and the British too broke to afford their services.[43] The life scientists acted as individuals, dispersing during the 1950s and 1960s to academia, industry, other government agencies, and private medical practices, while the rocket team remained, for the most part, intact until retirement or death. Among the aeromedical specialists, only psychologist Siegfried Gerathewohl went to work for the space agency as late as the 1960s. Whether it was that *unvölkisch* individualism of the autoexperimenter or a mistrust of the civilian government involving itself in medicine—after what had happened at Dachau—all of the other Paperclip physicians stayed away from NASA.

ORGANIZING FOR SPACE MEDICINE

After the war, a free exchange of personnel between the Wright Lab and the School of Aviation Medicine began, due primarily to the fact that Armstrong and Benson had both headed the lab before coming to the school. While most of the Heidelberg Paperclips went to Texas, several were assigned to Dayton, including biomedical engineer Hans Mauch and physiologist Otto Gauer. They were charged with conducting practical research into matters directly related to air corps operations. Thus the lab personnel tried to determine what new human-engineering measures would be required to integrate acquisitions from the Luftwaffe—jet- and rocket-powered aircraft—into their arsenal.

The task called for a quantum leap ahead of the work done by Armstrong and Heim and even Randy Lovelace. For one thing, the speeds the new aircraft could reach were nearly double what the United States had been able to achieve thus far. This increase created correspondingly greater hazards for the pilots and crews. Bailing out could not be accomplished by simply crawling out of a hatch or standing up in one's seat and then jumping because the force created by the velocity of the airplane, equivalent to a seven-hundred-mile-per-hour windblast, could tear facial skin and even blind a pilot. The accelerative and decelerative forces were also much greater than anything previously encountered in propeller-driven aircraft. Reaction times would be critical at the speeds these vehicles reached, which meant that a redesign of cockpit interiors was necessary in order to allow pilots to reach particular buttons and switches easily. Jets were noisy, too. Improved hearing protection was obviously required.

The higher altitude capability of the new planes also created immediate and novel hazards for pilots and crew. The low air pressure at one hundred thousand feet necessitated pressure suits that covered the entire body. Pilots who bailed out at such altitudes could begin to spin so fast that they would die from the centrifugal pressures on their heart, lungs, and brain before they reached an altitude where there was enough atmosphere for their chute to work or oxygen to breathe on the way down. Enough was known about the atmosphere at that level to cause worry over the exposure of aircrews on long-duration flights to cosmic rays, a potential long-term health hazard.

Four different Wright Lab directors between 1946 and 1954 added a number of new facilities to enable needed research. These included a downward-ejection tower, a vertical accelerator, a Link Trainer facility, an animal surgery room, a spin table, a third human centrifuge, acoustical chambers, an instrumentation laboratory, a bioelectronics laboratory, a clothing-fabrication facility, a hundred-foot vertical-ejection tower, a shop for sculptors working on ergonomic design issues, a remote manipulator, and a speech-recognition lab.[44]

A key effort was finding the human tolerance levels for the forces encountered during high-speed ejection. Working first with dummies and animals, then with human beings, lab personnel duplicated the conditions created during bailout, when both pilot and seat would rocket up and out of the aircraft or be propelled out and downward—through the bottom. Windblasts during these tests measured between 80 and 300 miles per hour.

The first live test in the United States of an upward ejection was performed (satisfactorily) in 1946, and downward tests were conducted in 1948. Both were survivable, although by the end of 1955, 23 percent of the air force's 757 ejections would be fatal. Another 14 percent would cause major injuries.[45] Obviously, the aircraft design, seat technology, and safety training needed major retooling.

After 1946, the school became part of the Air University, a postgraduate institute for training officers. Its departments included aerobiology, pathology, physiology/biophysics, radiobiology, biometrics, pharmacology/biochemistry, and psychology.[46] Although he was named commander of the same in 1946 and would never return to the Wright Lab and the materiel command, Harry Armstrong followed the activities of his old lab very closely while at the school, particularly the work with experimental aircraft at a new field lab at Muroc, California. His efforts at Wright Field had taught him that the lag time between an experimental craft such as the X-1 and a workable aircraft was from ten to twenty years. In his estimation, however, enthusiastic engineers would want to send someone up in one of the V-2s before anyone knew. The school and the lab really needed to put things into overdrive if the air force were to be ready to launch someone into space within a decade.[47]

Newly promoted to brigadier general in May, 1948, Armstrong appointed Hubertus Strughold and another Paperclip, Heinz Haber, to define the types of medical problems that a manned space program could expect to encounter. Haber, who held doctorates in physics and astrophysics and had been head of the Department of Spectroscopy at the Kaiser Wilhelm Institute for Physical Chemistry, would describe the physical environment. Strughold would develop theories about the likely effects of that environment on the human organism. Both were very interested in the theoretical and scientific implications of life—human and nonhuman—in space, but as a more immediate concern they wanted to safeguard the lives of air force personnel who might ride a von Braun rocket.[48] The first task they undertook was surveying the existing scientific literature—in other words, examining everything that had been published on the physical environment above twenty thousand feet or that had a bearing on survival at extremely high altitudes.

Centrifuge tests in Germany and the United States had already demonstrated that human beings could survive the expected ten Gs to which a capsule's occupant would be subjected. Temperature extremes, radiation exposure, toxic gases in the cabin, and the mental pressures of isolation and confinement were all problems that Haber and Strughold identified but had already been examined to some extent using high-altitude balloons, isolation chambers, and other means.[49] Low air pressure would require a full-body pressure suit that would enable the blood to circulate and other physiological functions to happen. The lack of oxygen meant a survival time of less than five minutes without proper breathing equipment. What was more challenging than had been expected, they reported to Armstrong, was extended weightlessness. While a handful of pilots had experienced a few seconds of zero gravity, there was concern that hours, days, or weeks of such conditions could cause physical and mental problems ranging from muscular weakness to psychosis to death. There was no way to create a long-duration weightless condition on Earth, so they were left with theories they had no way to test.[50]

SPACE MEDICINE GOES PUBLIC

Strughold and Haber worked through the summer and fall and found enough material that Armstrong felt ready to have a panel discussion at the school in November 1948, cosponsored by the air surgeon, the National Research Council, and Wright Lab. It was the first professional conference on biology in space, and the panel members, besides Strughold and Haber, included seven physicians from the military and academia.

Haber opened with a description of the means by which a capsule could be placed into orbit, drawing on his knowledge of celestial mechanics and propulsion. This was completely new information to his audience, so he went slowly, explaining the liftoff and the speeds a craft would have to reach to enter various orbits, depending on the location of the launch site and the angle of flight. He then described the escape velocities that would be required of a craft to reach each body in the solar system, depending on its distance from the Earth, the angle of departure, and the gravitational pull of the target body.[51] Strughold's talk centered on travel to Mars.

The panel was an unexpected hit, with seven hundred attendees crowding the Randolph movie theater to hear the Germans. The *Journal of Aviation Medicine* printed transcripts of the speeches in its 1949 issue.[52] The enthusiasm was enough for Armstrong to ask the school scientists to submit detailed plans, by department, of the approach they would take in tackling these medical problems.[53]

Strughold had a slightly different plan in mind. One evening in January 1949, he called Haber into his office, and over glasses of bourbon the two talked about the study and about the opportunities it offered the school and the scientists. They decided that the matter of human space travel was something that required much deeper study, far beyond what they could do in their free time. They needed an official platform from which to speak about their findings, too. Creating a new department would be a good plan, provided they could count on the air force to back them up in public. In the end, both agreed that Strughold ought to broach the subject with Harry Armstrong. Not only had he known Armstrong longer, but both were medical doctors and both had headed military research labs and could discuss the ins and outs of getting the necessary funding and approvals.

Historian Clarence Lasby surveyed 165 Paperclips who had worked for different government agencies in 1960 and found that they "were nearly all disappointed in the failure of the military services to utilize their abilities during the 'lean years' of the 'ice-box policy' when they were in 'cold storage.'"[54] Whether Strughold or Haber at that stage felt frustrated over the pace at which work was proceeding or with the Germans' share of the leading-edge research, no record remains. What is certain, however, is that Strughold saw this as the chance of a lifetime. The next day, bright and early, he made an appointment to talk with Armstrong and at ten o'clock went into the general's office.

"He was wondering what I had in mind," Strughold recalled later. "Perhaps I wanted to quit and go back to Heidelberg. But when I told him that we had come to the conclusion that a project was not enough, that we should have a *department* for these extraterrestrial studies, he was very relieved and pleased. Immediately he asked how many people do you need, how many rooms, and what budget." Happy that the transaction had gone so well, Strughold left Armstrong's office very satisfied with the whole situation. He had gone in as a former enemy working on a short-term contract and come out as the world's first "professor of space medicine."[55]

Founding the Department of Space Medicine was one of Armstrong's last official acts at the school. Two months later, in July 1949, he was sent to the Pentagon to replace Malcolm Grow, who was serving a courtesy tour of four months as the first surgeon general of the air force before retiring. Otis Benson, who had replaced Armstrong at the lab, then had served as surgeon of the Fifteenth Air Force and surgeon of the air forces in the Mediterranean during World War II, would again step up as Armstrong's successor. With the job at the school would come a promotion to brigadier general.[56]

The Department of Space Medicine was officially established on February 9, 1949, with Strughold as its scientific head, Armstrong as temporary administrator until Strughold was ready to take charge, and Haber as a staff member. Soon they were joined by meteorologist Konrad Büttner and Haber's older brother, Fritz, who held a doctorate in aeronautical engineering and had worked for the Junkers aircraft company designing, among other things, piggyback air transport systems.[57]

In spite of the new department, only Armstrong and a very small number of higher-ups associated with the school felt they could use the word "space" in grown-up company. For those at the Wright Lab, surrounded by practical-minded aeroengineering types, it would not be until the end of the decade and the deployment of planes capable of reaching the edges of the atmosphere that the term was accepted as anything but fantasy. Space was the place the air force dared not go, at least in public.

Struggling for acceptance by the other services, the newly created U.S. Air Force knew that the "experts" considered interplanetary travel, at least in the near term, as merely science fiction. Paul Campbell arranged the school's first space symposium that was open to the public at the University of Illinois, where he was teaching in 1950. He cautiously advertised it as only a talk on "weightlessness." The plan was to approach the subject warily, beginning with a simple review of the literature on the workings of the inner ear. Wernher von Braun had been invited, too. It would be his first appearance at a medical symposium.[58] The university expected to attract only a couple dozen people given the minimal publicity they had given the event, but students packed the auditorium, eager to devour anything on space, rockets, and interplanetary travel. The published proceedings went through three press runs before the printer was finally able to send a set off to each participant. Too many teenagers had been snapping them up, he told Campbell.[59]

The event's success may have convinced some of the air force brass that they were right about space and its appeal to teenagers. Harry Armstrong, by then surgeon general of the U.S. Air Force, felt that the time was right to host a full-scale conference that would be open to the public. The location would be the school, he decided. By the close of 1951, six hundred people were working there, one hundred of them in research and teaching.

Still not quite brave enough to use the word "space," the school titled the November 1951 event "Physics and Medicine of the Upper Atmosphere," but no one was fooled. The conference attracted coverage from major print media and included the participation of thirty-five scientists and engineers from all over the United States, including von Braun and several members of his organization, plus three hundred military and civilian guests. These included Chuck Yeager, Clayton S. White of the Lovelace Clinic, Generals Carl Spaatz and Ira Eaker, geneticist H. J. Muller, the navy's aviation-medicine expert, Ashton Graybiel, physicist James Van Allen, and astronomer Fred Whipple. The press had representatives from the *Saturday Evening Post, Reader's Digest, Aviation Age,* and the Associated Press wire services.[60] The editor of *Colliers* magazine, Cornelius Ryan, attended with one of his illustrators, Chesley Bonestell. Both liked what they heard and saw and decided to do an illustrated series on von Braun's vision of space exploration.[61] The published proceedings would become "the Bible of scientific medicine" for the next decade.[62]

Aerospace Medicine as a Military Mission

Armstrong's biggest challenge in the early 1950s was the Korean War, an interlude that serves as a reminder that the military component was a vital part of the careers of the American aerospace-medicine specialists. In the foreword to *Physics and Medicine of the Upper Atmosphere,* the proceedings of the symposium held in November 1951, Armstrong discussed the relationship between aviation medicine and space research. It is obvious that he was writing it with Korea, the first armed conflict of the Cold War, as the backdrop:

> The effectiveness of the United States Air Force, in its primary role of preserving peace, is measured in terms of the deterrent effect its combat striking power has on potential aggressors. . . . The skill and ingenuity of the aeronautical engineer in designing aircraft with increased speed, endurance, and altitude performance have currently projected our flying personnel into the immediate vicinity of an environmental frontier beyond which our knowledge is incomplete, and in some respects, totally lacking. . . . [T]he

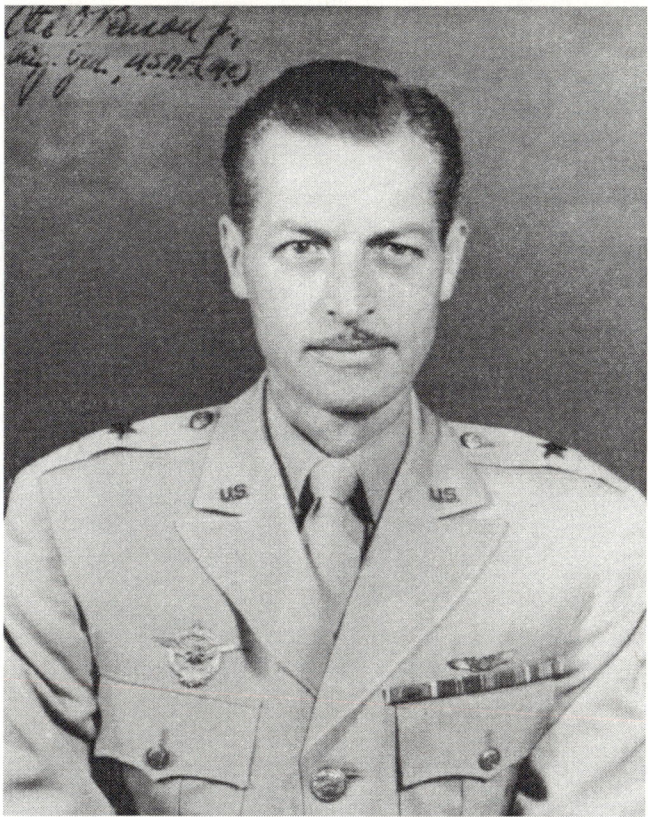

*The new brigadier general and commandant of the School of
Aviation Medicine, Otis O. Benson Jr., around 1949. National
Library of Medicine photo.*

practical aspects of the matter at hand . . . derive their immediate
importance from their relationship to the preservation of world
peace, or, if that should fail, the preservation of our nation and the
other free nations of the world.[63]

Armstrong, Benson, Lovelace, Stapp, Campbell, and the others were all
career military officers or physicians with long periods of active and reserve
service. All had been volunteers. Soldiering was a vital part of their personalities and could not be separated out.[64]

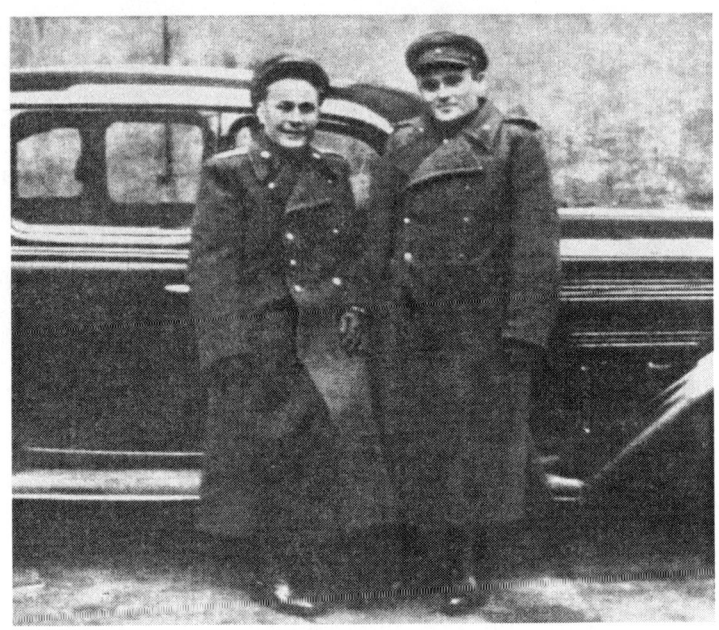

Soviet rocket designers Andrei Tupolev and Sergei Korolyov retrieved German rocket parts at war's end but no aeromedical personnel. NASA photo.

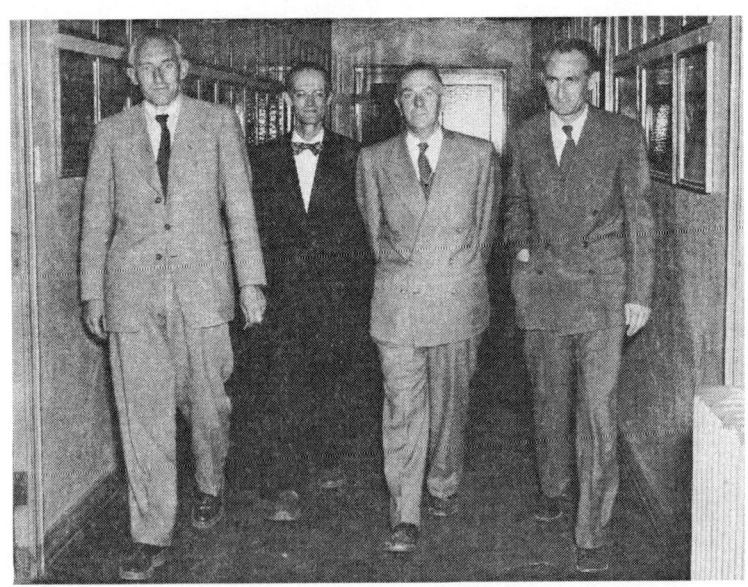

The faculty of the SAM Department of Space Medicine. Left to right: Fritz Haber, Konrad Büttner, Hubertus Strughold, and Heinz Haber. USAF photo.

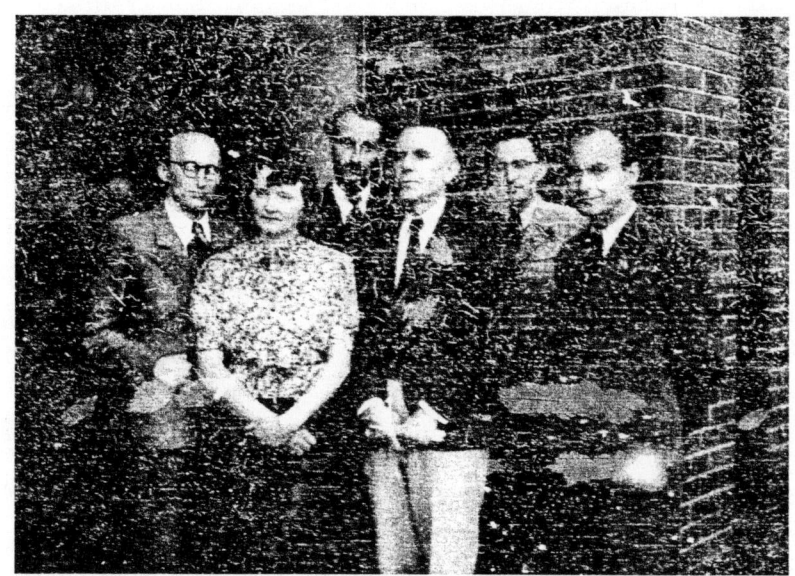

Part of the German staff that worked for the U.S. Army in Heidelberg after World War II. From left to right: Johannes Prast, Ingeborg Schmidt, Heinz Haber, Hubertus Strughold, Siegfried Gerathewohl, and Heinrich Rose. All were sensory physiologists except for physicist/astronomer Haber and psychologist Gerathewohl. U.S. Army photo, reprinted from the Report from Heidelberg.

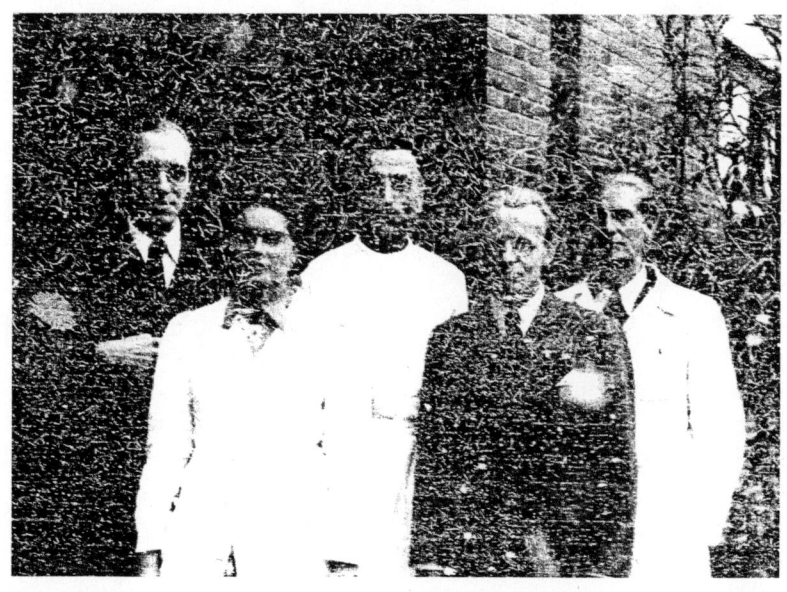

These rare images depict the Heidelberg teams of Benzinger and Ruff. Benzinger team, left to right: Heinz Maier-Leibnitz, Charlotte Kitzinger, Benzinger, engineer Henry Seeler, and Helmuth Beinert. U.S. Army photo, reprinted from Report from Heidelberg.

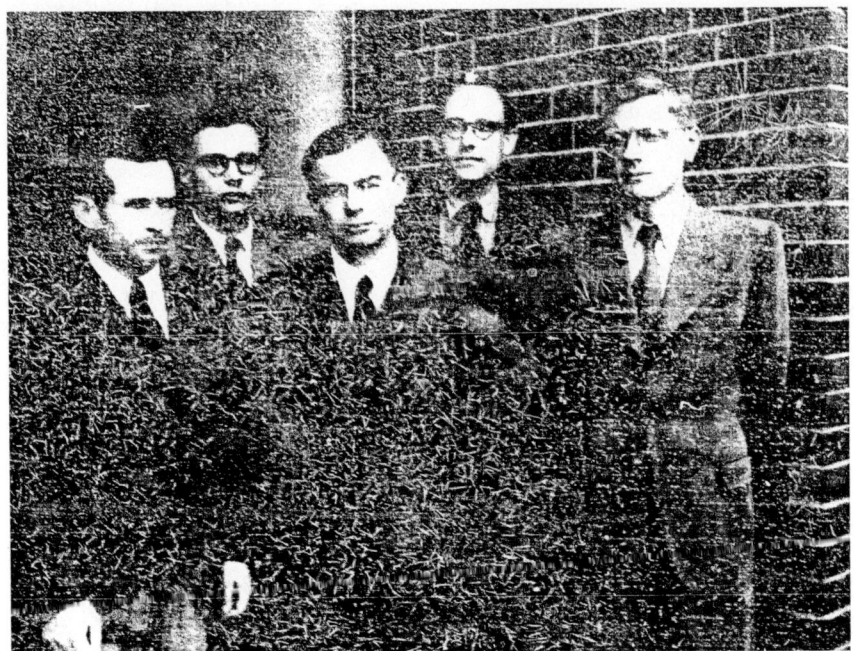

Ruff team, left to right: Hermann Becker-Freyseng, engineer Karl Hausser, Ruff, Konrad Schäfer, and Otto Gauer. U.S. Army photo, reprinted from Report from Heidelberg.

THE NEW AMERICANS

By 1953, the Lufts were well enough established that Ulrich was able to help a mountaineering team making an attempt on K2 (the second-highest mountain in the world) buy oxygen equipment and to send a hundred-dollar donation to the Deutsche Cordilleren Rundfahrt as they set out to combine climbing and science in the Peruvian Andes.[65] The family had built a home in the hill country between San Antonio and Austin, not far from several other Paperclips, including master technician Oskar Lange and his wife, the Roses, and the Clamanns. Bruno Balke had arrived two years earlier, although without his family at first, and was staying on a farm where he could run and ride to his heart's content. The Lufts' son Friederich was in fourth grade and had friends among Texas youngsters and the other Paperclip kids. Alice Luft, also a former LMFI employee, stayed at home in spite of her scientific training, as did Marie Clamann.[66]

At the time, though, some of the Paperclips felt that they were no longer wanted.[67] Some of them believed Otis Benson was not as sympathetic toward them as Armstrong had been. Others thought he was efficient and very competent at dealing with Washington but that, perhaps given his education, Benson simply gave the impression that he was not as much in awe of the Germans as his more rustic predecessor had been.[68] Whatever their reasons, after their five-year contracts were up, several of the German doctors left. Ingeborg Schmidt moved to the University of Indiana. Konrad Büttner, who had worked as a section chief at Rechlin for Theo Benzinger and been a professor of biophysics at the University of Kiel, left in January 1952 for UCLA and a research fellowship in bioclimatology. Physiologist Werner Noell moved to Buffalo, Heinrich Rose to southern California, and Fritz Haber to aviation manufacturer Avco Lycoming in Connecticut. Otto Gauer went from the Wright Lab back to an academic career in Germany.

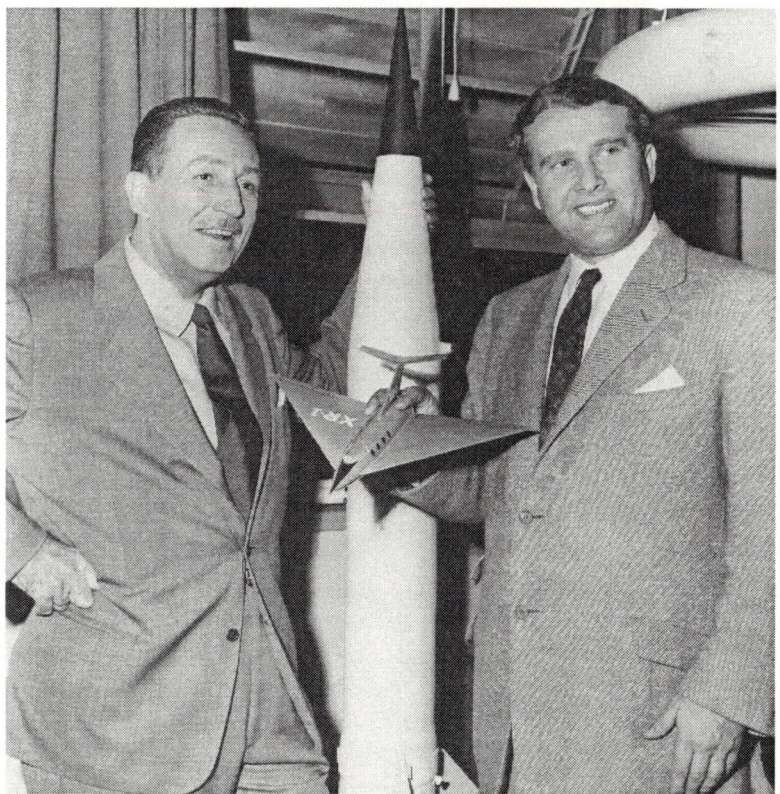

Walt Disney consulted with Strughold and Heinz Haber of the SAM as well as German rocket designer Wernher von Braun (right) for his television shows, films, and theme park. NASA photo.

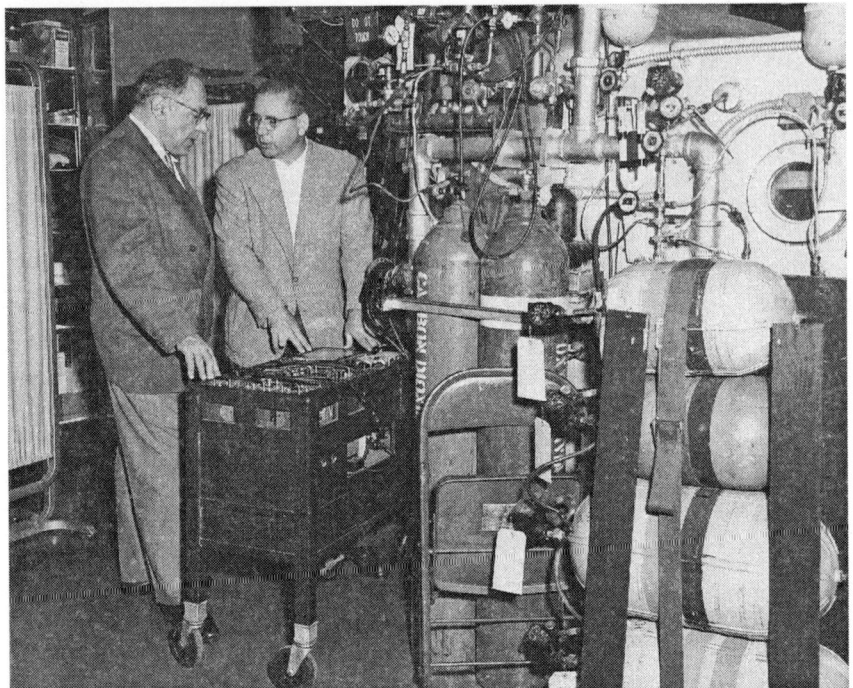

Willy Ley (left) was a visitor to the SAM in the 1950s. USAF photo.

Ulrich Luft and his wife decided they wanted to stay in America, where their young son could continue to chide his father about his Scottish accent. He had begun to feel some disquiet about the momentum and trajectory of his career at the school, however. He was unlikely to be leading any Himalayan expeditions there and had missed out on a chance to go to the Andes. The work in San Antonio was interesting but in a way becoming too routine, and he knew he could put his knowledge of high-altitude respiratory problems to work much better somewhere other than the Texas lowland. Through the grapevine Luft had also heard about the expansion that Randy Lovelace was planning for the clinic he owned with his namesake uncle in Albuquerque. Lovelace's old Mayo mentor, Walter Boothby, had even come to work for the school and then left for Albuquerque, partly for his health but also because the work there promised to be innovative.[69]

Then, out of the blue in 1953, Clayton S. "Sam" White of the Lovelace Clinic wrote that Boothby had decided to retire. Would Luft like to have his job?

White and Lovelace dangled what they knew would be tempting carrots: climbing in the Rockies and the chance for Luft to apply his skills to both government aerospace contracts and the respiratory problems associated with living and working in the mountains and desert southwest. Luft knew that Lovelace was genuinely interested in respiratory research in the high mountains, having been present for the official opening of a research station at Marocochan, Peru, in 1949, which Luft had not been able to attend.

Luft jumped at the opportunity, and his family moved to Albuquerque in January 1954.[70] Even as those who stayed in the United States felt themselves to be settling in as Americans, the U.S. Justice Department, specifically the FBI, was keeping them under surveillance. The Germans knew this, and it actually came in handy when someone received a threatening note, as Strughold did in 1958.[71] The watchdog treatment was given in part to verify that the scientists had no contacts with any Communists and were not engaged in espionage and also because some of them had relatives and friends still in the eastern zone and therefore were considered subject to pressure from Moscow. They had to make full reports of any conversations with Eastern European scientists at conferences, and existing friendships were scrutinized with and without their knowledge. Mail coming from Germany was either intercepted or handed over to the base commandant, copied, and translated for governmental review.

The letters were invariably innocuous but provided U.S. intelligence agencies with glimpses of social conditions in the East. Konrad Büttner's sister, for example, wrote in 1951 that she and her husband and children had finally been able to emigrate to West Germany after moving through a Kafkaesque series of government obstacles. Her husband, Karl (a middle-aged civil servant), had been fired because the East German government could not afford to keep anyone on the payroll who was anywhere close to pension age, she reported, so he had gone to the West "in the black market manner" and found work there. Büttner's sister had to wade through months of red tape to be able to leave and take the family's belongings with them.

First she had to prove they owed no back taxes and had no bank debts, then the husband had to return (again, surreptitiously) to verify that there was no work for him at home. The police were reluctant to put this fact in writing because, by official decree, no one was unemployed in East Germany. The wife, meanwhile, accumulated a whole book of documents, including lists of the family's belongings, which she had copied by hand seven times. Then both the administrative district office and the mayor had to approve the paperwork. Husband and wife had to sign an affidavit saying that they owned the furniture and that it was not then in use by any refugees. Finally, they had to secure testimony from two other tenants verifying the information. As they finished with these requirements, the Bureau for Culture issued a new regulation: A list of all of the books they planned to take out of the country had to be turned in, showing the title, author, publishing house, and publication date of each. Again, seven copies of the list had to be written out by hand. The family's belongings were finally loaded into an unpadded railroad car, and when the family reached the border, they were quizzed by four young East German policemen about their furnishings in order to identify them as being truly theirs.

The culture shock they experienced in what was then West Germany was greater than what six years of separation had prepared them for. Their children were unable to attend school at the appropriate grade level because they lacked training in Latin and English, among other subjects. Fat, meat, sugar, marmalade, linen, and stockings were not rationed, as they still were in East Germany. The couple was astonished at the number of well-nourished, even fat, people they saw in West Germany. The sister was rather bitter, too, that all of the West Germans who could pay for a vacation got one, while those in East Germany who desperately needed rest and better food could not afford such luxuries.[72]

Letters such as these probably contributed to the decision of Luft, Strughold, Büttner, Schmidt, Rose, Clamann, and many others to stay in the United States permanently. All of the Paperclips and their families who remained accepted citizenship in the 1950s. Those who did not do so went back to Europe, in some cases never feeling completely at home in either the United States or the new Germany.[73]

Chapter 5

THE FASTEST MAN ALIVE

E ven as the war was winding down, the scientists and engineers at Wright Field were experimenting with their German "acquisitions" and beginning the process of melding them with their own designs. One outcome would be the X-1 rocket plane, the first aircraft to take its pilot faster than the speed of sound. At the isolated test station in the California desert where pilots were wringing it out, a solitary flight surgeon was using himself as a guinea pig on the ground to make such brutal flying, with its inevitable crashes and ejections, survivable. He, too, would go faster than the speed of sound.

Civilian scientists had found new organization and purpose through their wartime associations and approached the army with plans to use captured V-2 rockets to explore the physical nature of the outer reaches of the atmosphere. In the process they would give the military's medical experts the data they needed on the space environment. The success of the rocket as a vehicle for sampling the edge of the atmosphere led to its incorporation into plans for an upcoming International Geophysical Year and even to the quite far-out notion of a permanent scientific station in Earth orbit.

Confident in the knowledge that their expertise and facilities were the best in the world when it came to space medicine, air force flight surgeons accelerated and augmented their research programs throughout the 1950s. Personnel at the School of Aerospace Medicine, the Wright Lab, and Holloman Air Force Base in New Mexico carried out weightlessness studies, balloon flights, laboratory work, more rocket-sled tests, and even high-altitude parachute jumps. Working on the very edge of space, they looked for and found the limits of human endurance, ingenuity, and courage.

JOHN PAUL STAPP

By 1947, given its wartime victories, the mastery of some amazing new technology, and recognition as an equivalent branch of the armed services, the air force was feeling decidedly frisky. Its experimental work on aircraft and the human-machine interface emphasized readiness for the next war; every airplane had to go higher and fly faster than the last one. There were speed and altitude records to be broken, and the air force went after them with gusto.

One of these was the sound barrier, the air resistance met by objects attempting to travel faster than the speed of sound. Some people had thought it would be impossible to design an airplane that could move that swiftly and still maintain its structural integrity. In October 1947, air force Capt. Chuck Yeager became the first person to break the sound barrier, and he did it flying an X-1 rocket plane. Carried aloft in the bomb bay of a B-29 Superfortress to an altitude of twenty-one thousand feet, the X-1 was released, then blasted forth over the southern California desert at a speed of more than 660 miles per hour until its fuel was exhausted and Yeager could guide it to a dead-stick landing on the dry lake bed below. The aircraft he flew had been built by Bell Aircraft, which was under contract to the air force and NACA, and the suit he wore for the flight had been designed at the Wright Lab, an experimental T-1 partial-pressure suit that was a skintight cotton-and-nylon ensemble made even snugger by the use of inflatable tubing down the sides. Physiologist James Henry, who had joined the lab after WWII, was the chief designer of the T-1.[1]

The flight surgeon on Yeager's project was Capt. John Paul Stapp, known to his family as Paul. Born to Baptist missionary parents in Bahía, on the coast of Brazil, he and his siblings grew up speaking Portuguese and living in a forty-seven room "castle" that had been built in 1813. It had a reputation as being haunted, so its price was low enough to allow the family to start a missionary school there. His parents allowed young Paul to indulge his interest in zoology, which he did by catching and studying sea urchins, fish, and blind caecilians (legless burrowing amphibians) on the beach below their home. They also encouraged his interest in writing and music (he played the piano, organ, bassoon, and cello). The Stapp children went home to Texas to fill in any gaps in their home-schooled educations, and Paul arrived there at age fifteen. Aside from the educational advantage, the move allowed him to come in contact with relatives who were practicing physicians.[2]

Stapp finished high school at San Marcos Academy, a Baptist military boarding school, and enrolled at age seventeen at Baylor University in Waco, Texas, originally intending to become a writer. Caring for a two-and-a-half-year-old cousin who had been badly burned in a fire (the child died after several days) caused him to rethink his career path and decide on medicine. After earning his bachelor's degree, Stapp pursued that goal with what has been described by friends and family as missionary zeal. He had to be zealous because he was as penniless as the proverbial church mouse, and there were three younger Stapp brothers to help support and educate. Paul worked as a zoology instructor, a supplier of snakes and scorpions to a biological wholesaler (he had to catch them first), and a door-to-door salesman of cookware. He completed a master's degree in zoology and, still saving up for medical school, the coursework for a doctoral degree in biophysics from the University of Texas at Austin. The latter he somehow finished during his first year of medical school, while also working as an instructor there to help pay his tuition. His medical degree from the University of Minnesota was granted three days before Christmas in 1943, the perfect present. It had been a long, arduous, often frustrating process—and particularly difficult during the Depression years—for a young man without means and who was nearly ten years older than his classmates.[3]

Raised in a family whose ideal was service to the Lord, he later recalled becoming "angrier and angrier and more frustrated" because his medical career was being delayed. "I was willing to practice medicine and do research in medicine for the rest of my life for nothing if I could only go to medical school. I was willing to work in a charity hospital the rest of my life."[4] He had been put on this Earth for a purpose, ordained by God to help others as a doctor and to combat the enemies of filth and ignorance. Why couldn't anyone else see that?

The last three years of his medical studies were financed by the Army Student Training Program (ASTP). After serving nine months of an internship at a Catholic charity hospital in Duluth, he was assigned to active duty, starting with a three-month military internship. Stapp had hoped to go instead to the Mayo Clinic for further study, but by the time his tour was over, the clinic had a backlog of physicians whose promised fellowships had been delayed by the war, and Stapp was well over thirty-five. "I rationalized that the Mayo Clinic was *started* by the Mayo brothers. They didn't go there. Maybe *I* could start something." He decided to try to create opportunities in his army work for research.[5]

In August 1946, he was assigned to the Aero Medical Laboratory (AML) at Wright Field, where, six days after his arrival, he witnessed the USAF's first manned ejection-seat trial.[6] Stapp liked the lab right away. The researchers were definitely not ivory-tower theorists or academicians defending their petty turfs. The work was ground-breaking, and the open, creative atmosphere fostered there since Harry Armstrong's days would let him write his own rules. What the lab did was also necessary: It saved lives—a lot of them.[7]

The following March, the AML sent John Paul Stapp on his first mission: to establish a field lab at Muroc Army Air Base in California, where the X-1 was being tested. His assignment was to develop fresh ways to protect the human body when the new aircraft crashed, which they did all too often.

The stubbornness and can-do attitude that had gotten Captain Stapp through his thirteen years of college and graduate study served him well at this point. Like Armstrong before him, he found himself alone and with no support from the higher-ups in Ohio. He didn't even have a building to work from until he made one himself from a few old, abandoned structures on the other side of the dry lake. Some airmen moved them for him on a flatbed truck, and he equipped the new field lab with the best that the salvage yard had to offer and whatever he could improvise, scrounge, beg, or otherwise obtain through "moonlight requisitioning."[8] The experience would serve him well in the future, when he would fly oddball stealth medical projects in under the radar and get what he needed by hook or by crook.

Along with his work as a flight surgeon, Stapp used a two-thousand-foot track at Muroc (now Edwards AFB) to commence the project that would ultimately put him onto the cover of *Time* and the set of *This Is Your Life* and inspire Hollywood to make a movie of his life.[9] This was the first of his rocket-sled studies, in which subjects were strapped to an ejection seat and propelled by rocket at several hundred miles per hour along a two-thousand-foot track and then abruptly stopped. The idea was to mimic a high-speed crash by accelerating and decelerating so quickly that the rider was exposed to extreme G forces. In addition to testing the effects of G forces on living organisms, Stapp hoped to determine the ultimate limit of endurance. Before leaving California in 1952 for an assignment back at the Wright Lab, Stapp performed around 180 animal and dummy experiments and 73 using humans—26 of them on himself.[10]

Although Stapp's work at Muroc (and later at Holloman) contributed greatly to both aircraft and automobile safety, it was also responsible for defining one of life's great truisms: Murphy's Law. It happened in 1949, when Stapp and his helpers were still learning the ins and outs of the rocket-sled test protocol. An assistant to Capt. Edward A. Murphy Jr. had designed a harness with sixteen accelerometers to measure the G forces. There were two ways they could be installed, and the assistant, naturally, installed each and every one the wrong way. Consequently, all sixteen failed to switch "on" when the sled started, and Stapp's body-blasting, teeth-jarring, bone-breaking ride that day was all for nothing. Captain Murphy concluded that "If there are two or more ways to do something and one of those results in a catastrophe, then someone will do it that way."[11] He was right.

STRUGHOLD AND THE SEARCH FOR LIFE ON MARS

Observations of the changing Martian color patterns had convinced late-nineteenth- and early-twentieth-century astronomers such as Percival Lowell of Flagstaff, Giovanni Schiaparelli of Milan, and Camille Flammarion of the Paris Observatory that Mars had channels or canals of some sort. Further observations of what appeared to be dark patches emanating from the poles led Lowell and others to conclude that these were man-made and that Earth observers were seeing crops growing in the Martian spring and then dying out for the year.[12]

Overall, planetary research entered a heyday after 1945 that has continued into the twenty-first century, thanks to wartime advances in physics. The techniques of polarimetry, infrared observing, interferometry, and radar all made it possible to look at other worlds with different eyes. Astronomers borrowed these tools to peer beneath cloud layers, to look for temperature differences on planetary surfaces, and to observe color and light reflections and thereby determine the chemical composition of a planet and its atmosphere.

Life on Mars was still a viable area of research in the early 1950s and, for some planetary scientists and astronomers, remained so until the Viking Lander missions of the late 1970s. The American Astronomical Society devoted its eighty-ninth annual conference, held in August 1953, to the idea of a possible manned Mars landing by 1980. Long before NASA became the patron of exobiology research, the search for life on Mars had attracted Hubertus Strughold and Wernher von Braun; astronomers Gerard de Vaucouleurs, Fred Whipple, and Clyde Tombaugh; exobiologist Wolf Vishniac; geneticist H. J. Muller; and about two dozen other prominent scientists.[13] Astronomers had found evidence that the planet lacked the atmosphere and climate to support advanced life and that the "canals" had been illusions. However, these researchers still held that it was possible, although not likely, that the shifting patches of dark and light, some of which appeared to be blue or green, might be an uncultivated variety of plant life. It was probably lichen, the thinking went, or maybe cactus, which would retain its water and was bulky enough not to freeze at night.[14]

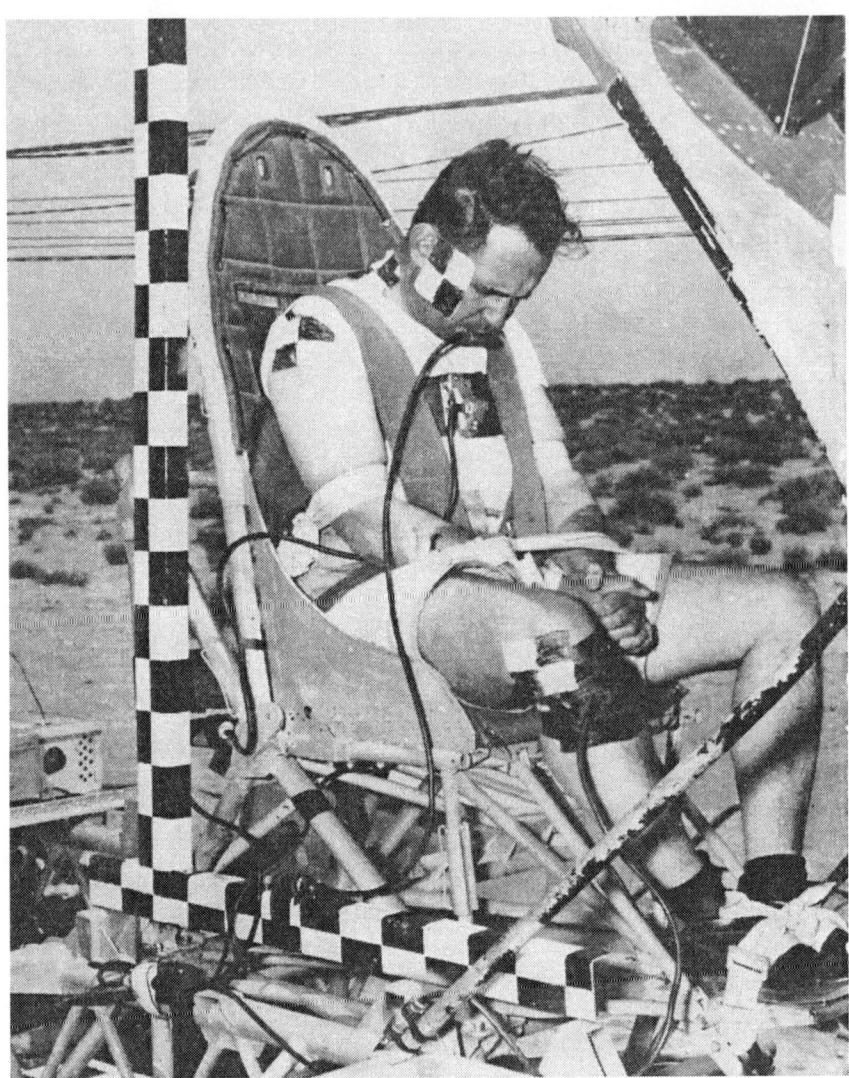

*John Paul Stapp, readying himself for a ride aboard the rocket sled
at Muroc. USAF photo.*

Strughold visited the Lowell Observatory in the early 1950s and spoke
with the director, V. M. Slipher and his brother, E. C. Slipher, who was
an astronomer also. They arranged for Strughold to observe the red planet
through the forty-two-inch telescope on Mars Hill there.[15] The observatory,
a private institution with connections to Harvard University, was famous not

only for the Mars observations of its founder but also for the discovery of Pluto by Tombaugh just twenty years earlier. Its specialty, in fact, was (and is) planetary observation within this solar system. Connecting with Lowell gave Strughold an opportunity to meet other planetary specialists in the Southwest, including Tombaugh, who by then was at New Mexico State University, and Lincoln La Paz, a meteorite specialist at the University of New Mexico.

In 1953, the University of New Mexico Press, which had published *Physics and Medicine of the Upper Atmosphere*, put out Strughold's book about life on Mars, *The Green and Red Planet*. Written "with editorial assistance" from the school's public-relations officer, Green Peyton, and dedicated to Harry Armstrong, it was a slim volume—it had fewer than one hundred pages—but it was comprehensive enough to present the lichen theory, offer the fairly persuasive arguments of astronomers who supported the idea, and then explain his own conclusions. Surprisingly, for someone so interested in exobiology,

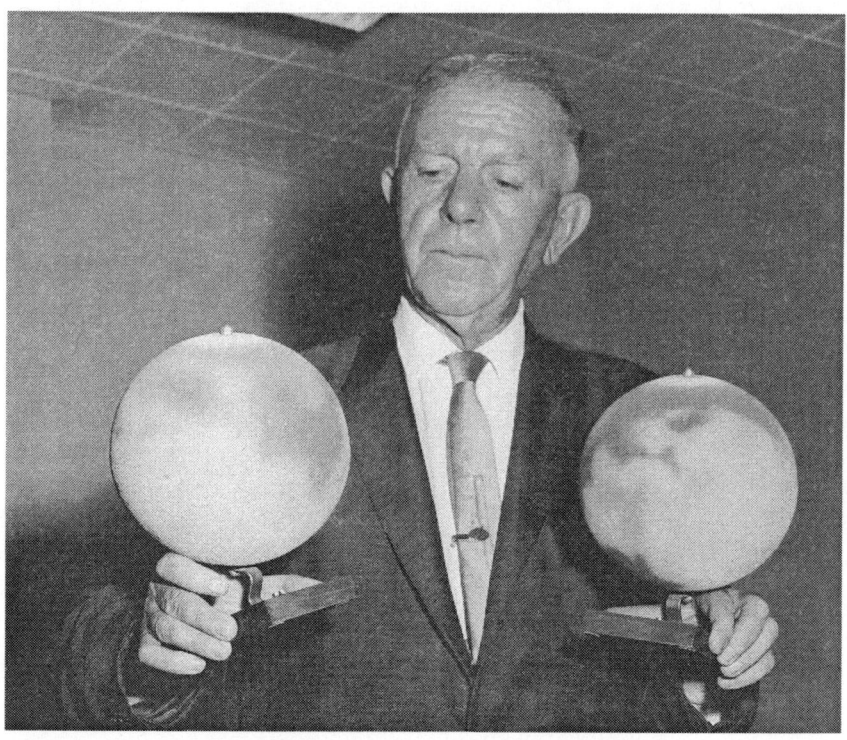

Strughold studied the likelihood of primitive plant life on Mars, a possibility he considered remote. USAF *photo.*

Strughold stated that the odds were very small that plant life was the source of the Martian coloration changes.

As a disciplined scientist who was able to separate conjecture and wishful thinking from reality, the German concluded that the planet's famous markings had been illusory. One explanation was that they had been a result of botany combined with the physics of astronomical observing and the physiology of human color vision. He cited the work of Soviet astronomer Gavriil A. Tikhov of the Alma Ata Observatory in Kazakhstan, who used chromatography to study the optical properties of plants on Earth and compare them to the colors perceived by observers of Mars. One of Tikhov's conclusions was that the colder the climate, the less the plants reflected the sun's rays in the portion of the spectrum between yellow and infrared. Thus, to the viewer, their color was optically shifted toward the blue end of the spectrum. The dark areas on Mars appeared to have a strong bluish-green tint compared to those on Earth, Tikhov was saying, but might not necessarily be blue.[16]

Strughold also became active in the International Mars Committee (IMC), founded in 1953 by E. C. Slipher and observatory trustee Roger Lowell Putnam. Originally an idea of Nobel chemist Harold Urey of the University of Chicago, the IMC was intended to organize observations of the red planet to be made during its close approaches to the Earth in 1954 and 1956. The committee was funded by the National Science Foundation, the U.S. Navy, and the National Geographic Society. Fourteen observatories participated worldwide, including facilities in the Soviet Union, South Africa, Australia, India, Java, Egypt, and Argentina.[17]

Drawing on these resources as well as his own research, Strughold also oversaw what he called "Mars jars" experiments at the school's Department of Microbiology. In the summer of 1956, a young lieutenant in that department, John A. Kooistra Jr., took a set of large glass jars, pumped the air out until the inside was as much like the Martian atmosphere as he could make it, and filled the jars with samples of soil believed to approximate the Martian surface. He also put into the jars bacteria native to the areas from which the soil samples had been taken and added just enough moisture to represent runoff from polar ice melt and subsequent moisture in the air. He put the jars in the refrigerator overnight and let them warm to room temperature every day. The only Martian feature not duplicated was the reduced gravity and cosmic radiation. The experiment showed that microorganisms could maintain life and even reproduce in the simulated Martian environment. These findings could not, of course, prove that there was life on Mars, but the vigorous multiplication of the bacteria led researchers to believe that the planet was at least capable of supporting primitive life.[18]

V-2S IN THE DESERT

Immediately after the war, the army had taken as many of the actual V-2s and spare parts as they could back to the States from Germany and sent the rockets, components, and von Braun Paperclips to Fort Bliss. Several groups of scientists had plans to use these as research platforms even as the army was starting to figure out how the things were manufactured and operated. Their goal was to learn something about the composition, chemistry, and physics of the upper atmosphere, which was a complete unknown. Both groups came together in what would be a fruitful collaboration of the armed forces and science.

When the end of World War II became imminent, scientists and engineers at the Naval Research Laboratory decided to continue the work they had been doing with smaller missiles and established a study group. By December 1945, the group had been approved as the Rocket Sonde Research Section and set about applying their knowledge of sounding rockets and missiles to the upper atmosphere. Shortly afterward, the War Department had established an Upper Atmosphere Research Panel to take advantage of the· V-2 and learn more about the composition of the region bordering space, including phenomena such as auroras, meteor showers, and solar and stellar ultraviolet radiation. The National Research Laboratory (NRL) had organized a panel from the military, industry, and academia in February 1946 to advise the Army Ordnance Department on ways to put the V-2s on hand to good use as research platforms. The V-2 Upper Atmosphere Research Panel, an informal, unsponsored group, would coordinate all of the experimentation.[19]

Between April 1946 and September 1952, contractor General Electric and the von Braun team launched sixty-four V-2s from the White Sands, New Mexico, proving ground.[20] These research rockets had new nose cones that were designed by the NRL to hold instrumentation and telemetry gear, a radar beacon for tracking, and a radio receiver for the abort signal, should it be necessary. The work they carried out included taking pictures of the sun's spectrum, collecting air samples at high altitudes, using mass spectrometers to evaluate the composition of the upper atmosphere, measuring the Earth's magnetic field and related current flows, and sending a Geiger counter aloft to determine the radiation levels in the near-space environment.[21]

The National Institutes of Heath (NIH) had been the first to take advantage of the V-2 rocket as a life-sciences research platform. NIH scientists tested the effects of cosmic rays on living organisms by sending tubes containing fruit flies *(Drosophila)* to a height of 106 miles aboard a missile and then parachuting them back to Earth for examination. The insects survived the journey and the radiation exposure with no problems.[22] In 1949, SAM Paperclips Heinz Haber,

Hans-Georg Clamann, and Konrad Büttner flew to Fort Bliss to consult with von Braun and requisition V-2 "warheads" for animal experimentation. The team was investigating the methodology for measuring and transmitting physiological data gathered from electroencephalographs, respiration and temperature monitors, accelerometers, and electrocardiographs they would attach to small test animals.[23] For several years, articles on the use of V-2s by meteorologists and physicists had appeared in the open scientific literature, and the medical people thought they could use the V-2s for physiological studies of small mammals in the space environment.[24]

The same year, James Henry of the Aero Medical Lab at Wright had designed a capsule similar to that used by the *Explorer II* balloonists of the 1930s but miniaturized to hold rhesus monkeys and mice. He was able to wire the animals to record in-flight data on their physiological responses to weightlessness and acceleration changes. The V-2 payload return mechanisms (explosives that would send the rocket into a flutter and a parachute for a soft landing) consistently failed, however, preventing Henry from getting a full picture of the effects of spaceflight on his small subjects. It was not until 1951 and the shift to the air force's new Aerobee rocket that he was able to bring a subject (actually nine mice) back alive.[25]

As the V-2s ran out, the United States turned to balloons. The navy made several manned ascents to 70,000 or 80,000 feet and used "rockoons" (balloon-launched rockets) to conduct cosmic-ray research on microscopic organisms and insects. Unmanned balloons went as high as 148,000 feet with similar payloads. In the early 1950s, USAF flight surgeons sent up more than a thousand balloons containing seeds, mice, rats, hamsters, rabbits, and a few monkeys, primarily to study the effect of cosmic rays on mammalian systems, reproduction, and the ability to survive such exposure.[26]

UNDERSTANDING THE ENVIRONMENT OF SPACE

Before the war, most of what scientists knew about atmospheric wind speeds below twenty miles in altitude they had learned using weather balloons, artillery-launched smoke shells, meteor trails, radar, and a few manned balloon flights.[27] The data had been sufficient for the researchers to create basic models that described the temperature layers of the atmosphere, its broad wind patterns, and essential electrical and magnetic features. They still did not know why the ionosphere even existed, how many ionized layers composed it, and why it behaved as it did, with its makeup and stability varying with the seasons, time of day, and the eleven-year sunspot cycle.[28]

Wartime research had led to substantial improvements in balloon construction, the sensitivity of photographic emulsions used to record high-energy particles, and the development of radiation-recording devices. Balloons could now take a fairly large and bulky apparatus from eighteen to twenty-five miles high. Meteorologists could observe noctilucent clouds, high-altitude formations that continue to glow from the sun's rays after local sunset, to determine wind speed and direction at an altitude of nearly fifty miles. By 1950, the Wright Lab was sending mice aloft to test the effect of cosmic rays on living organisms. With the exception of a few hairs that turned white, they survived in excellent shape.[29]

Rocketry enabled the scientists to make a huge leap in understanding about what goes on in the ionosphere some fifty miles above the Earth's surface. Physicists made one of the earliest measurements of atmospheric density and tentatively concluded that it was one-ten-millionth that of water. The new V-2 technology was also pressed into service to determine the air temperature at various altitudes. One method involved setting off grenades at various altitudes. Results varied by as much as seventy-five degrees Fahrenheit, causing researchers to wonder whether their equipment and technique needed to be improved or whether they had discovered unexpected seasonal or locational variations. In 1951, thanks to missile-research results, NACA had to rewrite the definition of a "standard atmosphere"—the unit of temperature and density at a given altitude—used to calibrate aircraft instruments. That same year, one physicist also proposed tearing up the existing tables on upper-atmospheric temperatures, likewise considered standard references. These obsolete tables had been written just three years earlier.[30]

THE INTERNATIONAL GEOPHYSICAL YEAR

Unbeknownst to the life scientists who were using the V-2s and Aerobees—and to most of the physicists and meteorologists—plans were already under way to repeat these sorts of experiments using a platform that could fly much higher than fifty miles. In April 1950, a group of American physicists and geophysicists had met at the suburban Washington home of James Van Allen to spend a social evening with English geophysicist Sydney Chapman. Van Allen had been a member of the original 1946 V-2 panel and was using modified rockets to capture and study cosmic rays. He knew as early as 1948 that "serious consideration" had been given to a "satellite missile" that would orbit the Earth. In talking shop, the conversation turned to rockets, missiles, and other new tools that had been placed at their disposal since the war.[31] The last time the scientific world had been able to get so much information on any one subject had been the 1932 International Polar Year (IPY). One thing led to another, and the group decided to approach their scientific peers with the idea of organizing another IPY for 1957, the silver anniversary of the last such event.

Within a few short years, the extravaganza would expand to become a global affair, and sixty-seven nations would agree to participate in what was renamed the International Geophysical Year (IGY). The idea's instigators hoped the occasion would persuade the U.S. military to put its new inter-continental ballistic missile capability to good use by sending a scientific laboratory into orbit around the Earth. Both the Defense Department and the air force had been examining the idea of an orbiting space lab since 1946, so why not?[32]

Since the organization of the National Research Lab's V-2 panel in 1946, interest in rockets as research vehicles had grown tremendously. Whereas the minutes of its first meeting had been distributed to only thirty people, by 1956 the mailing list had grown to 118 subscribers working at seventy-three different organizations. The military's policy of openness regarding the rockets fostered this expansion. Even though the launches were carried out on military bases, the vehicles and the information about them had always been deemed unclassified: launch schedule, rocket design, flight data, and the scientific results. Because of this growth in interest and experience with rocketry and the cooperation of the military, American IGY planners proposed forming what they called the Rocket and Satellite Research Panel (RSRP) as a research platform in 1957. Hubertus Strughold was a member, along with Wernher von Braun and at least two other Paperclips.[33]

Strughold's participation notwithstanding, the IGY did next to nothing in the way of direct life-sciences research, however. The year-long event added immensely to the understanding of the upper atmosphere and the transition area between space and atmosphere, though, particularly in the area of cosmic radiation. Without such knowledge, sending a human into space would have been a very foolish and risky endeavor.

During the first twelve months of the IGY, U.S. scientists launched 116 rockets over a range extending from 75 degrees north to 72 degrees south. Fifty-four of the rockets were ship-based rockoons. Sixty-two were from land bases: 6 from Holloman AFB, 15 from California, and 41 from Hudson's Bay, Canada. The New Mexico launches examined cosmic rays, electromagnetism, and plasma displays, plus water vapor, micrometeorites, airglow, and charge density at the edge of the atmosphere. Northeastern Canada was the only site where the structural properties of the atmosphere, its composition, pressure, density, and temperature were measured. Knowledge of these properties was vital for designing propulsion systems, steering mechanisms, and vehicles that would operate where the atmosphere was too thin to support conventional aviation.

Like they had with the V-2s, experiment designers used hand grenades atop more sophisticated rockets, adding newly designed, ejectable spheres that contained sensitive miniature accelerometers. They also employed sophisticated ground equipment to track meteor trails and luminous clouds they concocted from nitric acid, sodium vapor, or ethylene. Investigators examined the argon content of the upper atmosphere, looking for information about the glowing northern and southern lights. Although auroras are beautiful, as plasma energy they wreak havoc on the electronic components of a vehicle traveling through the upper atmosphere. The scientists also found that the hotter the air, the higher it expands, and so its density diminishes more slowly with height.[34] Discoveries such as these made the work of designing the launch vehicles and space capsules that much more complicated, but the changes were absolutely necessary for a successful mission.

These IGY findings added to the desire to put a satellite into orbit. One goal of importance to both physicists and life scientists was to trap actual cosmic rays. Much of what they had heretofore detected was not the rays themselves ("primaries") but by-products of their collision with particles in the atmosphere. Balloons were a relatively clean method of collecting primaries, but they could only go so high. Rockets reached well into the ionosphere, but they generated so many secondary rays that their data were considered unreliable. If knowledge was to advance, scientists knew they had to have a more capable platform that would go higher and stay up longer. From everything they heard though the grapevine, they thought they would get that platform before the IGY was out.[35]

SPACE MEDICINE MOVES AHEAD

Medicine is not a profession that is driven by fads or whims. Not until 1953—some thirteen years after the idea was broached with the American Medical Association (AMA), after much prodding by Harry Armstrong, and after four years of concerted effort by Otis Benson—were aviation-medicine practitioners able to become board certified. As it was, the AMA refused the Aero Medical Association's request for a certification system and bounced the group to the American Board of Preventive Medicine and Public Health. Late in coming as it was, board certification was the definitive peer verification that aviation medicine was a distinct specialty.[36] By the mid-1950s, space medicine was positioning itself for similar treatment. Through stepped-up publication in scientific journals, a series of symposiums, and increased visibility within professional organizations, space medicine began to take shape as a special area of expertise. It was a seamless blending of military and civilian activity.

Paul Campbell organized the first meeting of the Space Committee of the Aero Medical Association, which was held on May 31, 1950. He invited around thirty people who were interested in aviation medicine to an organizing lunch during the annual meeting of the association in Chicago. People came to the door, looked around to see whether anyone had observed them, then entered quickly, and slid into a seat at the table. Some sat there only a minute, then got up, and hurried out without having said a word. Campbell was sure that they were afraid of having their names too closely associated with an entity that had the word "space" in its title.[37]

Fifteen people ultimately stayed in their seats long enough to vote what they called the "Informal Committee on Space Medicine" into existence. Besides Campbell and the University of Chicago's Andrew Ivy, these included Hubertus Strughold, Otis Benson, Konrad Büttner, the Habers, two other Paperclip scientists, a navy researcher, and several Ph.D.'s and medical doctors from academia. To give the group some substance, they voted to include in absentia another 21 Aero Medical Association members they felt would probably have joined had they been in attendance. Harry Armstrong and Randy Lovelace were included in that group, as was former LMFI scientist Otto Gauer. Six navy flight surgeons, 4 air force flight surgeons, and 8 from academe made up the rest of the total 36-person membership. By 1954, the group had more than doubled—to 86 members.[38]

Before long, the new group had achieved enough stability that its parent organization was willing to devote sections of each annual conference to space-medicine papers. The *Journal of Aviation Medicine (JAM)* had begun publishing articles on space medicine in 1950; thus, information on the subject was reaching a larger audience.[39] It printed pieces by Paperclip scientist Hermann Schaefer on cosmic radiation and by Fritz Haber and Heinz Haber on ways to produce a zero-G environment on Earth. A paper on the boundary between the atmosphere and space, written by Strughold, the Habers, and Büttner, was in the works, as was one on the physics and physiology of weightlessness by Heinz Haber and Siegfried Gerathewohl.[40] The journal published seven space-related articles in 1952 and twice that number two years later.

One medical issue of particular interest was cosmic radiation. Passengers in a space vehicle that stayed up for more than a day—the physicians were anticipating a one- or two-person air force observation satellite—might need to be shielded if the cosmic-radiation levels proved to be damaging. Insufficient evidence existed as to how much radiation was too much. Physicists and biologists now had some—but not enough—data on the amount of cosmic-radiation exposure that could be expected. Furthermore, what they had recently learned changed existing ideas about the origins and mechanisms of radiation propagation and therefore continually altered the thinking about its possible effects on humans. Here was an area that required their concentrated efforts in both lab and field research.[41]

Weightlessness was a second major concern, and usable data would be critical for predicting whether it would be so disorienting that the pilot or astronaut would not be able to concentrate on necessary tasks and thus miss making a split-second maneuver. Would the vehicle controls and other equipment be too difficult to manipulate without the assistance of gravity? Would weightlessness interfere with the sleep cycle on longer flights? Would it be impossible for a person to swallow food or beverages and get them to stay down? Were there any other difficulties as yet unanticipated?

Several school researchers had been studying this issue. One of the leaders was a bespectacled Paperclip, Siegfried Gerathewohl. A glider pilot with a doctorate in psychology, he had managed an aviation-cadet selection program for the Luftwaffe during the war. Afterward he had sought a position at the army's medical-research center in Heidelberg and come to the United States with that group when the facility closed.[42]

Gerathewohl's work was of both a practical and theoretical nature. He and coinvestigator Herbert D. Stallings (a USAF pilot), along with dozens of other Randolph volunteers, made weightless test flights in 1956 and 1957, as did a bowl of goldfish and eight kittens from the school's vivarium, including one whose inner-ear mechanism Gerathewohl had surgically removed so that it had no sense of balance even under normal gravity conditions.[43]

The psychologist conducted very basic experiments, including the eye-hand coordination tests developed first in Germany by Strughold and von Diringshofen in the 1930s. He and his subjects also experimented with drinking, eating, and urinating in zero G. Although attempting to drink water from an open glass seems patently ridiculous today, it was the first time anyone had ever tried to carry out mundane tasks in the absence of gravity. The experimenters learned that water went every which way in the form of wobbling round globules of random size. They discovered that urinating in zero G made a surprising number of participants nauseous. Most—but not all—of them found the floating sensation of weightlessness exhilarating, but others felt disoriented or dizzy. Vision changed, too: Some participants observed that luminous objects appeared to move upward, a condition the school researchers termed "the oculo-agravic illusion," caused by the pull on the eye muscles when turning the head in the absence of gravity.[44]

These activities were ongoing and pursued vigorously by the people involved. They were pioneers, they felt, and space was their frontier.

THE HOLLOMAN FIELD LABORATORY

In 1953, the Aero Medical Laboratory at Wright sent John Paul Stapp, by then a lieutenant colonel and senior flight surgeon, to the gypsum desert of southern New Mexico to organize and head a second field lab. The near-perfect sunny weather at Holloman AFB was one reason the site was selected. Another was doubtless its remoteness. To Stapp, though, the big appeal was the leftover thirty-five-hundred-foot track, originally built to launch missiles. With this combination, he could carry on with his rocket-sled experiments and almost anything else that he or the Dayton lab could dream up. Their focus would be on saving the lives of pilots who might eject from experimental or future supersonic aircraft at the upper reaches of the atmosphere.[45] Before his reassignment to Ohio again in 1958, Stapp supervised the highest manned balloon flight ever, the advent of in-flight research on weightlessness, a series of rocket-sled experiments in which a human subject withstood the greatest number of Gs ever, and another series that set what is still the world's land-speed record for an unenclosed human body—his own.

The story of John Paul Stapp and his accomplishments in the desert outside Alamogordo would be incomplete without mentioning one group of test subjects he considered to be an indispensable part of the team: animals. In fact, all space-medicine endeavors relied on animal testing, something that did not and still does not sit well with animal-rights activists.

In the early 1950s, the aeromedical researchers from Wright had used the V-2 and Aerobee rocket-launching facilities at Holloman to send mice and monkeys into the upper atmosphere and space. These animals arrived with the researchers, and any survivors went home when the work was done. With a permanent outpost in New Mexico, the air force decided to build a small vivarium, similar to a bigger one used at the School of Aviation Medicine. The new facility housed large numbers of mice, a colony of chimps, and from time to time a few bears and pigs. Within a few years the population grew to more than four hundred creatures from nine different species.[46]

Guinea pigs and rats were often used aboard the rocket sleds, but the animal that Stapp and his team used for the most important experiments, those just before the first human rides, was the chimpanzee. These primates resemble humans in basic bipedal composition, although there are differences in muscular and skeletal construction, and chimps have much less adipose tissue (fat) than their human counterparts. They also have observable social behaviors that gave the scientists clues about the animals' psychological reactions to the testing. They could have been trained to carry out simple, repetitive tasks, but Stapp's primates were anesthetized and did not have to do anything more than ride the sled—unconscious.

Stapp was fond of the chimps and reportedly cooked liver and onions and other favorite dishes for them several times a week. However, the minister's son believed that in the hierarchy of creation, God had made human beings in His own image and likeness and placed them over all of the lesser life forms. Growing up in the malarial jungles of Brazil had also taught him that life was a constant struggle against plant and animal adversaries.[47] Consequently, Stapp took—and allowed—no risks to human life until the systems had been checked and rechecked and tested with animal subjects first, even if that meant that an animal occasionally died during the test or was "sacrificed" and autopsied afterward. When Northrop Aircraft built the sled it called the Sonic Wind (version number one) to ride the 3,500-foot track at Holloman, a chimp went first. When the track was lengthened to 5,000 feet, a chimp also made the initial run. Before Stapp made his own record-setting track run, several primates had ridden first, going nearly 600 miles per hour, and a dozen chimp runs were made at nearly 1,000 miles per hour.[48]

Some of the Aero Medical Laboratory animal tests seem unnecessarily brutal today, but at a time when air force pilots were dying and precise information as to why they perished was nonexistent, Stapp and others made the decisions they felt they had to. Most of the animals survived in good health, but some of them died as men searched for the upper limits of human survivability, a border area that had to be surveyed if vehicles and escape mechanisms were to be designed to accommodate pilots' tolerances. At some point early in the sled research, the idea arose that maybe a head-first ejection into the windstream might be best, the way a high diver hits the water. An anesthetized chimp was strapped aboard the sled in a head-first position and took a 270-G stop. It died a very messy death, and the test was never repeated on either man or animal. A few of the very small animals were literally vaporized by high G forces; others survived the tests but were killed for necropsies that would reveal hidden internal and cell-level damage. These sorts of incidents, fortunately, were in the minority.[49]

Animal tests gave Stapp a workable estimate of an upper threshold for humans' G tolerance. Early results showed that an animal would not be hurt if the number of Gs it received were kept under twenty-five percent of the number that would kill it. It did not take many sled rides to determine that the death point for the animals who were physiologically most like humans—chimps, bears, and pigs—was about two hundred Gs. Stapp reasoned that this meant that if what he termed the "point of beginning injury" was fifty Gs for those animals, it would likely be the upper limit of safety that the air force ought to seek for its human pilots.[50] Northrop's Gee Whizz decelerator sled at Muroc had given Stapp data only for forces approaching forty Gs, and, thanks to the animals, he knew he had to test the region closer to the fifty-G mark. It was time to get back to work now at Holloman. Time to go for a ride.

Stapp later claimed that he began using himself as a test subject accidentally. Oscar, the Muroc crash-test dummy, had done 32 runs, and chimps were supposed to be next, but the paperwork on the primates slowed things so much that the only alternative was to send himself down the "Grand Slam" test track. His supervisors at Wright were horrified to find out that he had made 16 such runs, pulling as many as 35 Gs, when "everyone knew" that the limit of human endurance was 18. Stapp got his chimps. He also got an order to stop performing the tests on himself and to stay under the 18-G benchmark. Mysteriously, the technicians and engineers from Northrop Aviation suddenly became very bad at math, the instrumentation used to calculate acceleration went all cockeyed, and all of the numbers Stapp reported from then on were off by fifty percent. Stapp made it to 40 Gs, but Wright knew only about the first 20.[51]

Over the course of Stapp's sledding career, more like-minded graduates of the School of Aviation Medicine came to work for him, increasing the number of human test subjects. Enlisted men also volunteered. Ultimately Stapp's researchers obtained data on men of all sizes, shapes, and ages and were able to produce a data pool that resembled the population of air force pilots fairly well.

As at Muroc, the subject he used most often was himself—and why not? He understood the project better than anyone else. He thought, acted, and expressed himself as a trained scientist. He could experience the results and simultaneously correlate them with the data from the other runs. He could make recommendations for altering the test the next time better than any sensing device, observer, or animal ever could. And, of course, he was a doctor. The second time he broke his wrist on a sled run, Stapp set it himself while walking back to the lab.[52]

Self-experimentation requires a certain amount of scientific detachment. Working on a shoestring, alone and essentially unsupervised while two thousand miles from the boss, requires a great deal of efficiency as well. Stapp had been born and reared for this job; he was the quintessential outsider who did whatever it took to accomplish his goal. He calmly accepted the broken bones, concussions, bruises, blisters, and lost dental fillings that his sled runs caused and used them as data in his crusade to save lives. He kept track of every injury and his own subjective impressions of the sled runs to chart both the physiological and psychological responses to this type of hyperstress.[53] If either he or the project were killed, there would be ample data for a fleshed-out analysis of the acceleration and deceleration experience.

Stapp made his first ride on the second-generation sled that Northrop built for him, the Sonic Wind, at Holloman in April 1954. He pulled twenty-two Gs, four more than he had officially achieved at Muroc. That run was number seven; an empty sled and chimps from the vivarium had undertaken the first six in what was to be a series of twenty-one runs. By winter Stapp felt that he, the team, and the sled were ready for a run at the upper limits of human endurance—as close to fifty Gs as he could get.

The End of the Ride

Every account of the career of John Paul Stapp contains the story of his most famous sled ride, the last one in the series, and usually tells it with great dramatic flair. A few pieces written much later, after Stapp had retired from the air force and could voice his opinions without angering the top brass, made it clear that this was no spur-of-the-moment stunt. Nevertheless, reporters and interviewers clamored for quotes from Stapp and anyone else at Holloman about all that might go wrong, about how great the risk was, and about how terrified all of them must be.

Terror was always the farthest thing from their minds. Like the engineer/test pilot who would not climb aboard a new X-aircraft until it had been checked and rechecked at every step from drawing board to wind tunnel to manufacture, Stapp and the other volunteers did not strap themselves onto the Gee Whizz or Sonic Wind until they had thoroughly tested every component for every possible outcome. They tested their theories for months, first on unmanned vehicles and then on those carrying dummies and animals. A flight surgeon was on hand for every test ride, as were other medical personnel, rescue equipment, and an ambulance. The attending flight surgeon examined the test subjects before selection and again just before allowing them to take their ride. Stapp even had someone drive a jeep up and down the length of the track, honking, to scare away animals that came to drink from the water brake. They might easily become a wet spot on the windshield—and they meant death or injury for the rider.

After so many months of planning, the actual record-setting ride, which was well attended by the press, was almost anticlimactic for the crew. It took place December 10, 1954, when the missionary flight surgeon blasted into the record books by accelerating to a speed of 937 feet per *second*, then stopping his 5-second rocket ride in only 1.4 seconds and 690 feet of track. He pulled 25 Gs in the acceleration phase and 43 during deceleration. The experiment was over in less than 8 seconds.

For anyone who wants to understand the psychic link between a test pilot and the kind of flight surgeon who routinely and repeatedly put his own hide in the hot seat, the best source on Stapp's ride is one not found in the newspapers and magazines. Instead, it is a scholarly article he wrote for the *Journal of Aviation Medicine* under the bland title "Effects of Mechanical Forces on Living Tissues." It is here that Stapp the applied scientist speaks; here is the fusion of his doctorate in biophysics, medical training, military background, and laboratory experience. In nineteen pages, he lays out in detached language the premise of the study, the methods he planned to use, the test equipment (rocket sled and track), the results of three of the fifteen test runs he had made in 1954, a discussion, and conclusions. There was no hyped-up prose. Like Armstrong's report of his bailout nearly thirty years earlier, one would not even necessarily know that the "subjective observations before, during, and after the run as noted by the human subject" were written by the author.

The reason for undertaking the studies, he wrote, was to meet the "urgent demand to find the ultimate useful limits of the open ejection seat." In operation, the military had found that the abrupt onset of high-pressure windblast, which blew past the pilot at more than four hundred miles per hour, was "capable of flailing the head and extremities during ejection with damaging force beyond the muscular strength of the victim to resist." In other words, it could break arms, legs, or necks. One way Stapp knew that, although he neglected to mention it, was that he had made all of his Muroc rides and the first eight at Holloman without benefit of a safety helmet. In fact, from available photos, he apparently made some rides at Muroc in an undershirt and shorts. This was to test the idea that the sudden force of the air pressure against the chest might lethally damage a pilot's lungs. Since pilots wore no protection on their chests, neither would the man on the sled.

In the article, Stapp next describes the means by which the Sonic Wind worked, noting that it consisted of a test unit and a separate propulsion vehicle on which from 1 to 12 solid-fuel rockets could be mounted at the rear. Typically 6 were used, providing 4,500 pounds of thrust for five seconds. The test sled was made of chrome-molybdenum steel tubing, with an onboard telemetry system that relayed data from accelerometers, tensiometers, EKG,

EEG, and wind-pressure sensors affixed to the subject. Onboard high-speed cameras were focused on the rider, and three-inch-wide, nylon-webbing straps that tested to 6,000 pounds functioned as a harness to hold him immobile. Additional restraints kept the arms together behind the back at the elbows and joined the legs above and below the knees. The ankles were tied together, and head and feet were fastened to the headrest and footrest. The subject wore telemetering devices inside and outside of his clothing, and a rubber bite block protected his teeth. Underneath the sled, a fixed-scoop water brake would "catch" the water in the 190-foot-long trough at the end of the track and eject it to the sides, stopping the vehicle. The windshield could be jettisoned during the ride to mimic the sudden onset of air at the time of ejection. On the December 1954 run, the windshield was removed to achieve as much acceleration as possible.

The protocol was for the attending flight surgeon to examine the subject shortly before the test and evaluate his circulatory, respiratory, and neurological well-being. He gave the subject an EKG and a urine test and took whatever X rays were needed. The subject had fasted for six hours before the test and had drunk no water for four hours. A full stomach, Stapp quipped once, made for a messy autopsy.

If the team's meteorologist gave the okay (more sunshine meant better pictures), the crew strapped the subject in and ignited the rockets from a control station in an underground blockhouse a few hundred feet from the track. The attending flight surgeon paid attention to the subject's physiological and psychological condition before and after the test, as did the subject himself, and wrote up a report afterward. As well as he could, the subject also reported his reaction during the brief ride itself.

Whenever Stapp was the subject, the attending flight surgeon was USAF Maj. David Simons, a Wright Lab researcher who had worked with James Henry on the V-2 animal launches a few years earlier. Simons reported in laconic fashion that after the test on December 10, the subject's "respiratory efforts were gasping, occurring approximately every 5 to 8 seconds." Twenty seconds after the end of the run, "the subject's face began to turn cyanotic"—blue—and there was a "marked, bilateral exophthalmos": Stapp's eyes were bulging out of their sockets. "Upon release of the harness," Simons wrote, "it was noticed that the subject was quite limp. . . . [He] was unable to support his own weight due to marked skeletal-muscular weakness and relaxation." At the hospital afterward, Stapp displayed confusion about the sequence of events, but his eyes began to return to their normal position. He had two magnificent shiners for a couple of weeks, and Simons described his reflexes as "hyperactive" for a day afterward.

Scientist Stapp quoted his own notes anonymously in the *JAM* article, calling his memories "the subjective report." He started with a description of the eighty-minute process of strapping him into the sled, noting that the chest strap "was pulled tight enough to restrain all rib motion in breathing." He could take only small, shallow breaths using his diaphragm muscle for the next twenty minutes. He mentioned "the subject's" mental condition, recording that during the last ten seconds of the countdown, he "tensed, bit hard on the bite block, braced his head against the padded head rest and concentrated on pulling the cord to start the motion picture camera."

At takeoff, Stapp began counting off the seconds in his head to correlate with the subjective results later. With great detachment he noted that "at about the count of two vision narrowed to the central fields only, and by the count of three there was a visual blackout." He recorded the feeling of his coveralls fluttering in the hypersonic wind and the sensation of being forced backward into the seat and then violently forward against the straps.

"On entry into the water brakes," he wrote, "the face immediately felt congested with severe pain around the eyes, as though they were being pulled from the sockets." They were. "Vision became a shimmering salmon-colored field with no images—evidently the pupils were impinged against the stretched upper eyelids." When the sled stopped, the salmon color remained even after he pried the helmet and visor off and forced his eyelids open over his bulging eyes with his fingers.

For several very scary minutes, Stapp and the rest of the team thought he was blind. Then, Stapp wrote, "[t]he congestion of the eyes . . . receded sufficiently to permit return of vision in an estimated eight and a half minutes after the run. Central vision returned first, then peripheral, by glimpses of intermittent patches of the sky which gradually persisted and coalesced into normal visual fields." He had double vision and pain for a few hours as well as sinus congestion, petechiae (blood blisters) from the acceleration, and "the usual burning sensation from the strap abrasion," but otherwise "there was only a feeling of relief and elation in completing the run and in knowing that vision was unimpaired."[54]

After this—his seventy-third run—the air force grounded John Paul Stapp, calling him too valuable a resource to risk again.[55]

When the sled tests ended, Stapp and the others at the AML's field facility concentrated on the instant of onset of force upon the body. They constructed a one-hundred-twenty-foot-long Holloman short track, informally known as the "Daisy Track" because it was fired by means of compressed air, like the popular Daisy-brand air rifle. In 1956, a chimp naturally rode the sled first, anesthetized and then strapped onto a couch that could be rotated to examine the effects of forces acting upon its body from different angles. Then a lieutenant made the trip, followed by a number of enlisted men and at least one captain. Four anesthetized bears, chosen because their pelvic structure is similar to that of humans, were used at a cost of a hundred fifty dollars each. The animals were "expended" and given postmortem examinations.[56] One of the project's chief scientists, Capt. Eli L. Beeding, rode the Daisy Track one day in May 1958 and accidentally pulled 83 Gs for .04 seconds. The laws of physics did not function as expected above 35 Gs. What should have been a 3:2 ratio of G forces leaped to a new plateau—2:1. Fortunately, Beeding was positioned backward, or he would not have survived. As it was, he went into shock and experienced severe spinal pain.[57]

Beeding's record-setting ride was a close call, but Stapp and his team chose to view the mishap as a serendipitous success because it established a limit of human tolerance in the backward-facing position. All told, the results that the team achieved successfully set the safe human limits of tolerance for the rate of onset, the magnitude, and the duration of G forces, particularly in the forward-facing position. Human beings could withstand 1 second of 25 Gs and up to 50 Gs for .2 seconds or less.[58] This was tangible information to pass on to the designers who were already at work on the air force's next generation of vehicles: airplanes that would fly beyond the atmosphere and into space.

Not all of the research at Holloman took place at supersonic speeds or even on the ground, for that matter. Three projects of note during that period also provided the designers of jets and space capsules critical data on the tolerances of their human drivers. Two of these took place aboard balloons and another in a jet aircraft.

PROJECT MAN HIGH

Between 1956 and 1958, flight surgeon David Simons was the project officer under John Paul Stapp on a high-altitude research program called Project Man High. This was a very low-budget endeavor designed to evaluate the physical environment of the upper atmosphere in terms of human surviv- ability. Simons and Joe Kittinger, a test pilot assigned to the program, acted as guinea pigs during the experiments.

After unmanned flights had tested the viability of their system, Man High took humankind to its loftiest altitudes ever: 96,000 feet for Kittinger and 101,500 for Simons, who stayed up for five hours, thus becoming the first person to see the sun set and rise again from space. Kittinger's flight proved the workability of the high-altitude weather balloon as a vehicle for manned exploration; Simons' was a more scientifically ambitious program that included some experiments in astronomical observation. Biological samples and emulsion plates were strapped to Simons's body as a means of detecting cosmic rays.

The final Man High flight took young test pilot Clifton McClure, screened from a pool of air force applicants, aloft for a brief flight in October 1958. The experiment was cut short when various malfunctions terminated communication with the ground controllers and sent McClure's body temperature to what should have been a lethal 108.5 degrees Fahrenheit. Frustrating as it was, the McClure flight proved the usefulness of an organized method of recruiting and screening candidates, a process that Randy Lovelace and John Paul Stapp would refine and use to select the first pilots to reach space by both aircraft and ballistic vehicle. McClure's ability to withstand tremendous physical stress and carry out his tasks as assigned also validated a theory that flight surgeons as far back as Harry Armstrong at Selfridge Field had always believed. In a critical situation, psychological strength—motivation—was more important than any technical skills a pilot possessed.[59]

ZERO-G RESEARCH

Between 1953 and the summer of 1958, the Wright team at Holloman conducted numerous tests on the effects of weightlessness under the supervision of flight surgeon Simons.[60] The scientist who conducted this research was Austrian physician-pilot Harald von Beckh. He had served in the Luftwaffe during the war and taught at their medical academy in Berlin, then left Europe in the late 1940s and emigrated to Argentina. There he had worked with Strughold's old friend Heinz von Diringshofen, who had found employment at the Instituto Nacional de Medicina Aeronautica. In-flight studies there on animal behavior in zero G earned von Beckh an invitation from the air force to conduct additional research at Holloman.[61]

Von Beckh developed a unique test protocol as a result of a serendipitous (for him) accident to a water turtle, *Hydromedusa tectifera*, in his Buenos Aires lab. While von Beckh was out of town, the animal's caregiver had neglected to control the temperature of its habitat; as a result the turtle became overheated, which destroyed its inner-ear mechanism. The physician observed that its resulting dizziness and inability to orient itself meant that the creature was severely hampered in its ability to eat. It simply could not strike out at food with its mouth and grab it. Eventually, though, the turtle adapted to its disability and was able to hit the target.

By then, von Beckh was familiar with the work that German aviation-medicine specialists had done during the 1930s and was intrigued by von Diringshofen's report of successful attempts at creating a weightless environment. The older man had flown repeated Keplerian trajectories—a steep climb followed by a steep dive—which produced nearly thirty seconds of weightlessness at the top of the parabola.

Von Beckh took several turtles up with him in a small Argentine air force jet and flew them in the same pattern. During the brief seconds of weightlessness he offered the turtles a bit of meat and watched to see whether they would strike at the bait. Like the damaged turtle, they tried but missed their targets over and over until repeated trips had taught them how to compensate for the scrambled visual and labyrinthine signals they were receiving. When the injured turtle went up for a ride, it adapted readily because it had already accustomed itself to its disability.[62]

Withstanding and adapting to weightlessness and the high G forces that immediately follow it during reentry became von Beckh's chief area of research. He perfected the parabolic flight pattern that Fritz Haber had meanwhile developed to create a longer period of weightlessness in flight, adding spirals that changed the G factor during the flight. He and his volunteers made more than two hundred experimental flights and captured on camera the effects of up to seven Gs and forty-five seconds of weightlessness on humans.[63] In one experiment, Clifton McClure kept himself awake for several days so that he could sleep through a takeoff and climb to altitude and then be awakened while in the weightless state. The result was total disorientation.[64] With such a sizable database, researchers could more confidently predict the human organism's response to spacecraft takeoff and reentry and know what sorts of parameters to use in selecting pilots to fly their spacecraft.

Von Beckh also used Stapp's Daisy Track to test a method of buffering the effects of sudden acceleration and deceleration by encasing the riders (two anesthetized albino rats) in a multiaxis device that changed direction with the force of motion.[65] His goal was to develop a means of shifting the G load on a pilot's body so that the accelerative and decelerative forces always moved at right angles to an imaginary line connecting the head and heart. Stapp's experiments had shown that higher G forces could be sustained if they traveled in this transverse direction. In addition, Heinz von Diringshofen had made prewar experiments in a dive bomber equipped with a tiltable seat on which a pilot could crouch or lie prone; he found that those positions greatly enhanced the pilot's ability to withstand G forces. Consequently, von Beckh developed a plan for what he called an "anti-G ejection capsule." This was a round, self-contained, pivoting ejection pod (rather than a seat) that the air force could use in airplanes flying at multiple Mach speeds and in its space vehicles.[66]

EVER UPWARD

In early 1957, the air force's visions of future spacecraft included a bailout capability. However, ejection seats for ordinary jet aircraft were still a serious concern even ten years after the air force had taken the first plane supersonic, so it was questionable how well such devices might function (if they functioned at all) in space or near-space environments. Statistics for ejection-seat use showed a twenty-three percent death rate at standard altitudes, most of which were caused either by the failure of the parachute or the seat to work in proper sequence or by ejecting at a low altitude—lower than two thousand feet.[67]

A second crucial concern was that even if the technical problems of seat separation and parachute deployment were solved, very high-speed or high-altitude ejections would result in "tumbling," which produced centrifugal forces that could kill the pilot. An astronaut would be exposed to an instantaneous and likely lethal combination of deceleration (from wind resistance), tumbling, spinning, windblast, temperature drop, and depressurization. Only one pilot had ever successfully bailed out at a speed greater than Mach 1, and he sustained a lacerated liver, concussion, and ocular hemorrhage. Six others had died.[68]

Researchers at the Wright Lab separated ejection into its components and studied each one in turn. Using a turntable, they found that a subject spinning on his side would become unconscious in ten to twelve seconds at 160 revolutions per minute. Even 90 revolutions produced vomiting and disorientation. In other experiments, they discovered that windblast of 650 pounds per square foot caused flailing of arms and legs beyond the pilot's ability to control them. The result was broken or dislocated limbs. In actual operation, windblast on one pilot whose face was bare—he had lost his helmet and face mask during the ejection—pushed three liters of air into the stomach through his open mouth and nose. The irony is that, although extremely painful, it kept him afloat until rescuers arrived when he landed—unconscious—in the ocean.[69]

In April 1958, engineer/test pilot Joe Kittinger, who by then was based at the Wright Lab, was given the job of solving the problem of high-altitude bailouts by John Paul Stapp, who was being reassigned to Dayton. Stapp named the project "Excelsior," which means "ever higher" or "ever upward," because his goal was to take a test subject, via balloon, to higher and higher

elevations and test his ability to parachute to safety. An earlier Wright program, called Project High Dive, had also studied high-altitude jumps using
a team of expert parachutists, but without success. The team of Kittinger and
Stapp decided to build on that work, particularly in the area of parachute
design. A test pilot would make three high-altitude jumps from an open gondola balloon using a new multistaged chute design. Although Kittinger was
jumping rather than ejecting and consequently was not strapped into a heavy
metal seat, with his reserve chute, oxygen equipment, telemetering devices,
and other survival gear, he still weighed three hundred twenty pounds.

Jumps one and two were from around 75,000 feet. The first one nearly
killed Kittinger, as both parachutes and a drogue chute opened and became

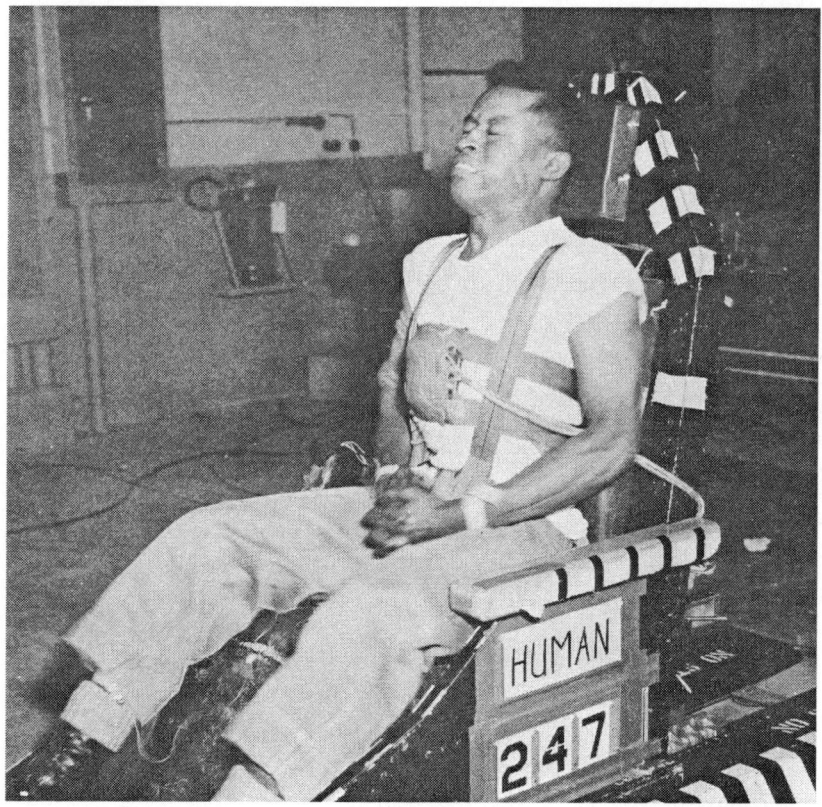

*Test subject "Human" (technician Alton Yates) grits his teeth as the Holloman AFB
"Bopper," a crash-restraint-system demonstrator, delivers a multiple-G jolt. Such
work led to consumer-safety measures such as seat belts and
automobile crash tests. USAF photo.*

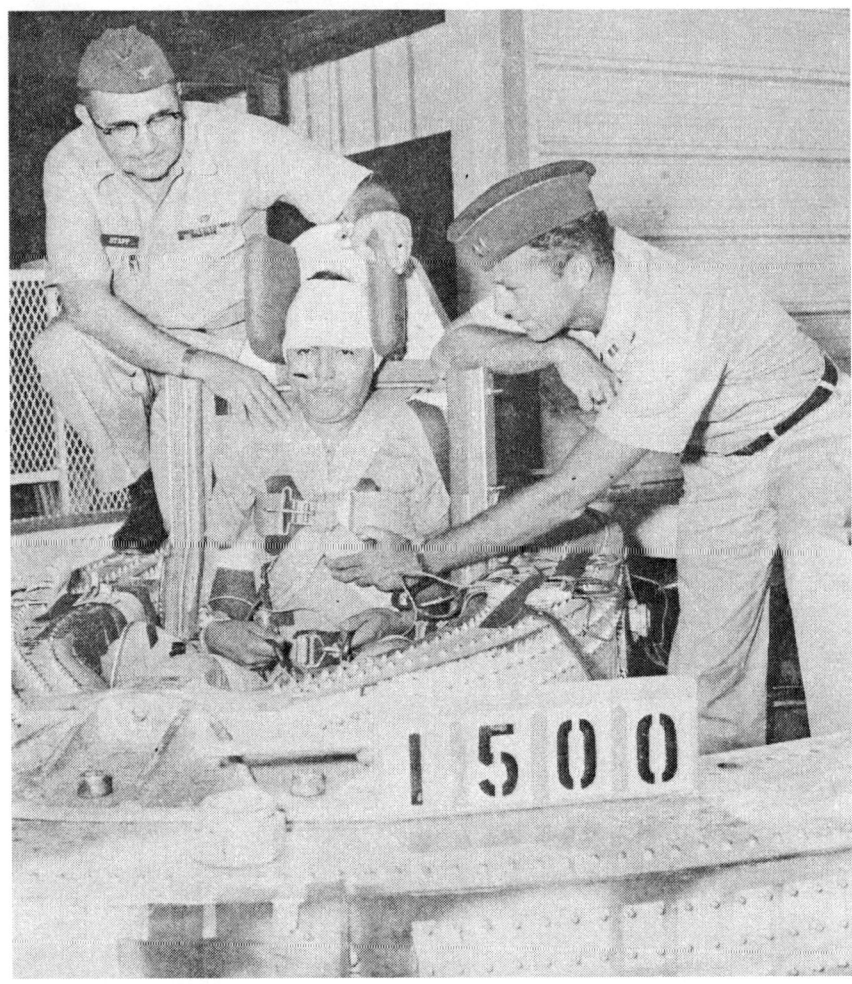

Stapp (left) and Eli Beeding (right) prepare another plucky Holloman volunteer with restraints and a bite block for his ride on the "Daisy Track." USAF photo.

entangled. He spun into unconsciousness, just as the lab experiments had predicted. Fortunately, a cutaway feature designed into the chute kicked in a few thousand feet above the ground, which allowed the reserve chute to open and drop the unconscious Kittinger heavily, but alive, onto the desert floor. The second jump went off like clockwork. After taking an hour to reach altitude, he jumped, free-falling nearly 50,000 feet and then floating to Earth and a gentle landing. The descent took thirteen minutes.

The third jump was from 102,800 feet and an unpressurized capsule. Kittinger would be well above the Armstrong Line, so if anything went wrong with his pressure suit or oxygen, he was too high to reach a safer altitude, even in free fall, before he would boil alive in his own blood. The fact that a few pilots' helmets had popped off in the lab during pressure-chamber tests and that his own had crept noticeably higher at the neck gasket during his first ascent was not reassuring.

Kittinger made his historic jump on August 16, 1960, and survived, breaking records and nearly breaking the sound barrier as his speed reached an unbelievable 614 miles per hour straight down. The chute's multistaged design gave him perfect stability the entire incredible distance, around eighty-four thousand feet—fifteen miles—before the main chute opened. The Excelsior team had found a way for a pilot to eject and survive from the very edge of space.[70]

Stapp made many loyal friends among the scientists, engineers, and technicians who worked under him at Muroc, the Wright Lab, and Holloman.

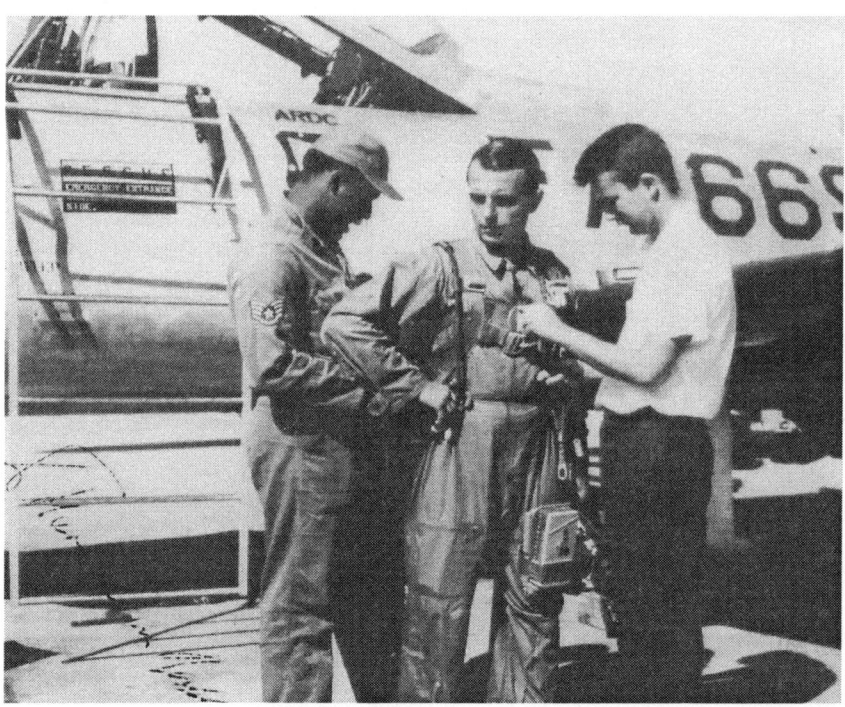

Harald von Beckh suits up for weightlessness experiments aboard a jet aircraft at Holloman AFB in New Mexico. National Library of Medicine photo.

Among the higher-ups, though, things were different. His irreverent, go-it-alone attitude—working around anyone who got in the way of his mission to save lives—had hardly gone unnoticed. Several times he was warned about the damage a death on one of his projects would do to the air force's image and his own career. Time and again he had to scrounge for funding. During the years when space was the place whose name no one dared to speak, he was often in competition with others who were also seeking the meager funds available for manned-spaceflight research.

Stapp felt that "the true worth of a scientist can be measured by the degree to which he's willing to do battle with the savages and cannibals of management." His greatest strength, he said, was "being very desperately stubborn about doing what I think should be done, what I think is right to do." It always paid off, he added.[71]

During Project Man High in 1957, he and David Simons had to argue and reargue the case for sending a man aboard a closed capsule into the stratosphere. It had cost just $10,000 to lift a hamster or mouse into the skies over Holloman a few years before, but to send a human up would cost more than $250,000. Stapp even diverted some of his rocket-sled money to the balloon program. He said that he thought the air force continued to fund his sled rides "because they hoped somehow I'd kill myself." If he killed anyone with Man High, though, he was warned that it would mean a court martial for him.[72]

The same admonition was made the following year regarding Project Excelsior and Kittinger, one of the air force's best (and best-known) test pilots. Finding money for the project meant both Paul Stapp and Joe Kittinger trekking to Washington to beg for funds.[73] By then, Stapp must have felt like the founder of a mendicant order of scientists.

There is another story, apparently true, about the time that the navy was looking for a name for a new unit of measurement: the force of gravitation on an object. They had been using an ad hoc nickname—a "jerk"—for the force of one G acting on an object for one second. Because Paul Stapp was such a jerk, someone suggested, why not name it a "stapp" instead? A reporter for a national magazine heard the remark and took it seriously enough to include the new term in an article. The taunt backfired; the name stuck, and the "stapp" went into the dictionary.[74]

Some of those who were close to Stapp detected a clash between him and Brig. Gen. Don Flickinger, who was the advocate for the Man in Space Soonest (MISS) project. Jealous of his popular success, the theory goes, "Flick" wanted Stapp run out of the service.[75] The tall, slim general had made his own share of news headlines years before. A secret flying mission to find a fast air route from Hawaii to the Philippines three months before war broke out earned him the Distinguished Flying Cross. He was medical officer of the day at Wheeler Field, Pearl Harbor, for the Sixth Pursuit Group on December 7, 1941, and during the war had made numerous parachute jumps into crash sites in Burma. There he had patched up wounded aircrew and passengers—including newsman Eric Sevareid—then hiked with them to safety, bargaining for safe passage by tending to the Burmese sick and injured. He tested early marker dyes for pilots downed at sea by having himself dropped off alone in the Pacific, hoping the search team would find him before the sharks did. After WWII Flickinger taught at Harvard Medical School and the School of Aviation Medicine. He jumped into new programs and used stealth and negotiation to accomplish his own personal and often eccentric goal: manned space flight.[76] He was one of the early believers.

There may be some truth to the rumors of a Flickinger-Stapp clash, but nothing other than anecdotal evidence has been found. Both men conducted themselves with bravery in the field and showed themselves willing time and again to put themselves in harm's way—for little reward—to help others. And it was Flickinger who got Stapp the money to finish the Man High project.[77] Perhaps the two were just too much alike. Flickinger, like Stapp, irritated a number of people. In 1961, he retired from the air force to emphasize the lack of support for military manned spaceflight, a topic no one apparently cared much about.[78] Someone also derailed Stapp. He went on to do crucial work in the selection of the first American astronauts, and he won national recognition for his invaluable contributions to the prevention of automobile-accident casualties. Colonel Stapp, however, never made general.

SETTING PARAMETERS

In March 1955, four years before NASA (formed in 1958) established its medical standards for astronaut selection, Flickinger, then in command of the air force's Office of Scientific Research, held a panel discussion on the topic at the Aero Medical Association's annual meeting in Washington, D.C. The panel members—six jet test pilots from the air force, NACA, and private industry—came to several conclusions: Desire and aggressiveness counted for ninety percent of a pilot's success (with formal education only a small factor); extensive ground simulation was crucial before a pilot could be sent to fly a completely new design; and the amount of safety gear modern pilots had to wear was so cumbersome and uncomfortable that it routinely hindered efficiency. Some members also expressed concern that simultaneously visualizing an airborne target, the instrument panel, and the terrain was a challenge above sixty thousand feet, particularly because the daytime sky became dark. All of them felt that a human being would never be completely replaced by a robot at the controls of a spacecraft or high-performance jet.[79]

By February 1957, the school's researchers had already been working long enough on selection standards for astronauts to have published on the subject in the *Journal of Aviation Medicine*. Their vision included a spacecraft whose "operating characteristics will not be radically new," suggesting that it would be largely an upgrade of current and anticipated aircraft design and "very much like a conventional rocket ship," meaning a German-inspired, rocket-powered aircraft. Their ship would be launched automatically, go into orbit, but make a conventional landing using wings and tricycle gear, "quite like the landing of a large jet aircraft." Bringing the vehicle back to Earth would require "essentially the same skills as those used in the pilotage of medium and large jet aircraft."[80]

The study was based at least in part on proposed Martian ferry vessels described by Wernher von Braun. Writing for the German and the American public in the early 1950s, the rocket designer had stated confidently that the third stage would be 15 meters long, 9.8 meters in diameter, with a wingspan of 52 meters and a wing area of 368 square meters. The medical writers decided to use these figures as likely estimates, even though von Braun worked for the army and drafted his spacecraft plans on his own time, not under contract with the air force. They also used his estimate of a 9-G takeoff, which would be much more rugged than actual Mercury, Apollo, or space-shuttle liftoffs proved to be. They even envisioned training their astronauts in "an actual spaceship either towed or carried to altitude, or powered by more conventional means."[81]

By February 1958, a year later and some five months before the formation of NASA, the school organized a working committee to determine the "requirements for crew members in extra-terrestrial flights." Bruno Balke served as chair, with Hans-Georg Clamann and five others as committee members. Their impetus was summed up in the first paragraph of a memo from Robert T. Clark, chair of the Department of Physiology and Biophysics: "As we are all aware a complete green light has been given the Department for research toward a manned space vehicle, the idea being that in the near future squadrons of high performance aircraft and missiles will be in use by the air force. It looks as though our present type of indoctrination in the low pressure chambers will soon be paralleled with indoctrination for 'space pilots' of these manned vehicles. This can conceivably in the future require training in extreme hypothermia." Clark noted, too, that their work over the past three years had provided them with the background information necessary to carry out their task.[82]

The group concluded that the best candidates for the air force's vehicles would be selected from the ranks of pilots and be slim, athletic nonsmokers aged thirty-five to forty-five. Greater age, they believed, would likely mean a man who was more emotionally stable, better trained, and possessed of better judgment. Physically, if cosmic radiation proved to be a health or reproductive risk, an older man might also have less to lose. Successful candidates needed to have demonstrated a tolerance for hypoxia, temperature extremes, G forces, and decompression, all of which a top military jet pilot would have acquired. They must be mentally stable and proven to be able to handle isolation, a restricted food intake, and extended periods of "complete relaxation," which could be interpreted as boredom, restriction of movement, or both. The group made no mention of height.[83]

Research was the next task. Balke and another scientist from the Department of Biophysics took a group of school volunteers to a site atop Mount Evans in Colorado to test their ability to acclimate to low-pressure, low-oxygen environments using exercise. He imposed a rigorous training program, with forced marches and relay races in which the volunteers ran up and down hills, carrying one another on their backs. The group did indeed acclimate.[84] Another committee member evaluated the human body's ability to adjust to extreme temperatures. A third studied the metabolic reserves in stressful situations—in this case water immersion (to simulate weightlessness).[85] All of these studies not only provided evidence of the feasibility of putting a man into space but also added to the school's already impressive credentials for carrying out the screening and selection of such a crew.

HUMAN FACTORS AND THE X-15:
ORGANIZING FOR MERCURY

In 1954, the air force, navy, and NACA pooled their talents and resources to create the first aircraft designed entirely as a research platform. Each entity had been separately considering such a project, hoping to explore the aerodynamics and physics of speeds at Mach 4 and higher.[86] To the Wright Lab, the human in the X-15 cockpit was the most important component in the system. The experimental aircraft was the first to incorporate human-factors design suggestions from the start.

Before the air force implemented any of its plans to put a human being into orbit, there were a number of questions the space-medicine specialists hoped the X-15 would answer. Two of these involved the person's reactions to the stresses of rapid acceleration and deceleration and to the weightless condition. Would a pilot lose the sense of orientation, that is, left, right, up, and down? Would the pilot be able to manipulate the controls, particularly during the crucial reentry period? Psychologically, would the pilot's overall sense of well-being, particularly on longer-duration flights, deteriorate to a point that precluded the ability to function as needed? The human-factors specialists at Wright also wanted data that would tell them which specific parts of the flight were the most difficult and therefore could best be aided (or accomplished) by mechanical or electrical devices.[87]

The researchers installed three control sticks—conventional, high-altitude, and high-stress—at the pilot's side rather than directly in front because they were concerned that the pilot might not be able to reach and manipulate a single center stick during weightlessness or extreme Gs. The cabin was hermetically sealed because normal pressure-breathing equipment would be insufficient. Designers also included an escape system. The pilot was to wait until the plane was below 100,000 feet. Then, devices on both sides of the seat would send the canopy hurtling away from the aircraft, and an automatic rocket catapult in the seat would fire and burn for half a second, long enough for the pilot also to be thrown clear of the plane. Two large fins and two booms would automatically extend outward from the seat as it began to fall, maintaining stability. At 15,000 feet the seat would fall away, and a parachute would open up, allowing the pilot to land safely. At the request of Scott Crossfield, the program's chief test pilot and member of the design review committee, the Wright people came up with a bailout bottle that contained thirty minutes of oxygen, enough to eject and land several times over.[88]

The premier achievement in terms of human-factors equipment was the flight suit. Called the MC-2, it was a full-pressure garment with built-in bladders that automatically expanded at a predetermined altitude, in this case just above 35,000 feet. The upward force they exerted on the lower extremities and torso kept enough blood going to the pilot's brain to avoid a blackout in flight. An experienced jet pilot was thus able to pull 7 or 8 Gs. Without the suit the pilot might have lost consciousness at 4 or 5. Such clothing, nicknamed "get-me-down-suits," had already proven themselves in flight. Col. Pete Everest's life had been saved by a T-1 partial-pressure suit during test flights of a rocket airplane when the canopy cracked in flight at nearly 80,000 feet.[89]

In order to produce the snuggest fit but allow for maximum flexibility, researchers fabricated the suit using nearly 160 body measurements. It took about twelve minutes to put on and was a task that could not be accomplished alone. Starting from the skin and working out, the layers consisted of thin long johns, a vent garment, the pressure suit, a layer of mesh, and, finally, a silvery outer layer. The vent garment was made of a rubberized material fitted with openings that permitted the circulation of liquid-nitrogen-cooled air. The pressure suit itself was a two-piece rubber affair, sealed at the waist. The mesh that went over it was a flexible green plastic, intended to prevent the suit from ballooning out once inflated. The outer layer, called the "sacrifice garment," was made from an aluminized fabric that possessed great tensile strength. It was not a part of the pressure suit per se but was disposable in the sense that it was designed to protect the wearer from windblast in the event of ejection, tearing if need be.[90]

Boots and gloves were pressurized, too, and attached to the suit by means of zippers. The helmet was pressurized with a separate, pure-oxygen system. To keep the nitrogen and oxygen apart, the helmet had a tight neck seal and was set at a slightly higher pressure than the body of the suit. An intercom was built into the helmet. A "back pan," a flat pack attached to the pilot's back, contained an anti-G valve for the bladders and two oxygen regulators, one of which was a backup.[91]

Live data on the in-flight performance of the aircraft had been transmitted to the ground during Stapp's X-1 project, but the X-15 was the first program to telemeter medical data in real time. The data gathering and relay were done with the aid of a small metal plate built into the suit and fitted with leads that were attached to the pilot. These picked up the heartbeat, respiration, blood pressure, and body temperature and transmitted them to Edwards AFB, where a flight surgeon monitored them constantly. Additional information, including feedback on the functioning of the MC-2 suit, and more detailed medical data were collected on board the aircraft for later analysis. Afterward, the flight surgeons used a whole-body radiation counter at Los Alamos National Laboratory in New Mexico to look for effects of the cosmic rays at that altitude. By the end of the program, physicians were also able to get an in-flight EKG on the X-15 pilots. Data on heart rates in particular would become useful in the first two Mercury flights, as their ballistic trajectories were similar to those of an X-15. By the time Alan Shepard was launched, the Wright aeromedical specialists knew to expect a heart rate of 145 to 160 beats per minute and that the pilot could function with full efficiency even beyond that.[92]

Crossfield and the human-factors specialists under Col. Burt Rowen at the Wright Lab worked out the bugs in the first model of the suit in late 1958, then tested the second version, the one Crossfield wore during the first flight in March 1959. Rowen was uniquely qualified for the job; he was a flight surgeon and jet pilot with parachute training and experience teaching at the School of Aviation Medicine. Crossfield rode the Wright centrifuge wearing the garment and saw that it raised his G tolerance by 2.5 Gs—to 7.5 or 8 Gs. He also tested it in the "hot box" at Wright nine times during 1957 and 1958. The normal test protocol was to go from minus 40 to 180 degrees Fahrenheit, but Crossfield accidentally wore the suit during an unbelievable 400-degree session. The cooling system worked so well that he did not know the room had been that hot until he touched something—and it sizzled. The team shipped the sacrifice garment off to Edwards, where a test dummy wore it while strapped to the rocket sled roaring along the track. It made ten runs at speeds of up to eight hundred miles per hour and was catapulted aloft in an ejection seat to check the likelihood of its tearing. The suit eventually took its wearers beyond the X-15 program's initial goals, reaching Mach 6.7 and altitudes higher than fifty miles.[93]

Chapter 6

ORGANIZING FOR SPACE

S enate Majority Leader Lyndon Johnson was genuinely concerned by the launch of *Sputnik,* although he knew a good political cause when he saw one and took immediate and forceful steps to get America into what was a space race from the get-go. The hearings he held into the status of space preparedness, the media and public response to the Soviet satellite, and concerns within the Republican White House came together to set off a debate about the nature of the national response to this Cold War challenge. A key question was whether the United States should continue its space research within the military agencies already charged with the task or put it into the public purview. The ultimate result was the creation of a civilian space agency, the National Aeronautics and Space Administration (NASA), and the reorganization of military space priorities and resources.

Because of the military's experience with the U-2 and X-15 experimental high-altitude aircraft programs and the multitude of other space-medicine and human-factors projects the air force had done at the School of Aviation Medicine, Wright and Holloman Labs, and Lovelace Clinic, the USAF aeromedical team was chosen to carry out nearly all of the testing and selection processes for the Mercury astronaut program. Their results would prove to be a complete success. What the air force thought would be a honeymoon period with the new space agency, though, turned out quickly to be nothing of the sort. They thought their role would continue to be one of mentor to the fledgling space agency and provider of services by its uniquely qualified staff at their state-of-the-art labs. However, NASA took on an existence and an agenda of its own, in large part due to the commitment John Kennedy made to put an American on the moon by the end of the 1960s. Under a new, able, and aggressive administrator, James E. Webb, NASA would establish a duplicate set of medical facilities just two hours from San Antonio at the new Johnson Space Center in Houston. The space agency requisitioned a handful of military medical personnel to jump-start things there, then over the next several years went its own way. The personnel of the school and the labs, who constituted nearly all of the country's qualified space-medicine researchers, were never asked whether it would be in the best interests of the profession, the astronaut corps, or the taxpayers to combine the resources of NASA and the USAF, to split the workload between the two agencies, or to support two parallel, manned space programs. They were completely out of the loop.

Plans that the air force was considering for an independent, manned space program would shortly come to nothing. The distance between the research facilities in Houston and San Antonio would become ever greater. The contributions of Armstrong, Strughold, Stapp, and others who had risked their careers and lives on behalf of the American astronaut would be forgotten to all but a few who knew their story.

THE AMERICAN PUBLIC, SPUTNIK, AND SPACE

Hubertus Strughold and flight surgeon David Simons were at the International Astronomical Federation conference in Barcelona, Spain, when the Soviet delegation announced the launch of the world's first artificial, Earth-orbiting satellite on October 4, 1957. The meeting was a drama in opposites, according to Strughold: jubilation on one side of the room, depression and irritation on the other. Once back in the United States, the School of Aviation Medicine held a press conference on the fallout of the *Sputnik* launch. The best guess was that perhaps four to six news reporters might attend. After all, the school had received a modest amount of attention from the national press in the last few years. A reporter from *Time* had come and spoken with Strughold and Haber, as had German-born science popularizer Willy Ley, a confidant of Wernher von Braun.[1] *National Geographic* had sent a team to do a feature, and CBS television had filmed two news stories there.[2] However, *Sputnik* hit the press office like a tidal wave. Applications to attend the conference flooded in from all over the United States and Europe, eighty or ninety requests in all, and the event was moved to a big hotel to accommodate the throng.

In the next six months the public-affairs office for the school handled sixty-eight inquiries from the public, twenty press briefings, and fifteen speaking engagements. Writers from *Time, Life,* the *Wall Street Journal,* the *Kansas City Star,* and the *Fort Worth Press* all came to the school looking for background and interesting features.[3]

Sputnik certainly made the average citizen believe in space travel. In 1949, a Gallup poll had found that just 15 percent of the public thought humans would reach the moon by the end of the century. After *Sputnik,* 41 percent thought we might get there by the 1980s.[4]

Moscow's coup and the reaction of the American press and public should not have shocked anyone who had given space serious thought. A 1946 RAND Corporation study had predicted a satellite for the USSR, and a 1952 report to President Truman said furthermore that Soviet propagandists would use the news to their greatest advantage.[5] The whole thing came as a terrible surprise, however, to Texan Lyndon Johnson.

As chair of the armed services preparedness subcommittee in 1957, Johnson was in a position to act on the news of the Soviet space triumph. Historian Robert Dallek argues that LBJ's motives in framing a response to *Sputnik*, at least initially, were pure when it came to national security and also for creating NASA as a civilian agency. Nevertheless, that did not necessarily mean that he did not also desire an enhancement of his own public standing in preparation for a bid for the presidency in the next election. In either case, LBJ picked up the ball and ran far with it. He called for hearings and dominated them, introducing and then cross-examining the witnesses personally, and acting as spokesperson to the media for the newly created Senate Special Committee on Space and Astronautics. He kept the hearings in session from nine A.M. until nine P.M. for two straight months. By the time they were over, the committee had accumulated almost twenty-five hundred pages of data, and Johnson had persuaded its members to make more than a dozen recommendations for action.

One result of this was that more money quickly began to flow to the air force for human-factors research, specifically in space medicine.[6] In spite of an overall increase in federal support for science in the immediate postwar years, which is evident in the creation of the National Science Foundation, RAND Corporation, the Atomic Energy Commission, and similar groups, the early 1950s had been very lean years for military science. The USAF had taken funding away from Atlas missile research and left unfilled numerous research jobs at the school as draftees returned to the work force. It had taken the air force and Congress eleven years to review, approve, and fund a request by Harry Armstrong in 1946 for $9.5 million to construct a modern complex, replacing the World War I–era facilities at Randolph.[7] Headquarters had cut the school's budget by twenty-five percent for fiscal year 1957.[8] Suddenly, however, almost any sort of equipment and raw material the staff wanted they could get—and quickly. They worked Saturdays and Sundays and were paid overtime for it.[9]

LBJ also began to pay more personal attention to the facility, which was not far from his ranch in Texas's hill country. Several years earlier he had suffered a major heart attack and so would come to the school for an occasional checkup with its cardiac specialists. Late in 1957, he witnessed an experiment there that he immediately put to good propaganda use for the American space effort: Hubertus Strughold's "space cabin simulator."

Back in 1953, the new professor of space medicine had suggested seemingly out of the blue that it was time to get "a proper kind of space cabin in the lab." He and Heinz Haber wrote up a research proposal, and once it was accepted, Haber created a blueprint of the desired specifications. They had built a wooden mock-up first and then given a contract to a Chicago firm, which delivered the actual cabin the following year. Due to the lack of staff, it had been used only for experiments of a few hours duration.

Now, two months after *Sputnik*, Strughold was ready to give the simulator a full-blown test. He would use it to emulate some of the conditions of a flight to the moon by isolating a human test subject for seven days and seven nights, the length of time Jules Verne had predicted for a round-trip lunar excursion. Airman Donald G. Farrell, a twenty-three-year-old from the Bronx, was selected from a rigorously screened pool of candidates. Farrell entered the chamber on February 9, 1958, only nine days after the United States achieved its first space success, the *Explorer I* satellite.[10]

The airman's task was to cool his heels inside the small sealed cabin while Clamann, Strughold, and Lt. Col. George R. Steinkamp and Maj. Willard R. Hawkins of the Department of Astroecology determined whether it was operating as they hoped, keeping the outside environment outside and maintaining the life of the man inside. That meant holding a constant air pressure and comfortable temperature; storing food, water, and solid waste; absorbing carbon dioxide; collecting and recycling water vapor; and allowing physicians to obtain cardiovascular and respiratory data.

The cabin's interior measured just ninety-six square feet, of which less than half was available as living space. To enhance the feeling of isolation and thus test the subject's ability to remain alone for a week in a cramped space, no outside visual or voice contact was allowed. Farrell was required to report the temperature and humidity and make other observations every eight hours with a microphone placed in the cabin, however. Two closed-circuit cameras allowed scientists outside to watch "events" inside the cabin, but they could make contact only via lighted panels displaying phrases such as "Meal Period" or "Begin Work." From his position in an aircraft seat inside the cabin, Farrell had to flip a certain switch before commencing each activity, demonstrating his vigilance in watching for new commands while performing other tasks. Researchers measured his attentiveness and judgment by noting his speed and accuracy in following a random series of tasks presented to him on a television screen and requiring him to press various buttons and manipulate gauges.[11]

To the press and public, the discovery of the Van Allen radiation belt was not nearly as exciting or meaningful as putting a living being into orbit, as the USSR had done with Laika, the dog, in November. Lacking an American pet in space, TV crews, photographers, wire services, and scores of reporters from across the United States came to San Antonio to see the next best thing: Airman Farrell, America's Earth-bound spaceman. This clamoring forced Otis Benson to set up a newsroom and scores of phone lines and to ration out his scientists to overeager reporters. "For want of a real expedition into space by an American flyer," reads an official air force history, "the press turned to the imaginary one scheduled at Randolph."[12]

Johnson heard that the simulator experiment was scheduled to wrap up while he was there for a checkup. He headed for the chamber and escorted Farrell out for the benefit of the news reporters and photographers and thanked him in the name of the American people. Benson thanked Farrell in the name of the school, and Strughold, in the name of medical science.[13] At Johnson's request, Farrell and the USAF team then flew to Washington for more interviews and congressional hearings. It was the first order of business for the Special Committee on Space and Astronautics, which LBJ had organized just six days earlier. He displayed Benson, Farrell, and Strughold at a lunch before fifty senators and representatives, generals, secretaries of the armed forces, and Jacqueline Cochran, who sat at Strughold's table. There would be a question-and-answer session for the three of them after lunch, Johnson said, and then casually added to Strughold that he was expected to give a five-minute talk "after the soup."[14] Space medicine had arrived.

AMERICA'S SATELLITE

Although a popular version of the history of *Sputnik* is that its October, 1957, launch took the United States completely by surprise and without a viable satellite program of its own, such was not the case.[15] There were many concepts for an American satellite, or artificial moon, as it was sometimes called. The U.S. Navy's Bureau of Aeronautics had briefly considered, then rejected, an idea for a navy satellite in 1945. The U.S. Army Air Corps had issued a request for a proposal for the design of a satellite early in 1946 and actually funded a million-dollar study of the idea by Douglas Aircraft, a contract that was later transferred to its think-tank spinoff, the RAND Corporation.[16] RAND had also conducted a study for the air force, concluding in 1954, that a satellite could be created and launched as an unmanned reconnaissance vehicle and that it made strategic sense to do so. In 1956, Lockheed was awarded an air force contract to design it.[17] In 1955, the Ad Hoc Advisory Group on Special Capabilities had reported to the assistant secretary of defense that the United States could launch a small scientific satellite in 1958 for a belated IGY effort.[18] In 1954, Wernher von Braun and his team at the army's Redstone Arsenal had made plans for a joint army-navy-air-force satellite as a contribution to the IGY in 1957.[19] The same year, the IGY organizing committee listed a satellite launch as one of the anticipated events on its official calendar, and the following year the U.S. committee formally announced that it intended to launch such a device.

President Eisenhower had decided by then that America's contribution to what was intended as a purely scientific event, the IGY, should not be associated with the military. Consequently, America's choice became Project Vanguard, a satellite based on a reworked navy sounding rocket and bearing the banner of the National Science Foundation.[20] By the time the IGY was underway in 1957, the United Kingdom, France, Japan, Australia, and Canada had also stated their intention of launching a satellite, and many other countries had signed on as observers, looking and listening for them once in orbit.[21]

It is also untrue that the United States had no understanding of the Soviets' space capability or of that country's plans to launch something in 1957. In its January, 1952, newsletter, the American Interplanetary Society printed a brief report on Soviet rocket research (which, although accurate, placed orbital and planetary missions as still somewhere vaguely "in the future").[22] Soviet scientists revealed in 1955 that they intended to launch a satellite as part of the IGY, and the Moscow evening paper ran an article on the plans for the device, reportedly listing its designer by name.[23] The IGY committee for the USSR formally announced the country's goals the following year.[24] In its June and July, 1957, issues, *Radio*, a Soviet magazine for ham-radio operators, published a call for all amateur listeners to report the reception of any signals they might pick up broadcast from satellites *launched in the USSR*. The magazine gave the frequencies for the broadcasts, described the sound the signals would make, and stated the power of the transmitter.

Radio also published data on the proposed American satellite, which was available in the open literature.[25] Ironically, the *Journal of Aviation Medicine* published an article in its October, 1957, issue that was based on a paper given at the Aero Medical Association's annual meeting that May, titled "Visibility of Artificial Satellites of the Planet Earth." The author was Ingeborg Schmidt, whose opening paragraph states that her calculations were "based on data available in the literature about the first satellite of the project Vanguard, which will be launched from the east coast of Florida during the International Geophysical Year." In the next paragraph, Schmidt describes the dimensions of the American satellite and its orbit.[26]

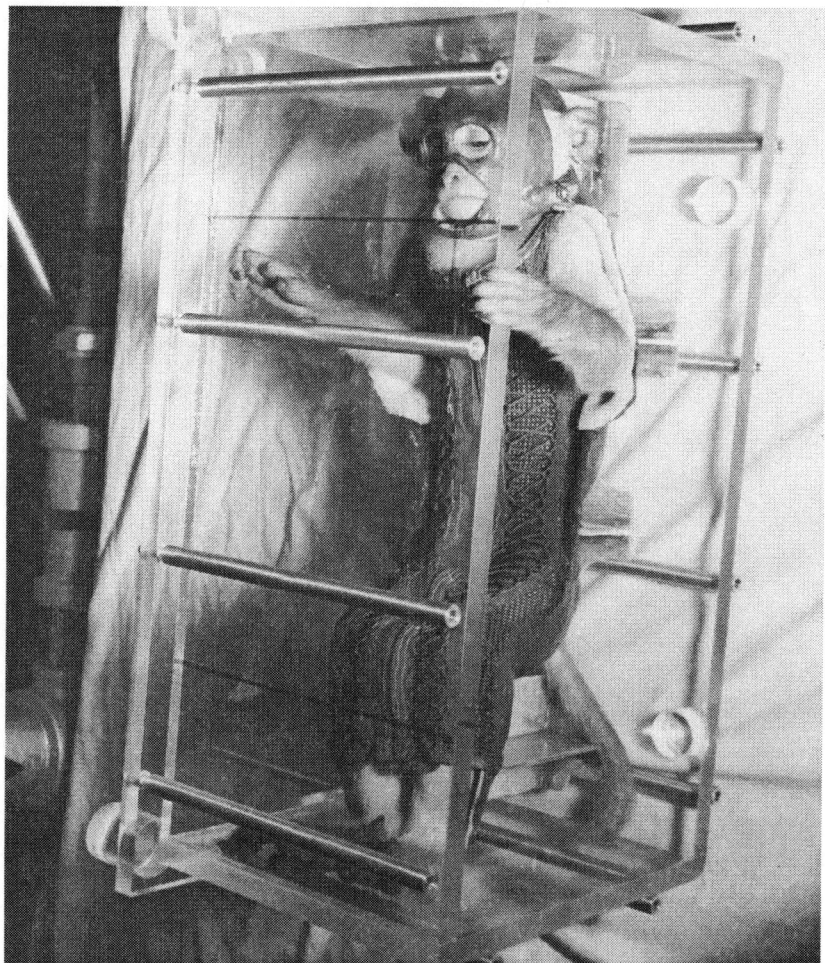

"Sam," named for the School of Aviation Medicine, training in his simulator. Paperclip craftsmen at the school made the animal compartments, training devices, and life-support systems. Photo courtesy of Roland Dornes.

What may have caused those who were knowledgeable about America's space capabilities and plans even greater consternation than *Sputnik 1* was *Sputnik 2*. It was launched just a month later, in November, 1957, this time with a living creature aboard: the small, female, mixed-breed Laika ("Little Barker.") Not only had the USSR shown itself capable of launching an object that could—the theory went—rain down death and destruction on the American people, but it also could and would send people into space soon.[27]

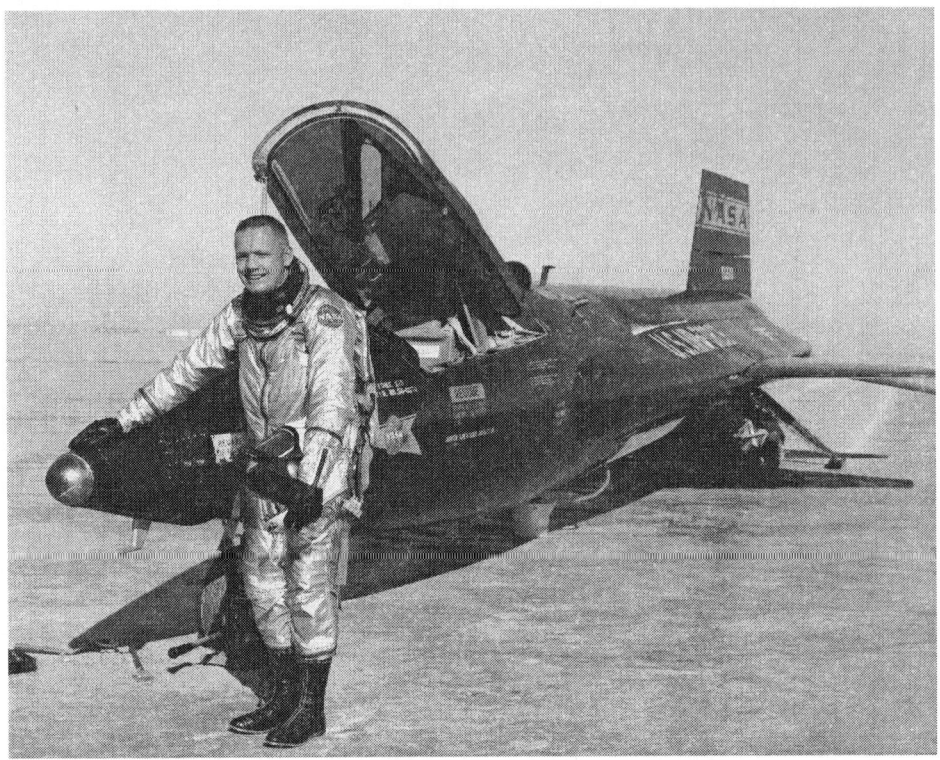

NACA test pilot Neil Armstrong and others who flew the experimental X-15 aircraft in the late 1950s benefited from the human-factors expertise of the School of Aviation Medicine, Wright Lab, and the Lovelace Foundation in the design of their flying suits and cockpit environment and controls. NASA photo.

Manned space capability had hardly reached the conjecture level in the United States when suddenly it seemed as though the Communists were poised to claim the next high ground.[28]

However, the air force had already begun formulating a plan as early as 1956 to send a military astronaut into space atop a rocket, Don Flickinger's Man in Space Soonest (MISS) project. It had come about in response to a request by the head of the Air Research and Development Command (ARDC) for ideas on advanced vehicle designs that could follow the X-15, a joint NACA-military project still two years away from flight. A manned ballistic missile would at least help the air force get more R and D funding, the thinking went. Consequently, the ARDC made two proposals: the Manned

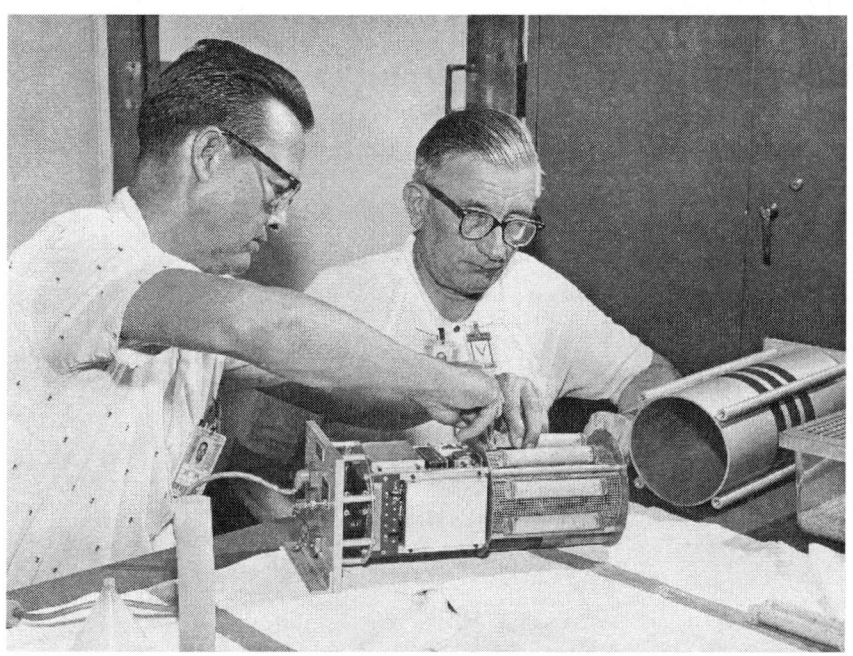

Hans-Georg Clamann (right) oversaw the design and construction of the containers used for animal space launches, including this mouse habitat. Photo courtesy of Roland Dornes.

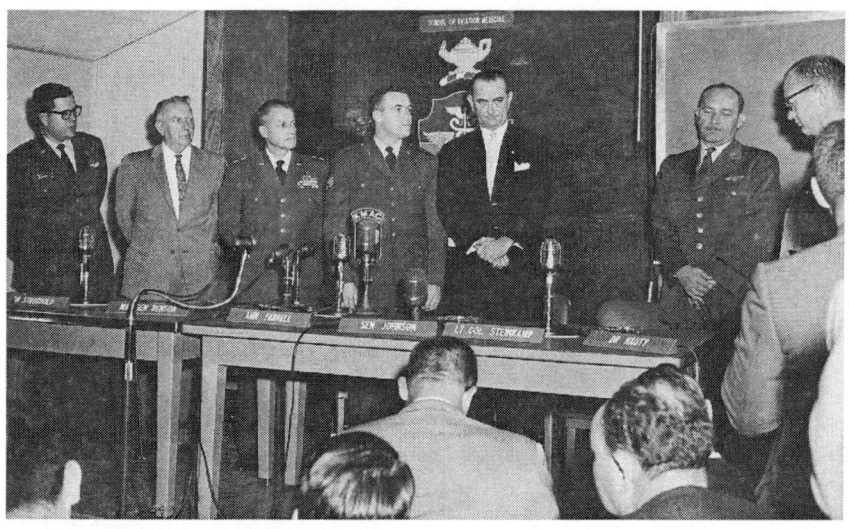

The press conference immediately after Airman Farrell's stay in the simulator. Strughold is second from left, and to his left are General Benson, Farrell, and a grim-looking Sen. Lyndon Johnson. USAF photo.

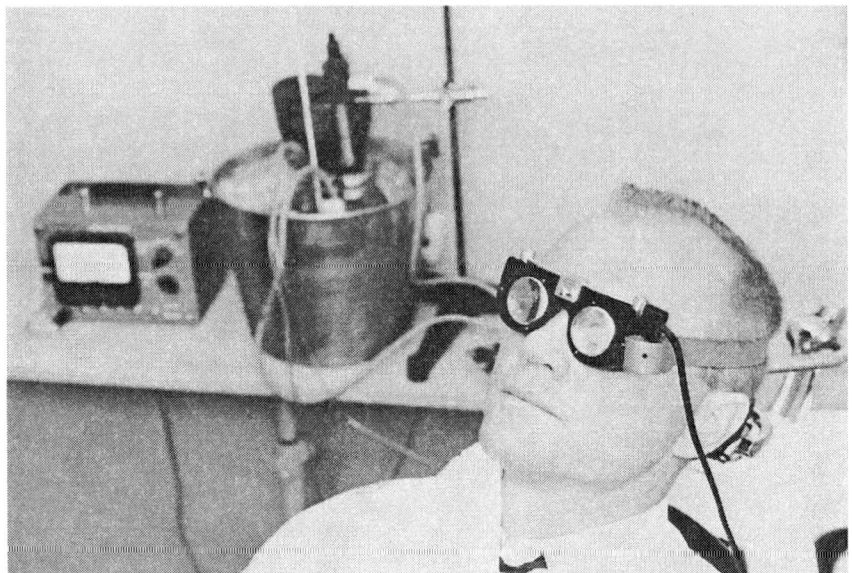

Mercury astronaut screening included tests of balance, similar to this 1961 caloric test, in which cold water was run into a subject's ears and the corresponding effect on eye movement was measured. This photo shows astronaut John H. Glenn Jr. undergoing the test. NASA photo.

Glide Rocket Research System, which would go Mach 21 and operate at four hundred thousand feet, and the Manned Ballistic Rocket Research System, which would launch a human atop a separable nose cone attached to an ICBM. By the end of December, 1957, perhaps urged on by the dog in orbit, air force headquarters ordered Flickinger, director of human factors at the ARDC, to set up a comprehensive astronautics program that would include these projects. Former Wright test pilot Donald Putt, then deputy chief of staff for development, requested NACA's help in supplying data for the manned space glider and man-atop-an-ICBM projects.

Medical and human-factors expertise would be especially necessary for the ballistic program, which was an eleven-step project that included animal and human orbital missions. Moon passengers would ride on a rotatable couch already tested by Harald von Beckh and could expect to experience up to 9 Gs and a cabin temperature of 150 degrees. The aeromedical people suggested that about fifteen primate test flights be made before they okayed a manned shot. They also recommended that, because passengers would require continuous telemonitoring, a television camera be included in the cockpit. Moreover, in expectation of a possible 12-G ride, the medical team also suggested a solid safety margin on the cockpit's interior design.

By March, 1958, two months after the request for cooperation by the air force, space enthusiasts within NACA had already convinced its leadership that they, too, needed to be looking into manned spaceflight. After some waffling, they agreed to cooperate on the ballistic-missile project but backed out in mid-May when it became known that they were to be tapped as the new civilian space agency. In August, as NASA, they would be given full responsibility for manned space flight. NASA's first manned program, Mercury, in effect killed Flickinger's MISS since the money for it was taken out of the Department of Defense (DOD) budget and assigned to the new space agency.[29]

NASA

Johnson had wasted no time back in October in clarifying the objectives of his special committee. They were to determine who in the executive and legislative branches would have jurisdiction over each aspect of space and astronautics; how such units would be established, what their function would be, how much power each should have; and finally, "how to deal with the international aspects of space."[30] The international policy role was a crucial one. If the United States wished to establish a permanent, ongoing space presence, it had to decide—and let the world know—whether any or all of it would be for military purposes. Whether from a heartfelt desire for peace or with an eye to the next election, Johnson made an opening statement at the first convening of the special committee and reminded the group that the decisions they faced were not those of choosing how to control atomic weapons or keep peace in the immediate aftermath of a world war. Instead, he explained, "while space adds a new dimension to the technology of weapons and the strategy of security, the ultimate opportunity of space is not that of a final battleground. Free men have no intention of rattling sabers among the stars."[31]

From the beginning, many people also considered space science a vehicle for bringing nations together and, for this, felt they needed a strong, civilian space authority that could operate on the world stage and be quite detached from the defense functions they wanted the military to carry out. In a statement before the special committee, State Department legal advisor Loftus E. Becker called for the separation of military and civilian space research because a civilian agency "would provide a means by which many nations would participate in this new venture" and also ensure that the study of space was "carried on in the classic tradition of scientific openness." Becker even called for a "suitable and necessary relationship with the United Nations," asking whether it might be good to put the new agency under the UN rather than make it a federal government affair.[32]

The question of creating a separate civilian space agency was debated when the National Aeronautics and Space Act of 1958, sponsored by Eisenhower and helped along by Johnson, was submitted for House and Senate approval. The act created NASA out of the National Advisory Committee for Aeronautics. NACA's name had come up most often when policy advisors looked about for an organizing center for the space effort. It had always been a slow, conservative organization ever since its beginnings in 1915, but it was greatly respected for the quality of its research, and it employed some of the best minds in aeronautical engineering. Users judged it unbiased, serving military and civilian interests equally well. The organization did all of its research in house at laboratories in Langley, Virginia, and Cleveland, Ohio, and had also trained many aeronautical engineers who went on to industry, academia, and the military. It had also done all of those things on a shoestring budget.[33]

In 1957, NACA had eight thousand employees. Thirty-five percent of its work was in support of space technology, the remainder in aeronautics.[34] That same year, NACA and the military, represented by the U.S. Army's Ballistic Missile Agency and the DOD's Advanced Research Projects Agency (ARPA), had established a special committee on space technology. By February, 1958, they were floating plans for travel to the moon and nearby planets.[35] Consequently, if a new agency were to be created with NACA as its foundation, it would be able to get its manned spaceflight program up and running fairly quickly.

Space historian Robert A. Divine asserts that it was the scientific community that pushed the hardest to make NACA into the new space agency. The engineering organization had balanced the interests of the military, industry, and science consistently and fairly. Technically, no other government agency under consideration—the Atomic Energy Commission, the National Science Foundation—could claim to be as qualified for the job.[36] The president's science advisor, James Killian, was NACA's biggest booster, claiming that it was directed by "some of the best civilian talent in the country" and functioned "with freedom from political influence and unencumbered by government bureaucracy and red tape."[37] Additionally, it had begun formal studies of the altitudes above fifty thousand feet and speeds ranging from Mach 10 to escape velocity six years ago, in 1952.[38] When all was said and done, there was no existing government agency better qualified to take on the management of a space program.

Johnson's committee held hearings into the matter of creating a civilian agency, and every person who testified favored its formation. All of them stated that they expected that such a move would not diminish the military's space effort and that the military and NASA would advise each other as needed. However, they felt that America needed to demonstrate to the world that science must be conducted in an open way, in contrast to the Soviets' near-paranoid secrecy. Whether it be a progressive outlook on their part, religion, fiscal prudence, or an elevation of science to a high pedestal, they emphasized the peace-making possibilities of a national space program.[39] "The simple fact is," NACA Director Hugh Dryden testified, "in addition to being a peaceful nation composed of citizens who hate the thought of war, we must so conduct ourselves that our friends around the world—and our enemies as well—will know beyond mistake that although we are amply strong as our national interest requires, we are striving by word and deed for peace."[40]

Dryden further testified that a civilian space agency could coexist with the military, a position supported by witness Donald A. Quarles, deputy secretary of defense. In its forty-three years, both men stated, NACA and civil aviation had not been bullied or coopted by the military but had enjoyed a symbiotic relationship. NACA's main committee, in fact, had two representatives each from the air force, navy, and Civil Aeronautics Authority; one each from the Smithsonian, the Weather Bureau, the National Bureau of Standards, and the Department of Defense; and up to seven others from arenas related to aeronautical science. The new Space Board would have between eight and seventeen members, at least one of whom had to be from the Department of Defense.[41]

Likewise, U.S. Army Secretary Wilber M. Brucker testified that, even though his branch of the service had many immediate uses for space capability, it did not consider such applications to be exclusively military. Nor was America's technological know-how uniquely military. Although first consideration must be given in all planning to national security, he said, the army would back any plan to use civilian resources and meet civilian needs.[42]

The executive branch, in fact, had already begun making plans for America's role in manned spaceflight and considered civilian activities to be a significant component. In 1958, the president's Science Advisory Council produced a report that referred to manned orbital flight as a logical goal and speculated about the resources needed for a lunar landing. The National Security Council issued a policy statement calling manned spaceflight inevitable.[43] The president's Advisory Committee on Government Organizations did not see many military applications for space on the horizon and felt that the DOD had more than enough to do without taking on the civilian space program.[44]

Both Brucker and ARPA director Roy W. Johnson qualified their remarks by stating explicitly that the military must continue to have the scientific and technological capability it already had—and nothing less than that. For his part, Johnson saw any need for a civilian space agency as arising from research that went beyond the immediate needs of the military, not from any wasteful duplication of effort.[45] Alan T. Waterman, director of the National Science Foundation, predicted that "the opportunities provided by space exploration will be very strongly scientific in character and civilian rather than military, although, of course, military requirements form a part of any general program."[46]

In the end, the Senate and the House passed the National Aeronautics and Space Act of 1958, creating the National Aeronautics and Space Administration on October 1, 1958.[47] In spite of Eisenhower's misgivings about over-emphasizing a manned space program (he felt only reconnaissance satellites were truly necessary strategically), his new Space Council voted right away to designate Project Mercury as having "highest-priority" status.[48] Within days of becoming operational, NASA had obtained approval of its manned spaceflight program: an agenda that had been hammered out in anticipation by a joint NASA/ARPA committee and agreed to by von Braun's team at the army's Ballistic Missile Agency.[49] It was ready to go.

SELECTING THE SEVEN

In April, 1958, retired air force Lt. Gen. James H. "Jimmy" Doolittle was chair of the National Advisory Committee on Aeronautics. He was an outspoken advocate of space science and technology and a longtime friend of Randolph Lovelace. The general knew that, in addition to Lovelace's experience as head of the Wright laboratory from 1942 until the end of 1945, he had more recently done contract consulting and research for the air force, the air surgeon general, the secretary of defense, the North Atlantic Treaty Organization, and aircraft manufacturers and airlines.[50] Some of Lovelace's work, including the screening of the U-2 spy-plane pilots for the CIA in the mid-1950s, had been top secret. His Albuquerque group had also been conducting extensive studies for the Department of Energy since 1951 on the medical effects of atomic warfare and for the past few months had been developing a test protocol for the selection of the X-15 pilots or any pilot, for that matter, who might fly in and out of the upper atmosphere.[51] Lovelace was already serving on NACA's Special Committee on Space Technology, and Doolittle again turned to him to head the Working Group on Human Factors and Training.[52]

Everyone concerned was very aware that they were breaking new ground. No one, except perhaps the Soviets, had done what they were about to do. They were going to decide whether a human being could survive in space and, if so, make the best possible guess as to who would be the optimal person to send. Little was known in the late 1950s about the competition's experience with space medicine, as Moscow published nothing in the open journals.[53]

To make the decisions required, Lovelace chose eight others to serve with him, including Ulrich Luft, Don Flickinger, and Scott Crossfield. He relayed to the group Doolittle's very general instructions that they "'study problems associated with putting a man in space.'" They concluded quickly and unanimously that the basis from which they would work was aerospace medicine. Their reasoning was that it encompassed high-altitude physiology, sports medicine, industrial medicine, human-factors research, psychology, physics, and general medicine—in short, everything they would use to make a successful decision.[54]

In late 1958, the administrator of the new NASA, T. Keith Glennan, also turned to Lovelace, appointing him to head a third group, the Special Committee on Life Sciences. This body was made up of members from the military; the Atomic Energy Commission; the Department of Health, Education, and Welfare; and the private sector. He also asked for three aeromedical consultants to be part of the group, one from each branch of the military. Given the amalgam of its members' backgrounds, its responsibility was to provide Glennan and others at the top with objective advice on space medicine and human-factors issues and also to jump-start the agency's aeromedical capabilities, which naturally were zero. Historian Loyd Swenson says that the group was to provide NASA "intelligent liaison and some expertise of its own in dealing with military aeromedical organizations." Such a role would have put Lovelace across the table from the groups at Wright and the school, rather than on the same side.[55] This is what Glennan wanted, however: someone who was not interested in building his own empire within the space agency or within the military but who would work along the lines both he and Eisenhower envisioned. Their goal was to keep the agency trim by using existing resources, particularly in the military, rather than creating a duplicate space-medicine staff at the taxpayers' expense.[56]

Unofficially, the Space Task Group (STG), which would evolve into the Mercury team, was created within NASA on October 8, 1958, at the former NACA's Langley facility. Forty-five people formed the nucleus of this group, including thirty-five Langley staffers who had worked closely with the air force's MISS program at Wright Field. Lovelace and Don Flickinger were attached to the STG in November of that year as aeromedical consultants.

In January, the two flight surgeons and a half dozen other STG members, including George Low, NASA's chief of manned space flight, formed a group to consider the human portion of the engineering equation. They came up with a set of initial requirements for the Project Mercury astronauts. Their "job description" did not include much for the pilots to do since "the entire satellite operation will be possible, in the early phases, without the presence of man." Physically, candidates had to be male, aged twenty-five to forty, under five feet eleven inches (due to the capsule's space restrictions), hold a B.S. in science, and have five years' work experience in science or engineering or as an officer aboard an aircraft, balloon, or submarine. Personally, he must be willing to accept hazards "comparable to those encountered in modern research airplane flight," be able to tolerate severe environments, and react well under stress. Examples of the sort of person the STC sought included test pilots, arctic explorers, submarine crews, paratroopers, mountain climbers, or scuba divers.

Dwight Eisenhower nixed that plan and directed that the selection be made from among the nation's military test pilots. It would simplify much of the process, as they already met the qualifications by definition. Furthermore, their records and medical histories were readily available, they were not security risks and could be reassigned on short notice, and both they and their families already understood and accepted the dangers involved.[57]

No one knew how many of the military's best pilots would be interested in staking their career on this far-out venture, and in fact no one knew how many even fulfilled all of the job requirements. Candidates whose service records matched in terms of experience and education and who expressed a desire to participate would still have to be medically evaluated. It was a touchy situation; reportedly both Scott Crossfield and Joe Kittinger were talked out of applying by Don Flickinger and Paul Stapp because they considered them more valuable in their current flying jobs.[58] Other pilots held back, thinking the whole NASA project might be a dead end, any flying might be minimal to none, and if Mercury was a giant and very public turkey it could kill a man's career.

Bearing such sensitive issues in mind, the STG first considered several Washington institutes as sites with the expertise and facilities to test medical and psychological fitness plus physiological responses to various environmental conditions. The National Institutes of Health, the Walter Reed Medical Center, and the Bethesda Naval Hospital all had some initial appeal because of their central location. For privacy reasons, neither the USAF nor the naval schools of aviation medicine made the list. Impartiality required that they use an independent facility that would keep the men's medical records separate from their military performance files so that nothing in their exams could be held against them. The group gave the task to the Lovelace Foundation, the research arm of the Lovelace Clinic.[59]

It is not known whether the STG ever considered a facility for which there would be no appearance of a conflict of interest, such as the Mayo Clinic or the Harvard Fatigue Lab, perhaps. They likely made a handshake agreement based on Lovelace's credentials because the job was never put out for bid. If there had been a contract, it should have been in compliance with the Armed Services Procurement Act and would have been listed with all of the other contracts in NASA's semiannual reports. It is not. My conclusion is that there was either no written contract or one hidden in a military budget somewhere.

With the aid of Flickinger, three top NASA officials, and several other members of the STG, the selection committee boiled down the requirements to a manageable number. They kept the age and height specifications, the bachelor's degree or equivalent, and the physical fitness mandate and added the stipulation that successful candidates be graduates of a test-pilot school, have fifteen hundred or more hours of flying time, and be jet-rated. A group of physicians chosen by the STG checked more than five hundred service records to see who might match this description. Then they obtained the candidates' grades and class standings from the appropriate test-pilot training schools, and listened as a senior instructor from the schools rated each man. Finally, they came up with 110 fliers on active duty who qualified.[60]

Of the possible candidates, 5 were marines, 47 were naval aviators, and 58 were air force pilots. The evaluation committee decided to divide this group into three and so sent out invitations to the first 35. Of that group, 24 responded that they would be interested in participating, and each of the first 10 who were interviewed showed a strong interest in getting into the program and staying there. The high interest rate told the space agency that they would have few, if any, dropouts. Consequently, NASA decided to choose only six astronauts and to not even bother interviewing anyone in the third group of 35. Sixty-nine men wound up coming to Washington in two groups for preliminary written tests, medical and psychiatric reviews, and technical interviews with engineering and medical personnel. By February 7, 1959, 32 candidates were being sent incognito to the Lovelace Clinic in Albuquerque and then on to the Wright lab in small groups.[61]

A. H. Schwichtenberg, a retired brigadier general and USAF flight surgeon, had recently joined the lab of his longtime friend Randy Lovelace as head of its Department of Aviation Medicine and Bioastronautics. He would lead the study there.[62] Ulrich Luft, then head of the Physiology Department, would draw on earlier results obtained during similar tests of six hundred military and airline pilots to examine the men for pulmonary function and exercise tolerance. A second goal for Luft was to determine the upper limit of safety for physical exertion among the astronaut-candidate population.[63]

The tests at the Lovelace Clinic took seven and a half days and three evenings. They were divided into six components: a medical and flying history, a physical examination, laboratory tests, a radiographic exam, physical competence and respiratory efficiency tests, and psychological evaluations. Many of these tests were none too pleasant. The astronaut candidates underwent blood and sperm counts, barium enemas, and detailed vision and hearing tests. They had ice water injected into their inner ears to induce vertigo and to gauge their adaptiveness to changes in balance. They were weighed under water to determine body density and flown to Los Alamos to have the amount of potassium 40 in their bodies determined; in a twenty-four-hour period they collected all the urine they excreted as well as two stool specimens. They had proctoscopic examinations and X rays of their colon, spine, teeth, sinuses, chest, stomach, and esophagus. They had color photos taken of their retinas and moving-picture X rays made of their heart.[64]

Luft's contribution was a test of overall fitness and cardiovascular conditioning that drew on his mountaineering experience. He had candidates pedal a bicycle ergometer, increasing the load fourfold until either the heart rate reached 180 beats per minute or the subject began to show signs of an overload on the heart or lungs. Each man was connected to an EKG to monitor for heart abnormalities, and once each minute his heart rate, blood pressure, and respiratory volume as well as the efficiency of respiratory-gas exchange were measured. By determining the oxygen consumption at the peak workload, Luft could calculate the aerobic-work capacity and the efficiency of their breathing at rest and after exercise and also determine the size of their lungs. He then rated each candidate in terms of standard values for their age, height, weight, and body density.[65]

Schwichtenberg had created a system for storing medical data in computers by means of color-coded cards marked with a pen. This data-collection method was entirely new and placed Project Mercury on the leading edge of information management in the medical-research field. While seemingly primitive today, it foreshadowed technological advances that space medicine would bring to the private sector, including real-time electronic transmission of patient data and data processing in large population studies.[66]

After passing the Lovelace tests, thirty-one candidates went on to Wright Air Force Base in Dayton, Ohio. Beginning in 1952, the Aeromedical Lab had been conducting a program for Don Flickinger and the human-factors division of the ARDC to establish a prototype crew-selection profile for the MISS and other air force space endeavors. The lab, as a result, had collected a significant amount of baseline data from Wright aviators, student volunteers from the University of Dayton, and, reportedly, a dozen frogmen on loan from the navy.[67] For air force and aviation medicine, the heroic age of self-experimentation, when the lab's director and his few colleagues were the sole subjects for every test—tests that had never before been done by anyone—of necessity had passed.

The redoubtable Col. Paul Stapp, by then the Wright Lab director, put the candidates through physical-endurance tests on treadmills, stair steps, tilt tables, and the centrifuge; environmental stress tests, in particular for heat, noise, and vibration; and psychiatric tests, observations, and interviews.[68] The candidates had every possible dimension of their bodies measured by the Department of Anthropometry that Armstrong and Benson had set up during the Second World War. Nude photos were taken to determine body type (endomorph, mesomorph, or ectomorph), only to conclude that body size had nothing to do with ability and that because the Mercury candidates were older and shorter than the average military pilot, they were therefore a little chunkier.[69] Some of the tests were conducted with the candidates in underwear and sneakers; others, while wearing full pressure suits. Blood pressure was taken while the candidate had his feet in a tub of ice water.[70] Each man's response to isolation was determined by putting him in a dark, soundproof room for three hours. For the heat test, each subject spent two hours in a chamber in which the temperature measured 130 degrees Fahrenheit, while the candidate wore long underwear and a flight suit and had a ten-centimeter thermocouple up his rectum.[71]

NASA's designers expected the astronauts to experience a great deal of noise and vibration during takeoff (they were right on both counts) and consequently wondered whether they would be able to hear any audible feedback from the capsule's occupant. To test this, each man read the phrase "Tomorrow evening at this hour, the famous physician, Dr. J. O. Lee, will speak to you on a topic of vital importance" into a microphone. He read once under normal conditions and twice again while experiencing different degrees of vibration. A second audibility test was performed in the pressure chamber at sixty-five thousand feet. In addition, each man sat in a small room designed to echo and sustain sound vibrations while someone switched on a 145-decibel broadband siren, which was loud enough to induce coughing in some candidates and made others' teeth chatter. The Wright staff gave the candidates three minutes in which to do a series of math problems they had previously done in a quiet room. Perhaps not surprisingly, given their occupation, the researchers found that the men adapted rapidly and their performance showed no serious decline. As a further test, the candidates were placed in a chair designed to move about on all three axes like an airplane, with the added condition of a blindfold and vibration at any of six different frequencies. Research by the navy had strongly suggested that a man could be shaken to death by the effects of sympathetic vibrations on his vital organs.[72] Encouragingly for NASA, nearly three-quarters of the men were able to perform the task of keeping their "airplane" straight and level.[73]

Some of the tests were physically difficult even considering the fact that all of these candidates were experienced jet pilots who were thus familiar with G forces, extreme altitudes, and bulky protective equipment. The centrifuge rides, for example, consisted of two forward-acceleration tests (seated) and one done lying in a head-forward position, each time connected to an EKG device, a mouthpiece with tubing to collect exhalation gases, and an optical device for detecting the precise moment of unconsciousness. Each was compared to a normative group: Wright's centrifuge personnel who were experienced at riding in the device. The goal was to find out how the candidates fared during exposure to acceleration of up to 9 Gs and whether previous experience in jet aircraft gave a measure of acclimatization. It did; their average blackout level was 7 Gs.[74] Obviously, to test this, they had to spin each man until he passed out. No exceptions.

The men also attempted "ascensions" to 65,000 feet in the high-altitude chamber wearing partial pressure gear. Those who made it were allowed to visit the 100,000-foot level very briefly if the medical monitor gave them the okay. Only two-thirds of those tested were able to complete a one-hour stay at 65,000 feet, due primarily to abnormal heart rhythms or psychological causes.[75]

One unexpected component of the Wright experience from the candidates' point of view was the amount of psychiatric testing they underwent. Over time, this was the component of the selection process that would cause the most irritation among the astronauts. Initially it had good purpose, though, one of which was to resolve questions the selection group had about specific factors that had shown up in the New Mexico balloon flights of David Simons, Joe Kittinger, and Clifton McClure.[76] Could a man continue to function under extreme and debilitating stress levels? Could he tolerate a day or more in unbelievably cramped quarters? Would isolation cause him to experience what psychologists were calling the "breakaway phenomenon," which had been observed on some of the balloon flights, when pilots suddenly experienced nearly unbearable isolation and disassociation? And what might happen should two astronauts ever fly together under the same conditions?[77]

The psychologists were everywhere, watching every move. Two of them, in fact, moved into the candidates' quarters and lived with them. They gave the men thirteen personality and motivation tests and another twelve on intellectual functions and aptitudes. They also asked each pilot about the others in the selection pool. Whom do you like best? Which other candidate would you like to go with you on a two-man mission? Whom would you send if you could not go yourself? That gave them information not only about each candidate but also about the man who was answering. The candidates sensed this and struggled to give what they felt were good answers.[78]

The medical and psychiatric examiners agreed in their favorable impressions of the competitive, go-getter attitude displayed by several candidates in particular. One man who was performing the Harvard step test to a metronome thought that he could do better than the goal of 150 step-ups in five minutes and increased his pace during the last thirty seconds just to see whether he could do an additional five steps. He did. Two candidates, both ultimately chosen for the Mercury team, scored twice the mean time for holding up a column of mercury in a tube by exhaling forcefully into a rubber hose connected to the bottom. Another lasted more than three times the average—one hundred seventy-one seconds, or three minutes—holding his breath. Another man later chosen for the program voluntarily went sixteen minutes on the Balke treadmill test, which increased the angle of the treadmill by one degree every minute. His score was fifty percent higher than the mean.[79]

The STG back at Langley took all of these results into account when they made the final selection decision late in March, 1959. A committee consisting of Lovelace, Flickinger, Crossfield, two psychologists, two psychiatrists, and an engineer/manager, possibly NASA's George Low, sat down and correlated all of the data from Wright and the Lovelace Clinic. Interestingly, the first factor that would eliminate any man, the committee decided unanimously, was not experience or fitness but "character traits undesirable in the team effort." Eight such men were thus ruled out right away. Excellence in the physiological tests was not even mandatory. The remaining twenty-three applicants were classified as "outstanding" or "highly recommended," and the committee wrote that all of them "demonstrated excellence in maturity, intelligence, motivation, and emotional stability."[80]

The examiners felt they could recommend eighteen of the candidates without any medical reservations, and seven of those were ranked as "outstanding." To narrow it down to the desired six, the committee went back to the technical qualifications of the pilot versus the technical requirements of the project. They tried to come up with a combination of six men who would complement each other and contribute something unique to the program. The committee already knew some of the specialized engineering skills they wanted crew members to bring to the project and had been looking for those particular talents.[81] Unable in the end to settle on six men, they chose seven.[82]

The committee chairman phoned each of those seven candidates and asked whether he was still interested. All said yes. On April 2, 1959, Randy Lovelace announced the names of America's first astronauts: Alan B. Shepard Jr.; M. Scott Carpenter Jr.; John H. Glenn Jr.; Virgil I. "Gus" Grissom; L. Gordon Cooper Jr.; Walter M. Schirra; and Donald K. Slayton.[83]

THE SEEDS OF CONFLICT

The archives and the history books contain ample evidence of the hawkish rhetoric that was expounded in many arenas after *Sputnik*, and an analysis of the military implications of the political maneuverings involved would (and does) fill several books. Clearly, everyone expected the American military to have a presence, perhaps the only presence in Earth orbit. In support of this assumption, space historian Dwayne Day has pointed out that the military has always had an important, even leading, role in scientific exploration in this country. From Lewis and Clark to topographical surveyors, from the Corps of Engineers to military balloonists of the 1930s, army scientists and engineers have been protagonists. There was nothing inherently un-American about sending a military astronaut into space.[84]

Accordingly, Eisenhower's original request to Congress for legislation that would establish NASA had made it clear that he wanted the civilian and military space programs to be cooperative but not entirely overlapping. He had always opposed big spending on unnecessarily grandiose weapons systems, likening the burden they would place on taxpayers to "humanity hanging from a cross of iron."[85] America's strength lay not in its arms advantages but in its economic power, created by freedom and capitalism, as well as in its research and education.[86] The fiscally prudent thing to do, then, was to avoid duplicating the efforts of the school and lab with additional government-financed laboratories. In fact, Eisenhower stated, when introducing the Space Act, that he wanted "the skills and experience that have been developed within the Department of Defense to be fully utilized in support of the civil space programs."[87]

While LBJ wanted a separate civilian agency from the start, he, too, saw an important role for a separate military space program, quite likely a manned one. For one thing, it would lessen the appearance of weakness he felt the

United States was projecting on the world stage, appearing as it did to be following a Soviet lead in space. He and others perceived that the surprise of *Sputnik* confirmed what many already thought: that America's intelligence-gathering ability was laughable, particularly to the garrulous Nikita Khrushchev, who guffawed loudly and publicly at the United States every chance he could. Intelligence had already misjudged the Soviets' ability to create the atomic and hydrogen bombs a few years back, and the United States was now playing catch-up to them on launch capability. This was serious business; America needed a military that could take and hold the new high ground. The cosmonauts, it hardly needs to be added, were all Soviet air force pilots.

For the military's part, their interests consisted of more than simply wanting bigger and better hardware. They wanted to put their own pilots into space and to hold what they saw as strategic ground: Earth orbit and the moon. They wanted control of their hardware and their personnel. They wanted the freedom that their laboratories had traditionally had to conduct broad scientific and technological research. They wanted to have the major voice in military-related policy decisions.

Smithsonian Air and Space Museum curator Roger Launius, formerly a historian for the air force and chief historian for NASA, has written that the space agency's mission "dovetailed nicely into cold war rivalries and priorities in national defense." It served as a tool to "sway world opinion about the relative merits of democracy versus the communism of the Soviet Union" and acted as an "excellent smoke-screen for the DOD's military space activities, especially for reconnaissance missions."[88] In the minds of the military chiefs who testified before Johnson's Senate Special Committee, the proposal to create NASA could be seen as a prime opportunity to clearly delineate their own territory and to demonstrate that the military had significant resources that the new civilian agency would not.

U.S. Army Secretary Brucker testified confidently that "military representation is particularly important to the over-all success of NASA since within the Department of Defense programs are to be found most of the talent, and most of the physical assets which are necessary to the immediate programs which would be carried out by the NASA. The NASA, therefore, will have major dependence upon the Department of Defense for a long time to come."[89] Both Brucker and Deputy Secretary of Defense Donald Quarles expected that the military would have the same relationship with NASA that it had had with NACA. The agency would advise the DOD when necessary, and vice versa. It would use military talent and facilities, yet develop its own resources for strictly civilian undertakings.

Both men might just have been presenting their "wish lists" to the committee—or whistling in the dark. Since early 1958, the air force had begun to worry that it might lose control of its existing space program in spite of the rhetoric about strengthening the military's space efforts. There was good cause to worry; the executive branch was not uniformly supportive of the military's position. Eisenhower would have liked to see more consolidation within the military. He thought, for example, that it had been a mistake to give individual branches of the service, rather than the DOD, authority for the missile program.[90] Two of his advisors, Nelson Rockefeller, chairman of the special advisory committee on government reorganization, and Percival Brundage, director of the budget, had recommended that all operational space functions be transferred to the presumably more balanced Joint Chiefs of Staff, which would allow the army, navy, and air force individually to have only supporting roles in the space program.[91] This did not sit well with the USAF, which foresaw its place on what it perceived as its turf being reduced to a very small sphere, where its opinion might carry no more weight than anyone else's.

Logically, then, when the Advanced Research Projects Agency was created within the DOD in February, 1958, to oversee both scientific and military space projects, the air force had seen it as a direct competitor for preeminence in space R and D and management. Several times Lt. Gen. Bernard Schriever, an aeronautical engineer, former Wright test pilot, and now air force Ballistic Missile Division commander, testified before Congress that any duplication of the air force's existing programs was wasteful in time, money, and experience.[92] He might as well have been talking to himself.

The turf grabbing and outright handing-over of military resources began as soon as the act creating NASA became law in the summer of 1958. When the space dust had settled, the USAF could only be grateful that it had not lost as much significant ground as the army and navy. Those branches had surrendered the army-funded Jet Propulsion Lab, the Naval Research Laboratory's Program Vanguard, and a large portion of the army's Ballistic Missile Agency to the new civilian agency. Of some small consolation, perhaps, ARPA was dissolved, and eighty percent of the military space projects in which it had been involved were given over to the air force. Significantly, all of these were unmanned.[93]

The new space agency had a mature set of experts devoted to human-factors and medical issues at its disposal as soon as it opened its doors in October, 1958. That year, the *Journal of Aviation Medicine* published the entire proceedings of a day-long symposium called "Aviation Medicine on the Threshold of Space," held as part of the twenty-ninth annual meeting of

the Aero Medical Association. In November, the international space-medicine and space-science communities gathered for the Second International
Symposium on the Physics and Medicine of the Atmosphere and Space. It
was held in San Antonio and jointly chaired by Benson and Strughold. The
three-day event was organized into several subjects: environment, vehicles,
medical problems, space rescue, planets, and, interestingly, medical issues
of time, including papers on time dilation, reaction times, and metabolism.
The entire first day was devoted to environmental issues, including radiation,
meteors, electromagnetic fields, gravity, and the composition of the upper
atmosphere.

Besides speakers from air force, navy, army, and former NACA (now NASA)
research centers, a number of people from private foundations and industry
attended. From medicine this included Randy Lovelace, Detlev Bronk of
the Rockefeller Institute for Medical Research, and E. J. Baldes of the Mayo
Clinic. The aerospace industry was represented by technical experts including
German rocket designers Walter Dornberger of Bell Aircraft Corporation
and Krafft Ehricke of Convair's Astronautics Division, Alfred Mayo of
Douglas Aircraft, and test pilot/aeronautical engineer Scott Crossfield of
North American Aviation. Astronomical observatories also took part, sending
Fred Whipple of the Smithsonian, Gerard Kuiper of the Yerkes Observatory,
and Gerard de Vaucouleurs from Harvard. Eleven of the forty-seven U.S.
residents presenting papers were former Project Paperclip immigrants, most
of whom were now naturalized American citizens. Scientists from Belgium,
West Germany, Switzerland, England, and Peru also attended, representing
the World IGY, the Max-Planck Institute, the University of Zurich, the British Interplanetary Society, and the Institute of Andean Biology. American
academia was represented by speakers from the National Science Foundation, five major universities, thirteen scientists from the School of Aviation
Medicine, and two from the U.S. Naval School of Aviation Medicine.

The medical specialists at the symposium envisioned themselves as con-
tributing more than just clinical research and care to the manned space effort.
They considered themselves scientists and researchers and thus a logical group
to undertake major efforts in basic theoretical research within the life sciences.
Furthermore, Otis Benson observed, that work would have to be interdisci-
plinary and come from government, academia, and industry alike. "Progressive
cooperation" between the physical and life sciences would be the hallmark of
research in what school scientists called "the vertical frontier."[94]

The military and the universities already had exobiology work under
way as well. Besides his Mars book, Hubertus Strughold published articles
on various space environments in the *Journal of Aviation Medicine* and gave

numerous talks on exobiology in the latter half of the decade.[95] Dietrich Beischer of the Naval School of Aviation Medicine reported at the Aero Medical Association's symposium on parallel studies of life in extreme Earth environments, including scalding hot geysers, arctic ice, and the ocean floor.[96] School of Aviation Medicine biologist John Fulton presented a paper at the San Antonio symposium on the Mars-jars experiments, which by then had shown that at least three anaerobic bacteria types were capable of surviving in simulated red-planet conditions.[97] Independently, astronomers William Sinton, Clyde Tombaugh, and Gerard Kuiper were investigating the possibility of vegetative life on Mars.[98]

Plans to put air force astronauts into space aboard an airplane or orbiting vehicle would stay fairly viable into the 1960s. The USAF even selected a half dozen pilots and christened them astronauts. The politics of a military astronaut corps were not favorable, though, and history itself also conspired against such a group. The moon race and the Vietnam War would suck the funding out of the air force's minuscule manned space budget during the 1960s like a tornado pulls oxygen from a room. Continual behind-the-scenes scuffling for control of space life sciences would be resolved only late in the decade, when both the air force and NASA's post-Apollo planners saw their manned space flight hopes wither to nothing.

Events would also take place that made the civilian NASA wary of hiring any astronaut without a military background. That meant robbing Peter to launch Paul for the whole duration of the moon race, anyway, and the thinking was that the air force's program would be redundant, at least from the medical and human-factors standpoint. And, after all, by the mid-1960s, anything the air force wanted to do in space, they could hire NASA to do for them. All they had to do was grovel.

Chapter 7

"DETAILED TO NASA"

I t is puzzling that a civilian space agency, conceived to demonstrate that American weapons-delivery systems could be beaten into the plowshare of science, hired only active-duty military pilots for most of its first decade. Because of the Cold War, however, they were the only group that had all of the credentials required for America's first astronauts. They could do the engineering, they could fly the machines, they were used to hazards, they were healthy, they took orders well, and they worked for peanuts. In addition, the space program also served a second, unspoken purpose—announcing to a watching world that the United States, not just the Soviet Union, could rain down destruction from the heavens. For the time being, it simply did not choose to do so.

This policy was unstated but supported by events that solidified this military-only strategy at the outset of the space race. Medical fitness thus moved down a notch in importance, further lessening the political power of the air force's space-medicine team. The first incident was the downing of an American spy plane over Russia at a crucial and embarrassing moment. Its pilot was civilian Francis Gary Powers, a former military aviator working for the Central Intelligence Agency and flying an ultrasophisticated vehicle that bore the word "NASA" on its tail. The second was a study of the feasibility of using women (all civilians) in space. The scientific results were favorable for the women, but the political fallout caused the project to be canceled.

Coming at a time when the infant NASA was taking its first steps toward becoming a respected space player, the latter incident especially strengthened the agency's resolve to stick with Dwight Eisenhower's mandate to hire only military, experimental-jet test pilots. Some version of that policy would remain in effect until the Americans had achieved the lunar high ground. The air force's space-medicine group began to fade from view.

By 1959, Don Flickinger, director of human factors and staff surgeon at ARDC Headquarters, had been fighting the good fight on behalf of USAF manned space efforts for half a decade. A new component of his work was the Manned Ballistic Rocket Research System (MBRRS), precursor to a small space station. A recent magazine article had touted women as astronaut candidates on the basis of their smaller size and consumption, and to Flickinger, that approach made sense.[1] There was nothing in the rule books to prevent it, either. The air force vehicle did not require any piloting, and work as a crew member was not envisioned as a combat job and thus closed to females.

That summer, Randy Lovelace had come back from a conference in Moscow, where it was rumored the Soviets planned to launch a female. Several women were indeed training at the cosmonaut center there, Star City, but no one in the United States knew whether to believe the story.[2] By this time Lovelace was chairman of NASA's Special Advisory Committee on Life Sciences, and the report, plus his friend Flickinger's interest in testing women for his own space project, piqued his scientific curiosity.

A long-time aviator, Lovelace knew that many women in the United States held pilot licenses. He also recognized that a number of them were employed in aviation, usually demonstrating propeller-driven aircraft or teaching others to fly, and that a handful with more advanced credentials competed in air races, test-piloted aircraft, and ferried planes to overseas buyers. During World War II, his friend Jacqueline Cochran had organized and directed the Women's Airforce Service Pilots (WASPs), which had trained more than a thousand female pilots to fly every make of military aircraft from the factories to bases on the U.S. mainland, to tow targets so that novice gunners could hone their shooting skills, and to test-fly new aircraft.[3] Because of postwar congressional restrictions on the role of females in the military, however, women were banned from flying further assignments.

Consequently, in 1959, no American woman (save Cochran) had access to jet aircraft, and therefore none had experience working and reacting at extreme speeds or against severe G forces or under weightless conditions. Still, the thought of evaluating a group of these elite female pilots the way he had the X-15 and Mercury candidates intrigued Lovelace. Where could he find a whole group of them willing to undergo the ordeal?

That September, Lovelace and Flickinger attended the annual convention of the Air Force Association in Miami. The two talked over the idea and, poolside, happened to meet Jerrie Cobb, a twenty-eight-year-old pilot who was there to be honored for her four world speed and altitude records. These achievements had won her the Woman of the Year in Aviation award from the National Aeronautical Association, the Pilot of the Year award by the National Pilots' Association, the Gold Wings award of the Fédération Aéronautique Internationale, and the Amelia Earhart gold medal of achievement from the Ninety-Nines, a national organization of women pilots.[4] Cobb, an Oklahoma native, had worked as a flying instructor, crop duster, ferry pilot on a South American route, and for the past year as marketing assistant to Thomas J. Harris, sales manager for Aero Design and Engineering Company in Oklahoma City. The firm made the multiengine Aero Commander, in

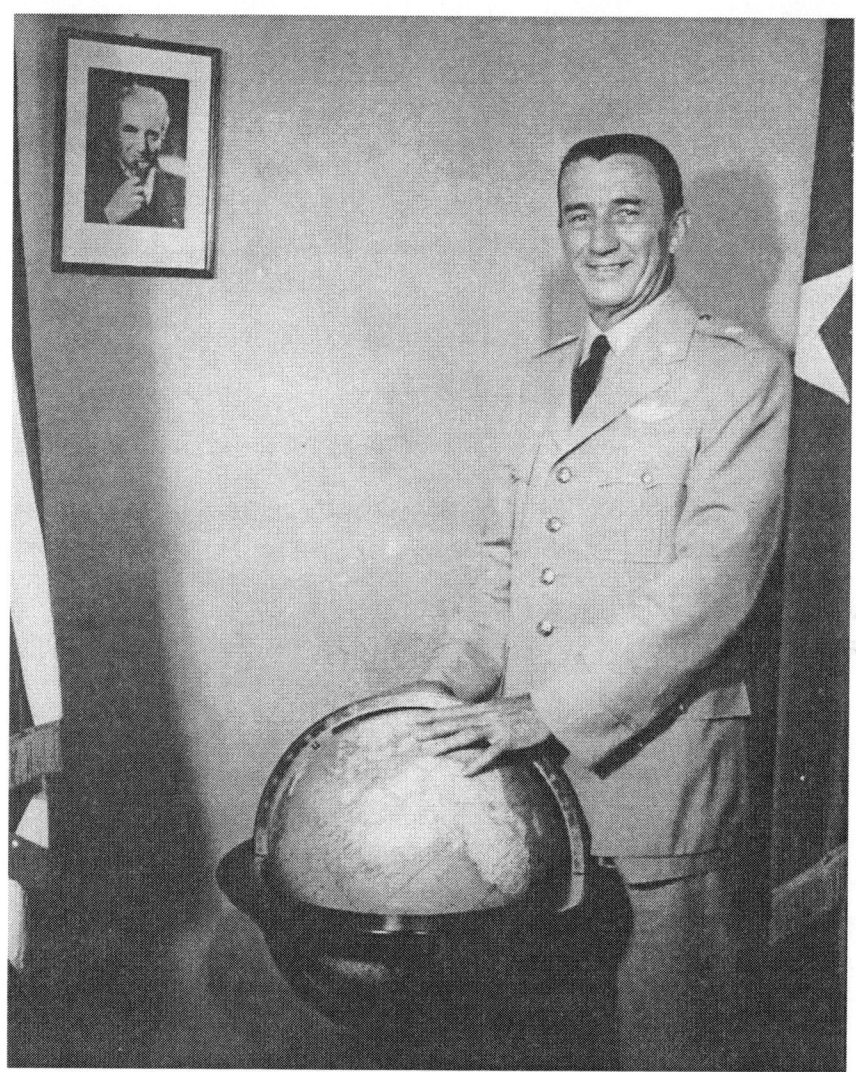

Brig. Gen. Don D. Flickinger, an outspoken supporter of a manned space program for the U.S. Air Force. Reprinted from Men of Space, *vol. 3, with permission of Shirley Thomas.*

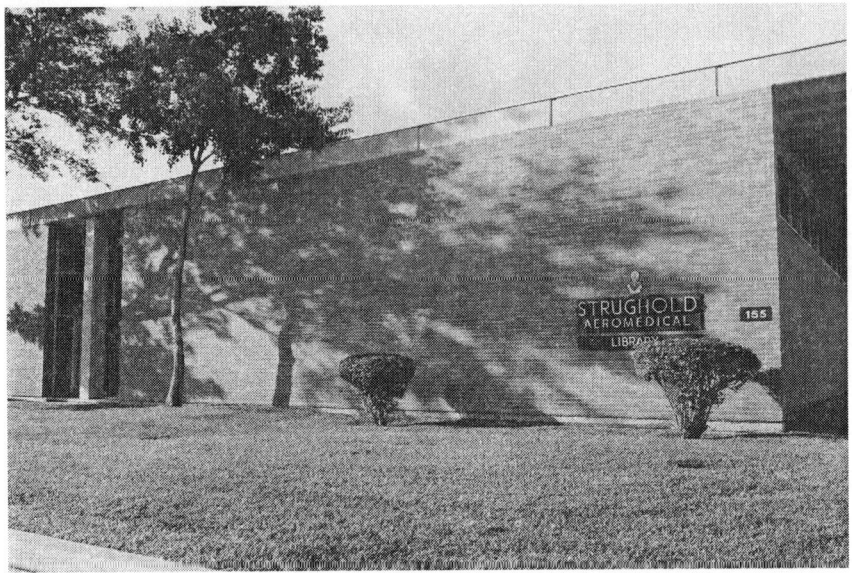

The Strughold Aeromedical Library at Brooks AFB, mid-1980s. Accusations that Strughold had been a Nazi and a participant in war crimes forced the removal of his name not long after his death. Base employees, who believe such charges ridiculous, have pointedly let the holes in the wall remain. USAF photo.

which Cobb set records in order to attract attention to the aircraft and its capabilities.[5]

A career woman in a male-dominated field well before the women's liberation movement of the mid-1960s, Cobb was also deeply religious and politically conservative.[6] When the two doctors spoke about the space program, Cobb envisioned herself championing America in the fight against godless Communism and broadening the role of women in public service. She volunteered immediately to be a test subject, and if she passed, to help them find other suitable female candidates.[7]

However, the air force canceled Flickinger's "girl astronaut" study before it even began. Consequently, he and Lovelace had to fall back and regroup, so instead they told Cobb to report to the Lovelace Clinic in February 1960.[8] There Luft and Schwichtenberg would put her through the same sort of test program they had given the U-2, X-15, and Mercury pilots. If she passed, Lovelace's connections in aviation medicine would facilitate further testing at military and NACA facilities elsewhere.[9]

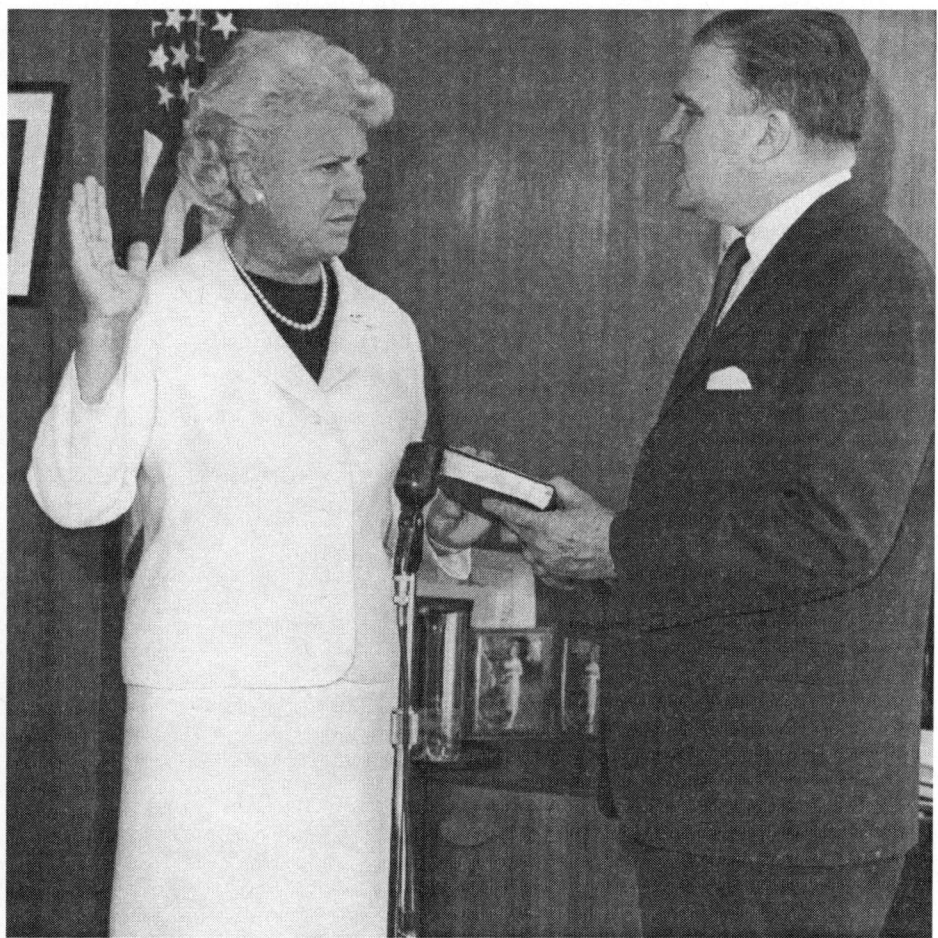

Jacqueline Cochran being sworn in by James Webb as special consultant to the space agency administrator. NASA photo.

Lovelace, Luft, and Schwichtenberg prepared a five-day regime for Cobb, nearly identical to the one the men had undergone, and she reportedly passed the seventy-five exams with scores equal to or surpassing those of the Mercury Seven. The entire time, she recalled later, the whole Lovelace staff had encouraged her, telling her that she was just as qualified as the males they had evaluated the previous year. They predicted she might even have a chance at being the first woman on the moon.[10] Given Lovelace's influential role as chief of NASA's entire life-sciences program, Cobb accepted such speculation at face value.[11]

Perhaps unwittingly, the surgeon furthered this misperception. He arranged for Cobb to be placed under the same publicity umbrella as the astronauts, which included an exclusive contract with Time, Inc., for their personal stories, which would be published in the pictorial *Life*.[12] Cobb and Lovelace were photographed at his clinic in Albuquerque, and *Sports Illustrated* pulled two pages on the Rome Olympics to update and expand a laudatory article they had written about her record setting in the Aero Commander.[13] When Lovelace went to the joint International Astronomical Committee (IAC) and Submarine and Space Medicine symposium in Stockholm that August, he gave a paper on the Mercury selection process coauthored by Luft, Schwichtenberg, and a fourth researcher, Robert Secrest.[14] He also chose that podium to announce the results of his studies on Cobb. *Time* magazine covered the story favorably.[15]

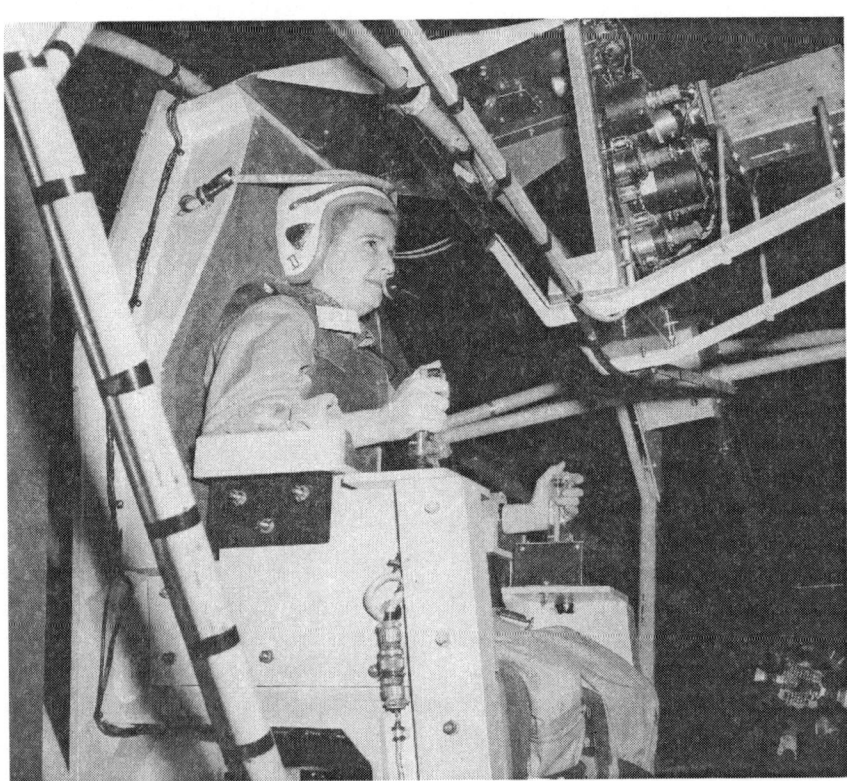

Jerrie Cobb "flies" the MASTIF *(Multi-Axis Spin Test Inertia Facility) simulator at* NASA *Lewis (now the John H. Glenn Research Center).* NASA *photo.*

Wire services abroad spread the word, and the American media picked up the story. The publisher held a press conference at their downtown New York auditorium to show off Jerrie Cobb and gave out advance copies of the feature they had written on her. Television's *Today Show*, network news, and national newspapers all wanted to get a microphone in front of Cobb. Arlene Francis interviewed her for a coast-to-coast radio broadcast, a half-hour talk covering everything from aviation to moon travel to Cobb's religious beliefs. When she returned to Oklahoma City, the governor declared her "Ambassador to the Moon." Lucrative advertising offers came her way from mattress manufacturers and cigarette companies, and fan mail and telegrams began arriving from Europe, Asia, and Australia. Publicity followed her on business excursions. On a trip to Pittsburgh, the site of Aero Commander's parent corporation, Rockwell-Standard, she was given a parade through the downtown and a country-club reception. That was followed by a trip to the West Coast for a television appearance. In between, friends and family screened her phone calls to help get her life back to normal.[16]

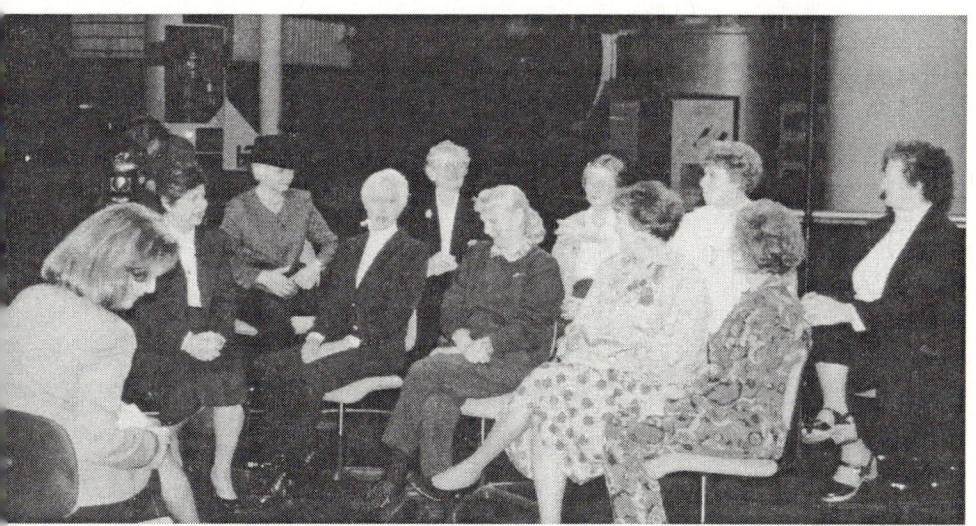

Most of the surviving Mercury women during an interview with NBC at the National Air and Space Museum in December 1994. From left to right, behind the news anchor: Sara Gorelik Rately, Rhea Hurrle Allison, Mary Wallace ("Wally") Funk, Bernice ("B") Steadman, Jerrie Cobb, Jane Hart, Gene Nora Stumbough Jessen, Geraldine Sloan Truhill, Myrtle ("Kay") Cagle, Irene Leverton. Photo by author.

Up to this time, talk about females in space had been conjectural, like the article in *Look* magazine that had described the first "space girl" as likely to be "flat-chested, lightweight, under 35 years of age and . . . the scientist-wife of a pilot-engineer."[17] The idea had its supporters and detractors, but now that an actual woman had been presented as a candidate for the job, some journalists and writers began covering the story more critically, fueling the debate. Both the *New York World Telegram* and *Science News Letter* ran stories that were not sympathetic to Cobb's efforts after checking with NASA and being told that there was no plan to put women into space.[18] A feature-length piece in *Space World,* the official magazine of the National Space Association, implied that using women was an inherently unscientific, impossible, and ill-advised scheme. The lead paragraph referred to "some psychiatrists" who had conducted "several exhaustive scientific studies [that] indicate that the best prospects for the job so far include schizophrenics, extreme introverts, Eskimos, aborigines . . . and even women!" The author quoted one science writer as saying that NASA ought to use "a female midget . . . from the Andes," due to her size and lung capacity, and cited a "high-ranking British scientist" who called for "a short fat woman" because she would be "best adapted to convert food into energy."[19]

Pleased with the initial results but unsatisfied with a test sample of just one, Randy Lovelace looked for more women to evaluate. His requirements were a commercial pilot's license with one or more special ratings (e.g., instrument flying), fifteen hundred hours of flight time, and younger than forty. He may have obtained the Civil Aviation Authority (CAA) records of the eight women that Don Flickinger had reportedly selected for his study.[20] Jerrie Cobb, with connections among the Ninety-Nines and women air racers, was also able to find fliers who met the basic requirements. In all, Lovelace wound up with thirty-one names.[21]

The Albuquerque physician also turned to Jacqueline Cochran. A lieutenant colonel in the U.S. Air Force Reserve, she was a past president (1941–1943) of the Ninety-Nines and current president of both the Paris-based Fédération Aéronautique Internationale (FAI) and its American subsidiary, the National Aeronautics Association.[22] She was still a record-setting pilot, too. In the 1950s, she became the first woman to fly faster than the speed of sound and the first to make a carrier-based takeoff and landing.[23] If anyone could go out and recruit women pilots, it would be Jackie Cochran.

Besides, both she and her husband, Floyd Odlum, were trusted supporters of Lovelace's medical work. Odlum, a very astute businessman, served as chair of the foundation's board of directors and was strongly supportive of aviation and the aerospace industry as a whole. As owner of the Atlas Corporation, the parent of Convair, he had invested twenty million dollars into the development of what would be the Atlas missile at a time when the air force had insufficient funds for intercontinental ballistic missile R and D.[24] Cochran flew all over the country and dropped in on Albuquerque as she pleased, sometimes bringing a new patient along for Lovelace. From time to time she asked her wealthy friends to help various causes, and in return for their financial support, they would receive an invitation to the Cochran-Odlum Ranch near Indio. Even Ulrich and Alice Luft were asked to the California date farm as thanks for translating a letter written to Cochran in Russian.[25]

Cochran had an ego to match her accomplishments. She was too old by a decade to join the program herself but vowed at the very least to head the first group of women to do so. She told Lovelace that she wanted to take the astronaut tests herself and apparently did so, claiming later to have "passed with flying colors." No record remains of her actual results, but as a longtime smoker with a history of abdominal adhesions, it is doubtful that she did as well as she claimed. The reason she stated publicly for not pursuing astronaut status herself was simply her age.[26]

Cochran started by going through the records of the Ninety-Nines and inviting members with the right credentials to take the tests.[27] She also had the executive director of the FAI, Ralph V. Whitener, search the NAA and FAA files.[28] Cochran also took the quest to the public arena and wrote an article for the April 30, 1961, issue of *Parade* magazine describing the results to date and soliciting more participants.

She took on the task of screening credentials for Lovelace and invited those she judged fit to the clinic for a round of physiological, medical, and psychological exams. Her most significant contribution, perhaps, was that at this point Cochran and Odlum began financing Lovelace's study.[29] Such an arrangement implicitly verified that the study had moved away from any official status with NASA.[30] The space agency had never asked for the study nor paid for any part of it, and now could rightfully disclaim any connection with a women-in-space project at all.

The clinic invited approximately two dozen women to be tested, and, in 1961, twelve of them passed phase one.[31] Lovelace forbade media access and kept their names secret. Even the candidates themselves did not know who, with the exception of their own roommate, had participated, let alone who had passed. Consequently, newspapers produced only terse articles describing the project as being much like any other air force, NASA, or general scientific study.[32]

During phase two, the protocol for evaluating the women began to differ more from the men's screening in that the isolation test now took place in a sensory-deprivation tank. This was a special swimming pool inside the Veterans' Hospital in Oklahoma City, known as the "dog dip," where the water temperature could be set to equal that of the air, and eight-inch steel walls made the room soundproof, lightproof, odorproof, humidity proof, and vibration proof.[33] Doctors observed Cobb through a two-way window and listened by microphone as she floated in the tepid water. Her only job was to stay sane in an environment that had as little sensory input as possible.[34] Earlier test subjects, males and females both, had lasted about six-and-a-half hours before lapsing into hallucinations. Jerrie Cobb remained in the water for nine hours and forty minutes and exhibited no psychological symptoms at all.[35]

In May 1961, Lovelace arranged for the navy to conduct the final phase of the testing.[36] For two days at Pensacola, Cobb underwent various strength and agility tests while wearing a high-altitude pressure suit, took part in underwater survival training, and passed a series of coordination tests in a rotating room. She flew faster than the speed of sound in the back seat of an F-102 while wired for an electroencephalogram that recorded her brain waves under varying G loads.[37] Once again, Cobb reportedly performed as well as or better than the men who had taken the same tests.

On a trip to NASA headquarters late that month, Randy Lovelace mentioned the study and the women's results to the new NASA administrator, James Webb.[38] He also told Webb that he would be speaking about the study at NASA's First National Conference on the Peaceful Uses of Space in Tulsa and introducing Cobb to the two thousand attendees. For eight years, Webb had run a Tulsa firm owned by Sen. Robert Kerr of the Kerr-McGee oil and power conglomerate. Extremely active in local civic and business organizations, Webb counted Tom Harris, Cobb's boss at Aero Design and Engineering, as one of his business acquaintances there.[39] An extremely skilled manager and bureaucrat, Webb saw in Jerrie Cobb the chance to accomplish several tasks at once in Tulsa—and at no cost to the space agency.

The conference had been intended to facilitate Webb's policy of involving private industry and universities with NASA, both as providers and recipients of space-related goods and services. He was heading there to kick off the event. Apparently without the knowledge of Lovelace or anyone else, Webb came up with a simple yet brilliant plan to bring attention to the conference, the space program, and Oklahoma and to link NASA with economic and social issues such as education and jobs, perhaps even gender equity. On the plane to Tulsa, he rewrote portions of his speech. When he rose to give the keynote address, he astonished everyone by naming Jerrie Cobb his special consultant.[40]

In a memoir published the following year, before the program was canceled, Cobb wrote that she was stunned but euphoric at her appointment.
"Here was a bonus I'd never even contemplated. I was actually to have a say
in America's move into space! It was too good to be true."[41] It might have
also seemed to Cobb that NASA was giving its imprimatur to the Lovelace
project after all. By April, she had been informed that the agency was not
sponsoring the program. Perhaps now this was going to change.[42]

Meanwhile, Lovelace asked the twelve other women whether they were
ready to move on to the isolation tank at Oklahoma City, with a trip to
Pensacola if they passed. Jacqueline Cochran was still willing to pay all of
their expenses. All of them were excited, but it was still a difficult decision
for some. Whereas the fifty male candidates had all been on active duty and
could be deployed anywhere, anytime, the women were private citizens. Some
had spouses and dependent children unaccustomed to having Mother gone
for long periods of time. Most of them had jobs in aviation, some by cobbling
together various freelance assignments, others by teaching flying, and one
by running a small airport and fixed-base operation. They held on to those
jobs by being "better than a man" or by flying for a company that specifically
wanted a woman, not because the playing field was level or because a pilots'
union or a seniority system had helped them along. Some had to quit their
jobs in order to take a gamble on NASA, and the gypsy pilots found themselves
giving up contracts and going without income. So it was with substantial
personal and financial risk that all of the women said yes.

Jerrie Cobb furnished a spare bedroom in her home for the women, who
would be coming in pairs. She began to think of herself as a leader, the prototype for a new astronaut corps. She corresponded with the others, securing
from them the signed waivers of liability the navy required. In July, Cobb met
with three women at the Transcontinental Air Race and spoke there with
several contestants who had taken the tests but failed to pass.[43]

The women looked on Cobb as a peer, albeit one who held four world
records and had already passed all of the exams. However, they revered
Jacqueline Cochran. All of the candidates were very grateful for her financial
support, and nearly all made it a point to meet and thank her in person.
They also knew she was a personal friend of Lovelace, not just one of his
test subjects.

Cochran began to complain to Lovelace about Cobb getting too much
publicity and taking on too much of the organizing herself. The two women
engaged in a long-distance sparring match, and each of them asked the other
for a meeting, but neither one freed up the time to do so. The result was a
clash of personalities that played a significant role in aborting an American

program for women astronauts. It probably also cost the women (or at least Cobb) Lovelace's long-term support.[44]

In a less vocal and more passive way, Jerrie Cobb had just as big an ego as Cochran, with an outright zeal for using the space race as a tool to win both the Cold War for Uncle Sam and souls for the Almighty. Sure that NASA wanted her as part of the astronaut team, particularly now as Webb's special consultant, she wrote up a plan for additional testing and the incorporation of women into the space program. Webb must have assumed he would never actually hear from the introverted Oklahoman because he shunted some of her correspondence to others, ignored it, or deflected her offers to be of more substantial assistance.[45] The only one who was sympathetic to her cause was Gen. Charles H. Roadman, a former department head at the School of Aviation Medicine under Harry Armstrong and now detailed to the space agency.[46]

In the meantime, the Soviet Union successfully orbited the world's first man in space, Yuri Gagarin, followed shortly by cosmonaut Gherman Titov. In the spring of 1961, America answered with two suborbital flights by Alan Shepard and Gus Grissom. The space race was on, and in May 1961, President Kennedy and his NASA advisors decided that a suitable national goal would be a moon landing by the end of the decade. The entire Mercury-Gemini-Apollo program became a crash project that absolutely had to end in an American attainment of the lunar high ground. Only practical engineering was to be part of the national effort: orbital flight, rendezvous and docking, a lunar module, piloted reentry, heavy launch vehicles, translunar insertion maneuvers, and so on. Social engineering was not on the agenda.

Perhaps Randy Lovelace was losing interest and wondering what he had gotten himself into. He contacted the navy and secured permission for the rest of the women to report to Pensacola, but when the navy suddenly rescinded the offer, citing a negative response from NASA to an inquiry about military necessity, Lovelace let the matter drop. By the end of summer, 1961, the study was dead in the water.

For the Albuquerque doctor and possibly for Jackie Cochran, the matter was over. For Jerrie Cobb, however, the denial served as a red flag. She responded by lobbying even harder—in effect, too hard. With evangelical fervor, she barraged Webb's office with written communiqués, swearing her willingness to give her life for her country: "I cannot help but believe that it is of the utmost importance to our country and I would willingly give my life for it," she wrote. "Please let me help." A dramatic death was only too easy for the space agency to visualize, considering its string of launch-pad failures. Webb felt that such a calamity would bring the entire American space program to a halt if an accident were to happen to a civilian woman.[47]

The granddaughter of an Oklahoma congressman, Jerrie Cobb either instinctively or in a shrewd political maneuver went around Lovelace, Cochran, and their NASA-military connections. She enlisted one of the women candidates, Jane Hart, the activist wife of Sen. Philip Hart (D-MI), to help her take their case public.[48] Hart had pull within liberal Democratic circles and had been Rose Kennedy's personal pilot when she stumped for her son John. Surely with a Democrat and friend in the White House, Hart could get the attention needed to show the administration just how important a woman astronaut program was to national prestige. The two paid a call on Vice President Lyndon Johnson. After politely hearing their plea, LBJ showed the ladies to the door and then dictated a letter to an aide, scrawling in his own hand across the page these bold words: "Let's stop this now!"[49]

The one success Cobb and Hart had was persuading Rep. George Miller, chair of the House Committee on Science and Astronautics, to hold special hearings into the astronaut-selection process in July 1962.[50] There Cobb and Hart testified in favor of incorporating women into the space program, the former urging immediate inclusion and the latter a go-slow approach with research first, launch later. Lovelace did not testify, but Cochran did, at her own invitation. She had mailed advance copies of her testimony to Lovelace, Webb, and high-ranking military friends. All of them had responded with a hearty thumbs-up.[51]

What Cochran said came as a shock to Jerrie Cobb. The older woman made NASA's own case, asserting there was no prejudice in a military hiring system that prohibited women from flying and thus from having access to jet aircraft. After all, there was no need to have women, specifically, to fly combat aircraft. That was the *duty* of American *men.* She stood up for her own wartime record and that of her WASPs by stating that they had performed seventy thousand hours of operational duty with a casualty rate slightly under that of males. However, females had one flaw that made them inherently unsuitable for careers as military pilots: They married. When they wed, Cochran said, they quit work. Forty percent of her WASPs had left to marry. She did not add that some left only after the military had announced plans to cancel their program.

Cochran argued instead for a space program that could quickly achieve the goal of the Cold War: the moon. The women must wait. Inserting even a Jerrie Cobb into the lineup on a crash basis could kill the entire space program if anything went wrong during her mission. Such testimony from the most accomplished woman pilot in the world clinched things for the committee.

Delivering a one-two punch to the women's case, on the second day of the hearings NASA fielded the team of George Low, director of spacecraft and flight missions, and astronauts John Glenn and Scott Carpenter, fresh from the orbital successes of the *Mercury 3* and *Mercury 4*. They testified that their experience in test-flying jet aircraft, where things invariably went wrong and at supersonic speeds, could not be duplicated in propeller-driven aircraft. Military schools were the only places one could go in America to get jet training, and, because Congress prohibited women from combat jobs—which included fly-ing—they could not enter those domains. That catch-22, they said, was the only reason no woman could be an astronaut for NASA.

Rep. James G. Fulton (R-PA) pushed and prodded Low, asking repeatedly why the agency could not have a separate female-astronaut contingent. He discounted the need for jet experience, a military background, or a college degree, instead seeing a female cadre as a public-relations move that would hike America's international credibility and do so much more rapidly than a moon landing. Low countered by saying that doing so would be enormously expensive, would not contribute to the engineering tasks, and would look amateurish at a time when the agency needed all the technical credibility it could get.

Subcommittee chair Victor L. Anfuso (D-NY) had no interest in pursuing the matter any further. He put words into the mouths of Low, Carpenter, and Glenn, phrased his questions (and rephrased their answers) to cast the agency in the best possible light, and periodically talked about how inspi-rational the two astronauts were to America's youth. He all but kissed the men while scooting the womenfolk out the door. Hart and Cobb had gotten what they asked for, but only that: a thrown-together hearing, done as a favor to a fellow senate Democrat. The hearings secured the status quo for NASA through the end of the Apollo program.[52]

The major newspapers and wire services covered the hearings, and the women's stories were reprinted in regional and local papers.[53] News is what drives editorial writing, and the reports of women "invading men's space," as it was sometimes expressed, generated quite a few editorials that overwhelm-ingly favored the women. The reasons given were emotional, ranging from the righteousness of sending a qualified human female into space instead of another monkey, to seeing NASA's objections as a matter only of male pride. After Valentina Tereshkova orbited the following year, a lot of resentment was expressed at being shown up once more by the Communists.[54]

Both the *Kansas City Star* and *Christian Science Monitor* picked up on a quote from Jerrie Cobb—"Now, if I were only a chimpanzee!"—made at an Air Force Association conference after the hearings. Referring to the SAM primates used in early Mercury test flights and to the "chimp college" at Holloman, which also bred and trained primates for NASA, she had expressed frustration that the United States had not taken advantage of her to "stage a propaganda spectacular and let her ride a Mercury spacecraft around the world a half dozen times or so."[55] Journalists were unfamiliar with the technological differences between American and Soviet spacecraft, for example, that cosmonaut and vehicle parachuted back to Earth separately. Instead, they wrote about what they knew: the physical and psychological qualifications for the job, which the women obviously possessed. Stumped to explain the rationale for downplaying a medical-selection process that had seemed so critical only two years before, some grasped for straws, announcing that sheer chauvinism was behind NASA's decision. Others tried to make the women's case on the basis of the irrelevant and unflattering assertion that if a monkey could do a task, so could a grown woman.

Before long, the fickle media turned its attention elsewhere, and the story was largely forgotten. The women resumed their lives, and most of them were still ignorant of the identities of their fellow "future lady astronaut trainees," or FLATs, their nickname for themselves. Based on the records, interviews, and correspondence they left behind, Lovelace and Flickinger seem never to have given the matter another thought. Never involved from the start, the School of Aerospace Medicine and the Holloman and Wright Labs took no notice of the events that had passed them by but that would permanently affect their role in space policy making.

On June 11, 1963, Jacqueline Cochran was sworn in as an unpaid special consultant to James Webb, a position she retained into the 1970s. She requested that the ceremony be performed quietly in Webb's office, with no notice given to the press.[56] Jerrie Cobb's contract had expired the same month as the hearings. It was not renewed.[57]

The space agency stuck with its policy of hiring only military men as astronauts, disguising them as civilians, and launching them aboard civilian rockets that were based on military technology. The first man on the moon, Neil Armstrong, was touted as a civilian astronaut, but he had learned to fly courtesy of the U.S. military in a school they called the Korean War. It was not until the very last Project Apollo mission in 1972, when geologist Harrison Schmitt landed on the moon, that a civilian with no military ties whatsoever flew for NASA.

OUT IN THE COLD

Randy Lovelace's friends and associates never stopped trying to figure it out—how the plane that was carrying him, his wife, Mary, and charter pilot Milton Brown home from Colorado wound up in a canyon that could be described in Ulrich Luft's mind only as "a death trap." The best reconstruction anyone could come up with, taking into account all of the elements of the equation that could be quantified, such as wind direction, altitude, temperature, topography, and size of the airplane, was that they simply wound up in the wrong canyon, and the aircraft just couldn't get up over the ridge in time. Talking it over with Sam White, Luft concluded that the plane had strayed from the usual air route between Aspen and Albuquerque for the simple reason that December 12, 1965, had been "a marvelous, cloudless winter day . . . and they just wanted to go joy-riding, enjoy the beautiful landscape."[1]

The canyon the aircraft had flown into wound around in snail fashion. A pilot halfway in would be unable to see the starting point behind the plane and barely be able to tell where they were going. If he was down below the canyon's walls, which were 12,000 to 14,000 feet high, there wouldn't have been time to climb up above the terminal wall, either. Even an aircraft like the one the Lovelaces had chartered, a twin-engine Beech Travelair, with an altitude range of 15,000 to 17,000 feet, needed extra time to climb at that altitude due to the thinness of the atmosphere. A U-turn had been the pilot's only option, but a wingtip had scraped the canyon wall and brought their plane down.[2]

It took two days for a helicopter to spot the wreckage and identify it tentatively as the Lovelace plane. The next day, several Forest Service personnel reached the site, moving with great difficulty because of the deep snow, and looked for survivors. The ski patrol and mountain rescue squad went in as well, but all of them were pulled back because of bad weather. No one wanted to "risk" taking an "inexperienced" climber along, Luft was told, even though he explained that he had "climbed the Himalayas once or twice." However, he found a sympathetic soul in an English television reporter who had rented a snowmobile that was being hauled by truck to a site near the crash. Hitching a ride on the back, Luft found when he arrived that the scene had been, as he phrased it later, "tampered with." Rescuers had been there about an hour and had already moved the bodies and disassembled pieces of the plane to try to fabricate stretchers on which the dead could be carried out.[3]

The Forest Service employee who was first on the scene drew a map of the site a few days later, at Luft's suggestion, showing the impact location, the major pieces of the aircraft, and the positions of all three bodies. What he drew showed that the airplane had bounced a good hundred feet and thrown the victims out, seats and all. The crash had been immediately fatal to the Lovelaces. The pilot had lived a short time, and footprints showed that he had tried to hike out for help, but minus a shoe and a sock. Perhaps feeling the effects of his injuries, he had gone back to try the radio but had died sometime afterward from his wounds, or the cold, or both.[4]

A week later Luft wrote the Forest Service to express his gratitude for the rescue workers' efforts and to ask about what he and the others had seen when they first arrived. The pilot seemed to have made no attempt to keep warm by using the clothing that was strewn about. Where had they found his body relative to the aircraft? The autopsy suggested that someone may have moved Mrs. Lovelace. Could she have done so herself, or did it appear as though the pilot had attempted to aid her? Who had covered Randy Lovelace with a coat? As Luft said in his letter, "Your answer to some of these questions might throw some light onto the sequence of events after the impact, which is still rather incoherent in our minds."[5]

"Rather incoherent." Had he thought about it in those terms, and he probably did, Luft might have used the same words to describe the decision someone in Washington had made to either junk or ignore everything he and the rest of the air force's aerospace-medicine team had done and to repeat it all at the space agency. No thought was given to the waste of time, money, facilities, and talent, and scant credit had been given, too, as the United States passed milestone after milestone of space "firsts."

Of course, if any entity were to blame, the USAF itself was certainly due its share. After the charismatic Harry Armstrong retired in 1957, there had been a power vacuum and a lack of cohesiveness. Some say that General Benson had taken the SAM's space efforts as far as required in the 1950s but that he had not personally supported a manned space effort by the air force.[6] In fairness, underneath Benson's spit-and-polish exterior was more spit and polish. Had he been directed to put an aviator on the moon, he would have done exactly that. Benson had had a heart attack in 1956, however, and in February 1961 he retired from the military. Paul Campbell had beaten the drum for the space program but was never in a position of either real power or authority. The only space-minded person left in the air force had been Flickinger, and he had left, too, the same year as Otis Benson.

Although no one really talked about it, many of the Paperclips had felt they were not used to their fullest potential in the air force. And whom could one blame? Strughold was hardly a Wernher von Braun in personality. Besides, they were all scientists, independent creative thinkers and, truth be told, did not want to be "organized" like the rocket engineers. Struggie had been gently pushed aside into the role of science advisor at the school and was now content to continue his esoteric, idiosyncratic, and highly theoretical studies, doing pioneer work on jet lag. Luft's old boss still lived alone except for a small dog and a very fat cat in an incredibly disorganized house. He still liked to cha-cha but had taken to prowling among his Paperclip friends in search of drinks and dinner invitations. Someone said he was even dating a very nice, pretty woman who worked at the school, at long last thinking about giving up the bachelor life.[7]

His other LMFI comrade, Hans-Georg Clamann, told funny stories about some of NASA's test launches just before Alan Shepard's flight in 1961, using the school's animals as the payload, like the one about his wife sewing tiny backpacks out of her kitchen curtains to hold the mice's instrumentation. The little things had chewed them off, and Clamann finally had to suture them to the animals' backs. Clamann represented continuity at the school. He was still researching, teaching, and working and would be for quite some time, as would Luft in Albuquerque. As with the other Paperclips, this was in part because the war and their contract status afterward had robbed them of any pension hopes until the last few years of their working lives. They worked because they had to, but no one ever heard a Paperclip complain about it.[8]

Of course, Lovelace had thrown his hat in with the space agency. Did he have anything to do with NASA's decision to distance itself from the air force? There would be no chance to talk about that now. Lovelace had resigned from his NASA consultancies six months before his death, anyway. Still, someone at NASA headquarters had written a press release announcing his death and expressing their deepest sympathy for the Lovelace daughters and for his friends and associates.[9]

The whole thirty-odd years that Luft, Strughold, Clamann, Benson, Armstrong, and all of the others in America and even Germany had spent working up to a manned space program had almost crystallized for an instant late in the 1950s. Within five years, military participation in NASA's space-medicine efforts had fragmented, and most of the pieces had blown away. In reality, it had been like trying to make a snowball on a high mountain peak, above the tree line, where it was too cold and dry and the snow was just loose powder. No matter how hard anyone had worked, it just wouldn't—couldn't—have stayed together. There had been a team, but it had evaporated into the rarefied air. There were still mountains for people to climb in space medicine, a human or two to put on the moon, but it would be another team that reached the summit.

NOTES

CHAPTER 1

1. Bob MacNaughton, "Doc Prescribes Medical Advances," *Talespinner*, May 22, 1981, p. 18.

2. Adrianne Noe, "The Medical Principle and Aeronautical Practice: American Aviation Medicine to World War II" (Ph.D. diss., University of Delaware, Newark, 1989), pp. 254–55.

3. MacNaughton, "Doc Prescribes Medical Advances," p. 18; Nancy Tomich, "Air Force Career Spans Decades of Progress," *U.S. Medicine* 17, no. 19 (Oct. 1, 1981): 3–5, 10–12.

4. Harry G. Armstrong, "War Department Air Corps Materiel Division, Wright Field, Dayton, Ohio, Engineering Section Memorandum Report on the Effect of Cold Temperatures on Personnel Flying Efficiency," in *Material Dated 1933–1939, Medical Studies: Material Contained Is of Medical Progress for the U.S. Air Force,* book 10, vol. 11, pp. 1, 8, Air Force Historical Research Agency (AFHRA) archives.

5. Tomich, "Air Force Career," p. 5.

6. Harry G. Armstrong, interview with John W. Bullard and T. A. Glasgow, "Oral History Interview of Major General Harry G. Armstrong (ret).," for Aerospace Medical Division, Air Force Systems Command, Brooks AFB, San Antonio, p. 6.

7. Institute for Research in Biography, *Who's Important in Medicine,* 2d ed. (Hicksville, N.Y.: Institute for Research in Biography, 1952), p. 51. Richard Gillespie, "Industrial Fatigue and the Discipline of Physiology," in *Physiology in the American Context, 1850–1940,* ed. Gerald L. Geison, pp. 237–62, provides an understanding of the relationship between industrial medicine and physiology.

8. Harry G. Armstrong, *Pilots Book, Air Corps, U.S. Army, Number 1,* box 2, Harry G. Armstrong Collection.

9. Freud Jung [Harry G. Armstrong], "A Special Form of the Functional Psycho-Neuroses Appearing in Airplane Pilots," in *Material Dated 1933–1939,* book 10, vol. 11, n.p., pp. 2, 8, 12–13, 15–16. The very last page of the report is signed "Freud Jung, Aug. 12, 1935," but within the text the author says that the study took three years. The only three-year span in which Armstrong could have surveyed any one population group was from 1931 to 1934, when he was at Selfridge Field, north of Detroit.

10. David H. DeVorkin, *Race to the Stratosphere: Manned Scientific Ballooning in America*, pp. 10–26, 159, 198–205, 207–14. Albert W. Stevens, an army captain and a Wright photogrammatist, went aloft with two others in the *Explorer*, which exploded and burst shortly after takeoff. Two men nearly lost their lives because they could not exit the gondola's narrow hatch without great difficulty. Harry Armstrong was named flight surgeon for the second attempt, the openings were enlarged, and other changes were made to the workload and layout. The successful *Explorer II*, launched in December 1934, brought back useful data on cosmic rays, ozone, the electrical conductivity and composition of the atmosphere, the variation of sky brightness with altitude, wind-direction and velocity changes with height, the distribution of microorganisms at different levels, the effect of ultraviolet light on small organisms, and the utility of high-altitude observation in mapmaking.

11. Armstrong, interview with Bullard and Glasgow, p. 16.

12. Charles A. Dempsey, *Fifty Years of Research on Man in Flight: Air Force Aerospace Medical Research Laboratory*, p. 1.

13. As of May 2000, the chamber sat outside Hangar Nine, the Brooks AFB aviation-medicine museum.

14. Armstrong, interview with Bullard and Glasgow, pp. 6–8, 13, Apr. 20, 1976; transcript, pp. 21–22, 24, AFHRA. No one had thought to mention that the device existed, let alone that it had been used as recently as August 28. Aviator Wiley Post several times tested models of a pressurized flying suit he was building with Phillips Petroleum and the Goodrich Company in Akron. See Lloyd Mallan, *Suiting Up for Space: The Evolution of the Space Suit*, pp. 28–32.

15. Armstrong, interview with Bullard and Glasgow, pp. 12–13. Original budget figures are not available, but after two years, the ARL's annual financial allotment was increased to $100 for supplies, $600 for lab animals, and a staff of one civilian physiologist.

16. Homer E. Newell, *Beyond the Atmosphere: Early Years of Space Science*, pp. 3–10. He labels this chapter a "substantial elaboration of a summary presented to Congress" in 1966 (the footnote says 1967).

17. Armstrong, interview with Bullard and Glasgow, p. 13; Gillespie, "Industrial Fatigue and the Discipline of Physiology," p. 255, and Alejandra C. Laszlo, "Physiology of the Future: Institutional Styles at Columbia and Harvard," both in *Physiology in the American Context*, ed. Geison, p. 85. Cecil Drinker, also a Harvard graduate, was head of the Department of Applied Physiology in the new School of Public Health there. He was also a noted industrial physiologist, which may explain how Armstrong, trained in industrial medicine, learned his name. His brother and fellow faculty member Philip Drinker is renowned as the inventor of the iron lung, another application of pressure-breathing research.

18. Dempsey, *Fifty Years of Research on Man in Flight*, p. 2.

19. Record 68 in *Dissertation Abstracts 1861–1980*, from vol. W1934 of *Dissertation Abstracts International*, p. 47. Computer file (Ann Arbor: University Microfilms); Boston: SilverPlatter Information Services.

20. Dempsey, *Fifty Years of Research on Man in Flight,* p. 6; Merriley Borell, "Instruments and an Independent Physiology: The Harvard Physiological Laboratory, 1871–1906," in *Physiology in the American Context,* ed. Geison, pp. 6, 293–321. Harvard was particularly noted for manufacturing and selling its own line of scientific apparatus, an idea that was imported from Germany in the 1870s. Heim no doubt had experience with designing and building laboratory equipment.

21. Dempsey, *Fifty Years of Research on Man in Flight,* pp. 4–6; Armstrong, *Material Dated 1933–1939.*

22. Otto Gauer, "The Physiological Effects of Prolonged Acceleration," in the U.S. Air Force Surgeon General, *German Aviation Medicine, World War II,* vol. 1, pp. 556–57.

23. Armstrong, interview with Bullard and Glasgow, pp. 29–30; photo and caption, box MG 1, Armstrong Collection.

24. Dempsey, *Fifty Years of Research on Man in Flight,* p. 116.

25. Armstrong, interview with Bullard and Glasgow, pp. 25–26. Very roughly, this is 1,000 mph.

26. Erik M. Conway, "The Politics of Blind Landing," *Technology and Culture* 42, no. 1 (Jan. 2001): 81–106. The U.S. Army Air Corps, Bureau of Standards, Civil Aeronautics Authority (predecessor to the Federal Aviation Administration), airlines, and universities were developing ways to navigate and land in inclement weather. Holloman was testing a method that used three signals broadcast from the ground, the Morse code for the letters A and N, plus a third tone. Holloman heard one of the letters in one ear of his headset and the other letter in the other ear. When he was on the right landing path, the two signals became one tone. Given that altimeters were accurate to only plus or minus forty feet, this was still a dicey method of putting a plane down; the third tone was added to indicate the glide path. Holloman AFB, where many early space-medicine research projects would be carried out, was named after this pilot, who died in a B-17 crash in Formosa.

27. Armstrong, *Pilots Book*; Maurer Maurer, *Aviation in the U.S. Army, 1919–1939* (Washington, D.C.: Government Printing Office, 1987), p. 354. Logbook entries are in Armstrong's hand, beginning when he was a second lieutenant in September 1931 and going through June 1940. Except for a gap from 1932 to September 1934, there were only four months in which he did not fly.

In the 1950s, Donald Putt would play a part in the air force's unmanned space effort. Jimmy Doolittle, later head of NASA's predecessor, the National Advisory Committee for Aeronautics, was then a test pilot at Wright. Another pilot was Bernard Schriever, who would head the air force's ICBM development program in the 1950s. Armstrong and Schriever appear not to have actually flown together but may have been acquainted.

28. Green Peyton [Green Peyton Wertenbaker], *Fifty Years of Aerospace Medicine, 1918–1968,* p. 83.

29. A. W. Hetherington and Don Flickinger, "Biomedical Instrumentation Requirements for Military Bioastronautics" (presentation at the American Rocket Society's fifteenth annual meeting, Washington, D.C., Dec. 5–8, 1960), Flickinger folder, Thomas Collection.

30. Armstrong, interview with Bullard and Glasgow, pp. 18–20.

31. Bob Benford, "Gen. Harry Armstrong Kept Early Research Secret," *Aviation, Space, and Environmental Medicine* 54, no. 6 (June 1983): 575; Tomich, "Air Force Career," pp. 3–4; Armstrong, interview with Bullard and Glasgow, pp. 1–2; Harry G. Armstrong, "Subjective Mental and Physical Reactions to a Free Fall in Space," in Armstrong, *Medical Studies*, pp. 4, 5, 10–11, 13.

32. Armstrong did have an article published in the *Journal of Aviation Medicine* in 1932, while at Selfridge. "Crash Tools for Airplane Crash Rescues" evaluates the army-issue rescue kit with its sledge hammer, tin snips, pliers, flashlight, axe, wrecking bar, hacksaw, and hunting knife. He also interviewed forty-five pilots and flight surgeons and reviewed eighteen years of crash records and found that *"not one single living person had ever been rescued from aircraft wreckage by means of crash tools"* (Armstrong's emphasis). Hardly anyone was ever "trapped" in an open cockpit—and in a fire there was no saving anyone. His final recommendation was simply a "¾-length, medium-bit fire axe."

33. Dempsey, *Fifty Years of Research on Man in Flight*, pp. 4–5.

34. Noe, *The Medical Principle and Aeronautical Practice*, pp. 193–96; Benford, *Doctors in the Sky: The Story of the Aero Medical Association*, pp. 115, 122–23; "David Bruce Dill/Harvard Fatigue Laboratory Reprints: Background," Mandeville Special Collections Library, University of California at San Diego, http://orpheus.ucsd.edu/speccoll/testing/html/mss0517d.html.

35. Roger E. Bilstein, *Flight in America* (Baltimore: Johns Hopkins University Press, 1994), pp. 53, 57, 64–65, 73, 78–79, 83, 86, 90, 91, 94.

36. Robert J. Benford, *Doctors in the Sky*, pp. 3–7, 15, 18–22; Noe, *The Medical Principle and Aeronautical Practice*, pp. 6–8, 12, 304. Noe links the creation of the association with increasing specialization at that time among doctors who relied on new technology. Keeping the knowledge needed to use their instrumentation within a small group let them function as gatekeepers in medical selection and classification.

37. Armstrong, interview with Bullard and Glasgow, p. 11.

38. Benford, *Doctors in the Sky*, pp. 53, 56–57, 75–78, 249; Strughold, interview with Shirley Thomas, audiotape reel 3, side 1, transcript, p. 6/36; Shirley Thomas, notes from Strughold interview, around Apr. 24, 1959, folder 1, box 8; Armstrong, interview with Bullard and Glasgow, p. 52.

39. Susan E. Lederer, *Subjected to Science: Human Experimentation in America before the Second World War*, pp. 73–74, 97–98; Albert Jonsen, *The Birth of Bioethics* (New York: Oxford, 1998), pp. 7, 132–33.

40. Hans-Martin Sass, "Comparative Models and Goals for the Regulation of Human Research," in *The Use of Human Beings in Research, with Special Reference to Clinical Trials*, ed. Stuart F. Spicker et al., pp. 50–55.

41. Gerald L. Geison, "International Relations and Domestic Elites in American Physiology, 1900–1940," in *Physiology in the American Context*, ed. Geison, pp. 134–35 and charts on pp. 129, 135. The Mayo Clinic became a major site of physiological research between 1918 and 1940, the bulk done by Boothby. Geison ranks Mayo seventh in the nation, after the University of Chicago, Harvard, Johns Hopkins, Washington University, Yale, and [Case] Western Reserve.

42. Boothby also graduated from Harvard Medical School in 1906 and taught there until 1916, when he left for Minnesota. Like Heim, Benson, and probably Lovelace, he had studied under W. B. Cannon, whom Geison calls "the single most important figure in twentieth-century American physiology." Cannon was one of the earliest of the American notables to complete his higher education in the United States (Harvard, 1900) rather than Germany.

43. Armstrong, interview with Bullard and Glasgow, pp. 17–18.

44. Cochran established more than one hundred international speed, altitude, and distance records for both jet and propeller-driven aircraft. She became the only woman flying solo to win the Bendix (1938), the first to exceed the speed of sound, and the first to make a totally blind landing. She won the Harmon Trophy, given by the International League of Aviators, sixteen times and was the first woman awarded the gold medal of the Fédération Aéronautique Internationale (FAI), which has oversight authority for all world-record attempts. She served two terms as FAI president, the only female to do so. She organized the Women's Airforce Service Pilots (WASPs) during WWII, which put more than one thousand women to work flying combat aircraft in the United States. She held the rank of lieutenant colonel in the air force reserve until her retirement in 1970.

45. Armstrong, interview with Bullard and Glasgow, pp. 16–17.

46. W. Randolph Lovelace II, interview with Shirley Thomas, Jan. 17, 1961, audiocassette 1, side 1, Thomas Collection.

47. Armstrong, interview with Bullard and Glasgow, p. 17.

48. Jacqueline Cochran, "The Oral Reminiscences of Jacqueline Cochran," interview with Kenneth W. Leish for the Columbia University Oral History Program, 1960, transcript, pp. 29–31; Margaret Weitekamp, "The Right Stuff, the Wrong Sex: The Science, Culture, and Politics of the Lovelace Woman in Space Program, 1959–1963" (Ph.D. diss., Cornell University, Ithaca, N.Y., 2001), pp. 50–63. Weitekamp provides a detailed description of Cochran's actions, an episode scarcely mentioned in historical writings elsewhere.

49. M. P. Lansberg, *A Primer of Space Medicine,* frontispiece, pp. 6–8, 17, 47n. 112.

50. Tomich, "Air Force Career," p. 10.

51. Ibid., p. 11; electronic communication with Margaret Opoku-Pare, student-services assistant at the University of Toronto, citing the university archives, May 15, 2001. No thesis supervisor is listed, but Armstrong acknowledges G. E. Hall, Alan C. Burton, and D. W. Lougheed (for Lougheed's assistance with the kymograph); David Salisbury, "History outside the U.S.," paper presented at the Aerospace Medical Association's annual conference, Houston, May 15, 2000.

52. Tomich, "Air Force Career," pp. 10, 11.

CHAPTER 2

1. Theodor Benzinger, "Personal Notes on Aviation Medicine in World War II and Relevant Organization of the German Luftwaffe," pp. 1–3, handwritten, undated (but 1980 or later); Benzinger, "Sketch of a Scientific Autobiography," 1975. Both in Theodore [*sic*] Benzinger Papers, FSC-76, Aerospace Medicine and Human Factors Engineering Collection.

2. Testimony of Erich Hippke, Nuremberg War Crimes Trials, case 2, *U.S.A. v. Erhard Milch*, microfilm B-17E, roll 2, pp. 106–108, and roll 3, pp. 759, 774.

3. Strughold, interview with Shirley Thomas, tape 3, side 1, transcript, p. 2/32, and transcript CC, p. 2/23.

4. No byline, *Aviation, Space, and Environmental Medicine* (Dec. 1986): 1220; Strughold, interview with Thomas, tape 1, side 1. Strughold learned of the burn in his forties, when he got his first pair of glasses. He liked to tell people that with his good eye shut, he could look at anyone, no matter what their rank, and see them with a hole in their head. He also had a photo taken of the burn to use during lectures.

5. Strughold, interview with Thomas, tape 2, side 2. The war ended on Nov. 11, 1918.

6. Karl E. Rothschuh, *History of Physiology*, p. 228.

7. Strughold, interview with Thomas, tape 2, side 2.

8. The German university system was the model for the emerging graduate-educational system in the United States. Students had long traveled there to train in science and medicine. The learning opportunities were excellent, based on the number of stellar researchers under whom they could study. Of the twenty-five years that Nobel prizes for physiology or medicine were awarded between 1901 and 1933, Germany claimed six, more than any other nation. In chemistry, Germans won the award fifteen times in twenty-nine years, three times as many as the closest contenders, the British and French. Eleven Germans were awarded Nobel prizes in physics on the thirty occasions the prize was given, twice the number of British and French scientists.

9. Strughold, interview with Thomas, tape 2, side 2.

10. In German, "Physiologie" is pronounced much like the English word but with a hard "g" in the last syllable. For whatever reason, in America Strughold always pronounced it "fizz-ology."

11. Hans-Georg Clamann, interview with Shirley Thomas, on Strughold tape 1, side 2, Thomas Collection.

12. Robert G. Frank Jr., "American Physiologists in German Laboratories, 1865–1914," in *Physiology in the American Context*, ed. Geison, p. 22; Geison, "International Relations and Domestic Elites in American Physiology, 1900–1940," pp. 115–20 in the same volume. Geison believes the war reversed the flow of American students to Germany because that country had sustained heavy casualties and damages, unlike the United States. In the 1920s, enrollment in American schools caught up with and surpassed that of German universities.

13. John R. Brobeck, Orr E. Reynolds, and Toby A. Appel, *History of the American Physiological Society: The First Century, 1887–1987* (Bethesda: American Physiological Society, 1987), pp. 2–4. When U.S. physiologists began to organize research labs in the 1870s, they followed the German model. As late as 1925, only seventeen physiology Ph.D.'s were granted per year at U.S. schools.

14. Strughold, interview with Thomas, transcript CC, p. 4/25. Strughold describes von Frey as "an aristocrat . . . very sharp-minded, learned, and very modest." Carl J. Wiggers, *Reminiscences and Adventures in Circulation Research* (New York: Grune and Stratton, 1958), p. 50. Wiggers knew von Frey (1852–1932) around the same time and

had met Strughold on a visit to the Würzburg lab in 1926. He describes the elderly physiologist as "an affable person, keenly desirous of imparting from his profound experiences anything that might be helpful to younger men. His criticisms, while acute, were always kindly." Von Frey treated him "as a member of his family" on the visit and "honored" him by sending him one of his assistants, "H. Strughold." Rothschuh, *History of Physiology,* pp. 254–56.

15. Strughold, interview with Thomas, tape 2, side 2.

16. There are many good histories that deal with Lindbergh and his historic flight, two written by the pilot himself: *We* (New York: Putnam, 1927) and *The Spirit of St. Louis* (New York: Scribner, 1953). A useful scholarly article that deals with him as a product of the age and includes his move toward environmentalism is "From the *Spirit of St. Louis* to the SST: Charles Lindbergh, Technology, and Environment," by Leonard S. Reich, in *Technology and Culture* 36, no. 2 (Apr. 1995): 351–93.

17. Strughold, interview with Thomas, tape 2, side 2; Peter Fritzsche, *A Nation of Fliers: German Aviation and the Popular Imagination,* pp. 2, 7–8, 12–13, 16–18. Two newer works on the Zeppelin and German cultural history are Dale Topping, *When Giants Roamed the Sky: Karl Arnstein and the Rise of Airships from Zeppelin to Goodyear* (Akron, Ohio: University of Akron Press, 2000) and Guillaume de Syon, *Zeppelin! Germany and the Airship, 1900–1939* (Baltimore: Johns Hopkins University Press, 2002).

18. Fritzsche, *A Nation of Fliers,* pp. 146–47. He believes Strughold was an anomaly. "[T]he world's best-known aviator, Charles Lindbergh, at first made little impression in Germany. [M]ost experts dismissed the flight as a matter of luck or ignored it altogether. [It] . . . was too much an affair between the United States and France for Germans to take much notice. . . . In the end, foreign records such as Lindbergh's did not add up to very much . . . compared to Germany's infinitely more valuable work laying the foundations of world air transportation."

19. Strughold, interview with Thomas, tape 2, side 2, and transcript CC, pp. 5/26, 6/27, and 9/28. The only adverse effect with the chamber was a headache that lasted three hours. The students were very enthusiastic about learning the results, however.

20. Samuel W. Mitcham Jr., *Men of the Luftwaffe* (Novato, Calif.: Presidio, 1988), pp. 25, 269–70, 275; Walter Zuerl, "Ritter von Greim: der Tank-Stößer," in *Pour le mérite: Flieger, Heldentaten, und Erlebnisse* (Steinebach-Wörthsee, Germany: Luftverlag Walter Zuerl, 1977), pp. 419, 420, 429–31. Von Greim was a general during the invasion of France and the Low Countries and led a flying division on the Russian front. Hitler replaced Göring with him just days before the bunker suicide. He was arrested but killed himself while in an Allied hospital jail, wounded while flying with test pilot Hannah Reitsch to be by Hitler's side.

21. Mitcham, *Men of the Luftwaffe,* p. 270.

22. "Early Space Pioneer," *San Antonio Express,* Sept. 19, 1971, Strughold vertical file, San Antonio City Library.

23. Strughold, "Die Höhenwirkung im Lichte nervenphysiologischer Betrachtung," *Zeitschrift für Luftfahrtmedizin* 2, no. 3/4 (1938): 241.

24. The Rockefeller Foundation's several fellowship programs allowed hundreds of young scientists to study abroad after WWI. Walter Sullivan also notes in *Assault on the*

Unknown: The International Geophysical Year, p. 24, that the first international group that was organized to conduct scientific research was the International Association of Academics in 1900, founded by the University of Göttingen. It fell apart during the First World War and was reestablished by groups in the United States, Britain, and France as the International Research Council in 1919. Germany and its allies were pointedly excluded.

25. Strughold, interview with Thomas, transcript CC, p. 8/29, and tape 2, side 2.

26. Fellowship recorder cards, NDW, record group 10, Rockefeller Fellowship Archives (RFA); Geison, "International Relations and Domestic Elites in American Physiology, 1900–1940," in *Physiology in the American Context*, ed. Geison, pp. 128–29 (charts), 134, 135, 138, 141, 147. Anton Carlson was the most productive American physiologist between 1900 and 1940, judging by publications, and Wiggers was number eight. Among labs, the University of Chicago ranked number one, with Western Reserve sixth out of twenty surveyed. Carlson trained fifty other fellows in addition to Strughold between 1920 and 1940, some coming from the Guggenheim Foundation and others from the National Research Council.

27. Edward Schneider to John Fulton, Middletown, Conn., May 3, 1941; A. J. Carlson to Fulton, Chicago, May 5, 1941; C. J. Wiggers to Fulton, Cleveland, May 6, 1941, Strughold, folder 3125, box 466, series 717, 1949, RG 2, RFA. Carlson wrote that he "impressed me as a first-class man, well trained in science, with a first-class personal character. What has happened to him since then I do not know. He may, for all I know, be a first-class Nazi. I hope not, because no first-class scientist can at heart be a first-class Nazi. But he is probably giving all that is in him for science in the interest of his own country."

28. Wiggers to Fulton, RFA. Strughold "devised a very clever procedure for determining cardiac output during anoxia" and "was always a painstaking, hardworking individual, and I predicted with von Frey that despite his quiet and retiring personality, he would some day be a leading man." Also, Wiggers, *Reminiscences*, pp. 292, 317; Strughold, interview with Thomas, tape 2, side 2; Strughold, "A Cinematographic Study of Systolic and Diastolic Heart Size with Special Reference to the Effects of Anoxemia," *American Journal of Physiology* (1930): 94, 641–55.

29. Joel D. Howell, "Cardiac Physiology and Clinical Medicine? Two Case Studies," in *Physiology in the American Context*, ed. Geison, p. 285.

30. Strughold, interview with Thomas, transcript CC, p. 8/29, and tape 2, side 2.

31. Ibid., tape 2, side 2, and transcript, p. 8/29.

32. Comments from "RAL's Diary," Aug. 28, 1929, on a form with the heading "Notgemeinschaft der Deutschen Wissenschaft," fellowship recorder cards, NDW, record group 10, RFA.

33. Strughold, interview with Thomas, transcript CC, p. 8/29, and tape 2, side 2.

34. One man Strughold met in Chicago was Paul Campbell, who would later contact Ulrich Luft amid the chaos of postwar Germany and help recruit him for Project Paperclip. Campbell would himself work with the Paperclips at the School of Aviation Medicine.

35. Strughold, interview with Thomas, tape 3, side 1.

36. Comments by "S-WSC" dated Apr. 26, 1929; comments by "S-FL," Aug. 19–23, 1929; and "RAL's Diary," Aug. 28, 1929, "Notgemeinschaft der Deutschen Wissenschaft."

Strughold also asked to visit the army's Mineola aeromedical lab, but it is not certain whether he did so.

37. "AG Diary" letter, Sept. 19, 1949, Heidelberg, folder 3125, box 466, series 717, 1949, RG 2, RFA. One interviewee noted, "Strugholz [*sic*] thinks the great advantage of his fellowship in America was that it gave him new horizons and a sort of liberated courage to follow his own bent in science when he returned to Germany. . . . It is interesting to note that I met two professors in one day who set such conspicuous and certain value on the traveling fellowships they held in the twenties. Strugholz thinks German professors are unreasonably distant from their pupils, and his own general demeanor is strikingly 'permissive' and undemanding." Wiggers, *Reminiscences*, pp. 126–27, 64–69, is a good source for the environment at Western Reserve and Munich, where Wiggers studied in 1912.

38. Brobeck et al., *History of the American Physiological Society*, pp. 141–42.

39. Strughold, interview with Thomas, transcript CC, p. 8/29, and tape 2, side 2; transcript DD, p. 45; reel 3, side 2; Hubertus and Mary Strughold, Christmas card to Ulrich and Alice Luft, Dec. 24, 1983, folder 19, box 8, "Strughold," Luft Papers. Spellings vary, but the doctor used "Struggie" during his 1961 interview with Shirley Thomas.

40. Strughold, interview with Thomas, tape 3, side 1. As a government employee, he had to return for two years. Strughold acknowledged that he had "a sore neck for three days" but that the inverted flight was a success because he got "more material for my lectures."

41. Rothschuh, *History of Physiology*, p. 255. Von Frey died on Jan. 25, 1932.

42. Thomas, notes from Strughold interview, p. 2.

43. Eloise Engle and Arnold Lott, *Man in Flight: Biomedical Achievements in Aerospace*, p. 66.

44. Strughold, interview with Thomas, tape 3, side 1.

45. Ibid., p. 1; Engle and Lott, *Man in Flight*, pp. 195–96.

46. Heinz von Diringshofen, "Vorläufige Mitteilung über Röntgenaufnahmen und Durchleuchtungen des Herzens bei Fliehdrafteinwirkung im Flugzeug," *Zeitschrift für Luftfahrtmedizin* 2, no. 3/4 (1938): 281–86; von Diringshofen, "Untersuchungen im Motorflugzeug zur Bestimmung der Erträglichkeitsgrenzen gegenüber Fliehkräften," pp. 322–32 in the same volume. He cites a 1928 NACA technical report in the second article. Von Diringshofen was both pilot and test subject, taking chest X rays of himself in flight to show changes in heart position and the endurance limits of centrifugal forces.

47. Oskar Schröder, "Organization of German Aero-Medical Research," chart, July 12, 1945, folder 519.6341-2, AFHRA. This chart, prepared by the chief of the Luftwaffe Medical Service while a British POW, was also used at the Nuremberg trials as evidence.

48. Strughold, interview with Thomas, tape 3, side 1; Thomas, notes from Strughold interview, p. 1.

49. Karl Baedeker, *Northern Germany: Baedeker's Handbook for Travelers* (Leipzig: Karl Baedeker, 1936), microfilm, card 2 of 9, 8–24; Baedeker, *Berlin and Its Environs: Handbook for Travelers* (Leipzig: Karl Baedeker, 1912), pp. 45, 54.

50. Alexandra Richie, *Faust's Metropolis: A History of Berlin* (New York: Carrol and Graf, 1998), pp. 409–48.

51. Photos, folders 22–24, box 1, series 1C, Luft Papers.

52. Baedeker, *Berlin and Its Environs*, pp. 5, 8, 10, 12, 14–15 (map), 177–79. The address of the LMFI was Berlin NW 40, Scharnhorststraße 35.

53. Strughold, interview with Thomas, tape 3, side 1, and transcript, p. 3/33; Luft, interview with Spidle, transcript, p. 1; Theodor Benzinger, "Sketch of a Scientific Autobiography," 1975, Benzinger Papers. According to Luft, Hartmann began working at the LMFI in late 1936, already planning the Himalayan expedition. Benzinger, an avid mountaineer, skier, and rock climber, said that he and Hartmann had become friends as classmates at Göttingen. It is likely that the Rein connection put his name before Strughold.

54. Hans Hartmann, "Experimentellphysiologische Untersuchungen auf der deutschen Himalaja-Expedition 1931," *Zeitschrift für Biologie;* "Das Bluthild in großen Höhen," *Klinischen Wochenschrift* (1932); article in *Zeitschrift für Biologie* 93 (1933): 391; "Physiologische Ergebnisse der deutschen Himalaja-Expedition 1931," no journal listed.

55. Paul Bauer, *Um den Kantsch: der zweite deutsche Angriff auf den Kangchendzönga 1931* (Munich: Verlag Knorr und Hirth, 1933). During the first expedition, in 1929, the German press gave Kanchenjunga the nickname "der Kantsch."

56. Luft, interview with Spidle, p. 1. It was Hartmann who actually hired Luft away from the University of Freiburg's pathology lab.

57. Ensign Ulrich Fischer, "Der Kreislauf unter Beschleunigung Röntgenaufnahmen beim Affen," *Zeitschrift für Luftfahrtmedizin* 2, no. 3/4 (1938): 1–13. This article also served as Fischer's doctoral dissertation, supervised by Otto Ranke of the LMFI. Also, L. Bührlen, of the Luftwaffe's medical staff in Erfurt, "Spitzenbeschleunigungen in zwei verschiedenen Lagen," *Zeitschrift für Luftfahrtmedizin* 2, no. 3/4 (1938): 287–90; Luftwaffe physician Hans-Karl Treutler, "Die Eigenreflexe der quergestreiften Muskeln während des Aufstiegs in der Unterdruckkammer," *Zeitschrift für Luftfahrtmedizin* 2, no. 3/4 (1938): 367–76.

58. "Hubertus Strughold, Ken Johnson Die," *Aviation, Space, and Environmental Medicine* (Dec. 1986): 1220.

59. For example, from Yugoslavia, Milivoy Kostitch, "Die Wahrnehmung der Gliederbewegung in Abhängigkeit von der Höhe," *Zeitschrift für Luftfahrtmedizin* 2, no. 3/4 (1938): 226–29; from China, Tsu-Te Chang, "Alter und Höhenfestigkeit im Tierversuch," *Zeitschrift für Luftfahrtmedizin* 2, no. 3/4 (1938): 239–42.

60. The *Luftfahrtmedizinische Abhandlungen* was published for the *Gemeinschaft der Lehrbeauftragen für Luftfahrtmedizin* (Association of Aviation Medicine Instruction), but it has not been possible to find further reference to the group. The Lilienthalgesellschaft was a prominent society for scientists and engineers interested in aviation. It survives today as the Institut für Luft- und Weltraumrecht (Institute for Air and Space Law). Strughold belonged to that association and to medical groups unrelated to aviation: the German Physiological Society, the Berlin Physiological Society, and the Berlin Medical Society. Hubertus Strughold, "Biography," undated, unnumbered box, Hubertus Strughold Papers, uncatalogued.

61. Strughold, "Development, Organization, and Experiences of Aviation Medicine in Germany during World War II," in the U.S. Air Force Surgeon General, *German Aviation Medicine*, vol. 1, p. 50.

62. At Nuremberg, many references were made to concerns about phone taps, particularly by Ruff and Romberg with regard to calls from Dachau to Berlin and to the office of Erich Hippke.

63. In 1927, Brauer had established the first aeromedical research institute at Hamburg, where he installed a large, up-to-date decompression chamber.

64. Ludolph Brauer, Albrecht Mendelssohn-Bartholdy, Adolf Meyer, and Johannes Lemcke, *Forschungsinstitute: Ihre Geschichte, Organisation, und Ziele* (Hamburg: Hartung, 1930). One of Brauer's coauthors and several contributors were apparently Jewish.

65. Strughold, "Development of Aviation Medicine," p. 3; Strughold, "Development, Organization, and Experiences of Aviation Medicine," p. 47.

66. Strughold, "Zur Frage der Höhenkrämpfe," and Hans-Georg Clamann, "Über die Möglichkeit von Augenschädigungen des Fliegers durch Sonnenstrahlung," *Luftfahrtmedizinische Abhandlungen,* n.d., ca. 1935. These are cited in *Zeitschrift für Luftfahrtmedizin* 1, no. 3 (1936–1937).

67. It was there that Strughold had earned his *Habilitation* in the late 1920s. Luft did a year of undergraduate work there and in 1936 completed much of the research for his doctorate in medicine.

68. Statement of Georg Weltz, *U.S.A. v. Karl Brandt et al.,* roll 2, p. 115.

69. Strughold, "Development, Organization, and Experiences of Aviation Medicine," pp. 49–51. The Kaiser Wilhelm Institutes were renamed for Max Planck after WWII.

70. Strughold, interview with Thomas, tape reel 3, side 1, and p. 5/35.

71. Clamann, interview with Thomas.

72. Hermann Becker-Freyseng, "Physiological and Patho-Physiological Effects of Increased Oxygen Tension," in *German Aviation Medicine,* vol. 1, pp. 493–514.

73. Paul Bauer, *Himalayan Quest: The German Expeditions to Siniolchum and Nanga Parbat* (London: Nicholson and Watson, 1938), p. 99. Bauer notes that "[Hartmann] afterwards wore short boots which gave his feet the appearance of horses' hooves." In his 1937 journal, which Luft and Bauer found later, Hartmann noted that even his decision to join a 1931 Himalayan expedition "was reached with difficulty, for I had to admit to myself that others with sound feet would probably be more useful than I."

74. Ulrich Luft and Paul Bauer, "Nanga Parbat 1937," in *Himalayan Quest,* pp. 97–150.

75. Bruno Balke, Fritz Bechtold, Rolf von Chlingensperg, Alfred Ebermann, Uli Luft, Herbert Ruths, and Lex Thoenes, *Nanga Parbat, Berg der Kameraden: Bericht der Deutschen Himalaja-Expedition 1938* (Berlin: Roth, 1943).

76. Balke had competed as a gymnast and fenced on the Czechoslovakian national team, winning medals in both foil and saber. He lost a spot on the Czech Olympic team because he was considered a pro, having earned some income as a coach.

77. Luft's papers on acclimatization were reprinted in the U.S. Air Force Surgeon General's *German Aviation Medicine,* vol. 1, as "Altitude Tolerance," pp. 304–20, and "Acute Hypoxia and Natural Acclimatization," pp. 409–13.

78. Cassidy, *Uncertainty: The Life and Science of Werner Heisenberg,* p. 314. Cassidy explains the professional atmosphere in which the Nobel-prize-winning physicist and

other scientists had to work: "[T]he social and political horizons of the individual German began to shrink from the global expanse of nation and profession to the private sphere of one's closest friends and associates. This privatization of public political experience entailed what Hannah Arendt has called the paradoxical 'atomization' of the new 'mass society' into isolated individuals, existing in a world of twisted reality, inverted ethics, and continual fear."

79. Affidavit of Siegfried Ruff, *U.S.A. v. Karl Brandt et al.*, roll 2, p. 62.

80. Sworn statement of Theodor Hannes Benzinger in the investigation of Theodor Hannes Benzinger, no. C7 303 348, Nov. 22, 1983, Department of Justice, Washington, D.C., pp. 54–57, papers of Theodore [*sic*] Benzinger. Benzinger claimed that his hospital employment made him a government worker, for whom party membership was mandatory. He added that, in protest of Versailles, he had joined the Sturmabteilung (Storm Trooper Division) at the same time to promote German remilitarization.

81. Statement of Georg Weltz, *U.S.A. v. Karl Brandt et al.*, roll 2, p. 115.

82. Helmuth Zebhauser, *Alpinismus im Hitlerstaat: Gedanken, Errinerungen, Dokumente* (Munich: Bergverlag Rother, 1997), pp. 91–101. "Record Check Information," U.S. Civil Service Commission, Oct. 21, 1954; "Security Investigation Data for Sensitive Positions," case serial number 77-55-11988, Oct. 18, 1954, U.S. Civil Service Commission. Both are in the Freedom of Information Act (FOIA) file on Bruno Balke, U.S. Office of Personnel Management.

83. Affidavit of Konrad Schaefer, *U.S.A. v. Karl Brandt et al.*, roll 9, pp. 8329–8330. Konrad Schaefer, who reported to Strughold, had trouble gaining entry to the state medical exam in Berlin in 1935 because of his lack of membership in any party-affiliated organization.

84. Cassidy, *Uncertainty*, pp. 300, 530.

85. Strughold, interview with Thomas, reel 3, side 2, and transcript DD, p. 43. In April 1945, at the very end of the war, Hitler declared that all engineers, doctors, and similar professionals who had anything to do with the German armed forces were henceforth officers in the regular army. By virtue of his civil-service rank, Strughold was commissioned a colonel literally overnight.

86. "Eidesstattliche Erklärung," Mar. 22, 1946, folder 5, box 1, Luft Papers. This was a required form in which signatories affirmed that they had not been members of the NSDAP, SS, SA, or similar Nazi organizations. Also, Ulrich Cameron Luft, "Testimonial for Franz Büchner," 1946 or 1947, folder 6, box 1, Luft Papers. In this affidavit for a University of Freiburg pathologist, Luft said that Strughold had, in fact, forbidden him to join anything Hitler had organized. It is difficult to tell whether this included the Deutsche Alpenverein.

87. Strughold, interview with Thomas, tape 3, side 1, p. 37/7.

88. *U.S.A. v. Karl Brandt et al.*, roll 8, p. 7780.

89. York [Hans-Jörg] Clamann, interview with author, notes, Round Rock, Tex., July 19, 2000.

90. "Record Check Information" and "Security Investigation Data for Sensitive Positions," FOIA file on Bruno Balke, U.S. Office of Personnel Management; Luft, interview with Spidle, p. 7; marriage certificate of Friedrich Luft and Mary Muir

Wilson, July 6, 1907, Edinburgh, Scotland, in box 1, folder 1; Lebenslauf (résumé), July 17, 1941, box 1, folder 2; Scottish driver's licenses 1931–1932, 1933–1934, 1935–1936; German passport, Dec. 14, 1938; and Wehrpass, 1937, box 1, folder 4, all in Luft Papers. Ulrich Luft's mother and her family were Scottish. He lived in Edinburgh for the duration of World War I, from age four to nine, and visited often in the 1930s.

91. Ute Deichmann, *Biologists under Hitler*, pp. 61–70. Deichmann offers copious statistics on membership among life scientists by specialization, gender, and age. Her review of party records shows that 45 percent of physicians and 58 percent of biologists joined. Among 41- to 50-year-olds, 53 percent signed up. Of scientists between 31 and 40 years of age, 63 percent became members. She also states that membership was never made an official requirement for the *Habilitation*, or appointment to a university teaching position.

92. Strughold, interview with Thomas, tape 3, side 1, pp. 37/7 and 38/8.

93. Ibid., p. 5/35.

94. This observation comes from reading the citations in *Zeitschrift für Luftfahrtmedizin*.

95. Strughold, interview with Thomas, tape 3, side 1, p. 35/5.

96. John B. West, *High Life: A History of High-Altitude Physiology and Medicine*, p. 251; *Bericht*, July 21, 1941, folder 2, box 1, Luft Papers. The LMFI backed both the 1937 and 1938 expeditions, probably only for Luft and Hartmann, however.

97. Richard G. Elliott, " 'On a Comet, Always,' a Biography of Dr. W. Randolph Lovelace II," pp. 360–61. Lovelace also went to the United Kingdom, Denmark, Switzerland, Norway, Sweden, Hungary, Holland, Belgium, France, Italy, and Greece.

98. Luft, interview with Spidle, p. 4.

99. W. Randolph Lovelace file, folder 1, box 5, Thomas Collection.

100. Erich Hippke, "Eröffnungsansprache auf der ersten deutschen Tagung für luftfahrtmedizinische Forschung in Berlin, 25 bis 28 Oktober 1937," *Zeitschrift für Luftfahrtmedizin* 2, no. 3 (1938): 148–57.

CHAPTER 3

1. Link and Coleman, *Medical Support of the Army Air Forces*, pp. 1–5, chart facing p. 38, pp. 47, 157–61, 166–70, 175–77, 210, 707–08.

2. Carlton V. Phillips Sr. (colonel, U.S. Army Reserve, ret.), interview with author, notes, Scottsdale, Ariz., July 30, 2001.

3. Link and Coleman, *Medical Support of the Army Air Forces*, pp. 62–63.

4. Ibid., pp. 310–12, 315, 318–25, 330–38.

5. Otis Benson, *Reminiscences of Brigadier General Otis Benson*, with Kenneth W. Leish, 1960, Columbia University Oral History Project, pp. 5–9. After Heim and Lovelace, then, Benson was the third former Harvard student among the Wright Lab leadership and at least the second to have spent time with Cecil Drinker. His period of study there was in 1940, and, like the other two, he was at Harvard when the prolific William Cannon was still department head.

6. Dempsey, *Fifty Years of Research on Man in Flight*, pp. 3, 30.

7. Link and Coleman, *Medical Support of the Army Air Forces*, pp. 257, 275–77, 303–310; Benson, *Reminiscences*, p. 5.

8. Dempsey, *Fifty Years of Research on Man in Flight*, p. 30; Link and Coleman, *Medical Support of the Army Air Forces*, p. 239.

9. Link and Coleman, *Medical Support of the Army Air Forces*, pp. 239–44. The U.S. military was not integrated until an executive order by Truman in 1948. Consequently, black, white, and Asian-descent soldiers were trained, deployed, and supervised in different ways and in different places.

10. Benford, *Doctors in the Sky*, pp. 151–53; Elliott, "'On a Comet, Always,'" p. 358. According to his biographers, Lovelace first became interested in a research career while at Harvard Medical School. Although it is not known what classes he took, he was there in 1935 and 1936, when Harvard was considered the premier physiology teaching and research institute in North America. The faculty included Cannon, aviation specialist Bruce Dill, and the Drinker brothers.

11. Scott Crossfield, interview with Shirley Thomas, notes, Thomas Collection.

12. Department of Defense Office of Public Information, Press Division, "Brigadier General Otis Otto Benson Jr.," Oct. 18, 1949, Otis Benson file, AFHRA; Dempsey, *Fifty Years of Research on Man in Flight*, p. 27. Benson flew five combat missions in B-17s and earned the Air Medal and several other decorations.

13. Link and Coleman, *Medical Support of the Army Air Forces*, p. 267; Benford, *Doctors in the Sky*, pp. 151, 154–56; Lovelace, interview with Thomas, tape 1, side 1. An experienced pilot, Lovelace said nearly twenty years later that he didn't think the risk had been particularly high.

14. Link and Coleman, *Medical Support of the Army Air Forces*, pp. 278–79, 282–83.

15. Ibid., p. 267; Tomich, "Air Force Career," p. 10.

16. Link and Coleman, *Medical Support of the Army Air Forces*, pp. 924–25; Benzinger, "Personal Notes on Aviation Medicine in World War II and Relevant Organization of the German Luftwaffe." Benzinger uncovered that fact about the same time.

17. Dempsey, *Fifty Years of Research on Man in Flight*, pp. 28–31, 39, 41–43.

18. Ernest A. Pinson, "An Address of Welcome and Dedication," W. Randolph Lovelace II Memorial Lecture, Eleventh AFOSR Science Seminar, Albuquerque, June 16, 1966, pp. 7–11.

19. Dempsey, *Fifty Years of Research on Man in Flight*, pp. 33, 51–52.

20. Link and Coleman, *Medical Support of the Army Air Forces*, p. 535.

21. Phillips, interview with author. Sometimes B-17s carried as few as two bombs. In 1944, the AAF used "grapefruit bombs" on a few missions; these were two P-38 aircraft filled with explosives and placed underneath the B-17's wings. Groups of bombers, escorted by P-38s, would go into a fast, steep dive, release the drones, pull up, and leave the area as quickly as possible. The drone was difficult to distinguish from the nearly identical fighter escort.

22. Link and Coleman, *Medical Support of the Army Air Forces*, pp. 618–19, 622, 628, 631–35; Phillips, interview with author.

23. Tomich, "Air Force Career Spans Decades of Progress," p. 11; Link and Coleman, *Medical Support of the Army Air Forces*, p. 551.

24. Link and Coleman, *Medical Support of the Army Air Forces*, pp. 548, 552–53, 559–60, 563, 585, 637–39, 642–44, chart p. 645, p. 646, chart p. 646, pp. 648–51, 653, 655; Phillips, interview with author.

25. Bryan Philpott, *Eject! Eject!* (London: Ian Allan, 1989), pp. 9, 10, 11. A Luftwaffe pilot made the world's first in-flight ejection in April 1941 at Rechlin.

26. Strughold, "Development of Aviation Medicine in Germany," p. 3.

27. Horst Zoeller, "Hanns Klemm Biography," Hanns Klemm homepage, Feb. 13, 1998, http://home.t-online.de/home/hzoeller/kl_bibl.htm.

28. Mitcham, *Men of the Luftwaffe*, pp. 301–302, 304.

29. Strughold, "Development, Organization, and Experiences of Aviation Medicine," pp. 13–15, 21. He wrote that "Most engineers were of the opinion that it would be impossible to man such a missile," but manned V-1 test flights were already underway in April 1944 for a proposed suicide group. See Hanna Reitsch, *Flying Is My Life* (New York: Putnam, 1954), pp. 214–19. Reitsch, a test pilot for that study, said the plan had received medical approval a year earlier and been carried out at Rechlin.

30. Strughold, "Development, Organization, and Experiences of Aviation Medicine," pp. 16, 21, 24–25, 28, 30–31, 38–40.

31. Siegfried Gerathewohl, "Psychological Examinations for Selection and Training of Fliers," in the U.S. Air Force Surgeon General, *German Aviation Medicine*, vol. 2, pp. 1027–52. Gerathewohl, who later worked for the SAM and NASA, described the situation tersely but gave no explanation for it in this article. He noted that hundreds of thousands of psychological examinations were given between 1928 and 1942, but the data were all destroyed "owing to the effects of the War."

32. Anonymous comments on Siegfried Gerathewohl in "F.B.I. Special Inquiry into 'German Scientists under the Protective Custody and Control of the Joint Intelligence Objectives Agency,'" file no. 62-1879, June 7, 1948, San Antonio, p. 2, FBI FOIA file on Gerathewohl.

33. Strughold, "Development, Organization, and Experiences of Aviation Medicine," pp. 38–40; Otto Graf, "Increase of Efficiency by Means of Pharmaceutics (Stimulants)," in *German Aviation Medicine*, vol. 2, pp. 1080–1103.

34. Benzinger, "Personal Notes on Aviation Medicine in World War II," p. 6; Benzinger, "Sketch of a Scientific Autobiography," p. 4; Strughold, "Development, Organization, and Experiences of Aviation Medicine," p. 45. Rechlin lost one employee to miliary tuberculosis ("galloping TB"). Another suffered tuberculosis of the ribs and knee, and a third, TB of the lung, but they survived. These occurred because the change in pressure burst open dormant tuberculin bacilli, which caused the sick person, in effect, to reinfect himself. A fourth employee was temporarily paralyzed by a small air embolism.

35. Testimony of Andrew Ivy, microfilm roll 9, pp. 9035–36, 9080; statement by attorney Fritz Sauter, roll 4, p. 2803, in *U.S.A. v. Karl Brandt et al.*

36. Testimony of Andrew Ivy, *U.S.A. v. Karl Brandt et al.*, roll 9, pp. 9127–32, 9159, 9162–63. American doctors used jail inmates and conscientious objectors as test subjects.

37. T. Forcht Dagi and Linda Rabinowitz Dagi, "Physicians Experimenting on Themselves," in *The Use of Human Beings in Research*, ed. Spicker et al., pp. 253–54.

38. Strughold affidavit, *U.S.A. v. Karl Brandt et al.*, roll 9, p. 8398; Strughold, "Development, Organization, and Experiences of Aviation Medicine," p. 37.

39. Affidavit of Rudolf Brandt, roll 1, p. 232; letter, Himmler to Rascher, Oct. 21, 1942, roll 1, p. 264; letter, Rascher to Himmler, Feb. 17, 1943, roll 1, p. 342; testimony of Wolfram Sievers, roll 7, pp. 5792–93, in *U.S.A. v. Karl Brandt et al.*

40. Testimony of Hans Romberg, in *U.S.A. v. Karl Brandt et al.*, roll 8, pp. 6789–90.

41. Testimonies of Siegfried Ruff, roll 7, pp. 6508, 6555–57, 6566–81, 6608, 6619; Romberg, roll 8, pp. 6795–97, 6801, 6803, 6805, 6811, 6824; Walter Neff, roll 2, pp. 623a–24, in *U.S.A. v. Karl Brandt et al.* Ruff refuted an allegation that Rascher killed sixteen at once as part of a legitimate research project. Neff, an inmate engaged to assist them, testified that Rascher killed between five and seventy inmates when Romberg was not in the lab. It was Neff who sabotaged the barometer, thinking it would make the machine inoperable.

42. Testimony of Romberg, in *U.S.A. v. Karl Brandt et al.*, roll 8, p. 6824.

43. Ibid., pp. 6821–22. Memo, Sigmund Rascher, roll 1, pp. 325–26; testimony of Romberg, roll 8, pp. 6729–30, 6736. Himmler later gave Romberg a medal for his work.

44. Testimonies of Konrad Schaefer, roll 8, pp. 7980–83, 8345, 8351, 8371–73, 8383–84, 8388, 8496, 8518–19; Hermann Becker-Freyseng, roll 8, pp. 7780, 7791–8009, 8237, roll 9, pp. 8518–19, roll 11, p. 11514; Franz Vollhardt, roll 9, pp. 8459, 8461–66; Fritz Pillwein, roll 9, pp. 8798–99, roll 10, p. 9903; Karl Hoellenrainer, roll 11, p. 10510; Wilhelm Beiglboeck, roll 9, pp. 8897–98, 8933, 8955, 8987–96, 9010–25; Andrew Ivy, roll 9, pp. 9039, 9051, 9061–62; Josef Tschofennig, roll 9, pp. 8871, 8873, roll 10, p. 9339; Joseph Vorlicek, roll 10, pp. 9389–91, 9402; Ernst Mettbach, roll 10, pp. 9720, 9722–23, in *U.S.A. v. Karl Brandt et al.* Pillwein, Hoellenrainer, Tschofennig, Vorlicek, and Mettbach were all inmates. Mettbach was also a test subject.

45. Sworn statement of Theodor Hannes Benzinger, pp. 87–94, 97–99, 113–14, 117; Linda Hunt, *Secret Agenda: The United States Government, Nazi Scientists, and Project Paperclip, 1945 to 1990* (New York: St. Martin's, 1991), p. 84. Testimonies of Oskar Schröder, roll 5, p. 3669; Georg Weltz, roll 8, p. 7147; Konrad Schaefer, roll 8, p. 8515; Vorwerk, roll 1, pp. 285, 311; Siegfried Ruff, roll 7, pp. 6591, 6620; Kurt Blome, roll 6, p. 4504, and cross-examination by McHaney, roll 1, p. 311, in *U.S.A. v. Karl Brandt et al.* Benzinger says that he and Rein simultaneously walked out of the October meeting in Nuremberg. He also says that some groups had little to do with others, that not all of the directors got along, and that he reacted to what he saw by retreating to his "splendid isolation" at Rechlin, never to discuss it with anyone.

46. Testimony of Erich Hippke, in *U.S.A. v. Erhard Milch*, roll 3, pp. 790–93.

47. Strughold, oral history interview with James C. Hasdorff for the Office of Air Force History, San Antonio, Nov. 25, 1974, p. 15, AFHRA.

48. Internal resistance has only recently received much attention from historians. Popular and scholarly writing has been limited primarily to two groups, the White Rose student organization at the University of Munich and the coterie of army officers and others who were in on the von Stauffenberg plot. Testimony at Nuremberg described

other smaller units: the Young Conservative Group of the Resistance movement, the Kreisau Group, the Wolf Group, the Wednesday Society, and various Christian, Socialist, and Social Democrat organizations.

49. Affidavit of Ulrich Luft, roll 9, pp. 8320–22; testimony of Konrad Schaefer, roll 9, pp. 8336–37, 8345, 8351, 8354–56 in *U.S.A. v. Karl Brandt et al.* Strughold thus employed a Freiherr von Romberg as a biophysicist. He hired Schaefer so that he might avoid the draft, and someone, either von Diringshofen or Strughold, put him on the Jüterbog payroll.

50. Jerry Deal, "Strughold Denies He Was a Nazi," *San Antonio Express,* June 7, 1974, p. 1; "Nazi Charges Resurface on Ex-Brooks Scientist," *San Antonio Express-News,* Oct. 26, 1993, p. 1; Debbie Nathan, "When a Nazi Walked among Us," *San Antonio Current,* June 15–21, 2000, pp. 10–11, 13ff.; "Ohio State Set to Remove Likeness of Alleged Nazi Doctor from Mural," *San Antonio Express-News,* Oct. 27, 1993, n.p.; Tamara Bubel, interview with author, notes, San Antonio, July 21, 2000.

51. Strughold, interview with Thomas, tape 3, side 1, transcript, pp. 37/7, 39/9; Thomas, notes from Strughold interview.

52. Ulrich Luft to Paul Bauer, Munich, Sept. 15, 1948, folder 34, box 3; Howard Burchell, St. Paul, Minn., Dec. 5, 1983, folder 16, box 3, Luft Papers. Luft finally received word of his mother and sister, but the three were not reunited until 1948.

53. Testimonies of Wolfgang Lutz, roll 8, pp. 285, 291; Hermann Becker-Freyseng, roll 8, pp. 7779, 7827–28, in *U.S.A. v. Karl Brandt et al.*

54. Mary Ann Jackson, "Bruno Balke Welcomes—and Creates—Avalanches," *Physician and Sports Medicine* (Sept. 1977), pp. 96–97, Bruno Balke Papers, High-Altitude Medicine Collection; Ulrich Luft, "Adventures in Hypoxia," folder 29, box 9, Luft Papers; Hedda Balke Marg, telephone interview with author, notes, Oct. 31, 2001; correspondence with Marg, Oct. 31, 2001, and Nov. 2, 2001.

55. Benzinger, "Sketch of a Scientific Autobiography," pp. 2, 4.

56. Ulrich C. Luft, "Interview with Ulrich C. Luft, M.D., Ph.D.," by Jake Spidle, transcript of sound recording, Oct. 11 and 16, 1985, p. 23, New Mexico Medical History Program; Benzinger, "Personal Notes on Aviation Medicine in World War II," p. 17; Konrad Büttner, "Heat and Cold in Aircraft," in *German Aviation Medicine,* vol. 2, pp. 757, 764–65; Büttner, "Physical Heat Balance in Man" in the same volume, pp. 766, 773–74, 776, 780–81.

57. "Tageszusammenstellung der Auswertestelle West," p. 103 (4.1.44); "Auszüge aus Gefangenenaussagen und Materialauswertungen," in *Records of Headquarters of the German Air Force High Command* (Washington, D.C.: NARA, GSA, 1961), microfilm roll 17. One second lieutenant, the navigator on a B-17 that was shot down over the sea near Bremen in December 1943 gave out numerous pages of detailed information, whether true or false.

58. Schwerdtfeger and Ulrich Luft, "Research Report 26/44: The Medical Care of English and American Fliers (Die aerztliche Betreuung der englischen und amerikanischen Flieger)," AAF-Library, translation no. 363 by Earl R. Hewitt, published by Oskar Schröder, air surgeon general; Oct. 31, 1944, Hans-Georg Clamann Papers, uncatalogued.

59. Richie, *Faust's Metropolis,* p. 531.

60. Testimony of Konrad Schaefer, in *U.S.A. v. Karl Brandt et al.*, roll 9, p. 8368.

61. Strughold, interview with Thomas, tape 3, side 2, transcript copy DD; affidavit of Ulrich C. Luft, in *U.S.A. v. Karl Brandt et al.*, roll 9, p. 8313; York Clamann, interview with author, notes, Round Rock, Tex., July 19, 2000. Welkersdorf (whose population in 1939 was 1,007) is today called Lwowek Slaski. Clamann speculates that the countess may have been Frau von Baranoff, who was also in Landshut when his family was detained there.

62. York Clamann, interview with author.

63. Strughold, interview with Thomas, tape 3, side 2, transcript copy DD.

64. Hans-Georg Clamann, interview with Thomas, tape 1, side 2.

65. Testimonies of Oskar Schröder, roll 5, p. 3679; Hermann Becker-Freyseng, roll 9, p. 8083; Wilhelm Beiglboeck, roll 9, p. 8895, in *U.S.A. v. Karl Brandt et al.*; Michael Foedrowitz, *The Flak Towers in Berlin, Hamburg, and Vienna 1940–1950* (Atglen, Penn.: Schiffer, 1998), pp. 3–14. The giant structure sheltered eight thousand civilians; several hundred inmate and POW laborers; and three hundred soldiers who ate, slept, and worked there. It also contained a ninety-five-bed hospital with two operating rooms and a whole air-conditioned floor with works of art from fourteen Berlin museums. Reportedly as many as thirty thousand Berliners jammed themselves inside during some of the raids. The zoo tower was built between September 1940 and April 1941 and was destroyed by the British in 1947 and 1948.

66. Strughold, interview with Thomas, tape 3, side 2, transcript copy DD.

67. Erika Lang Shofstal, interview with author, Tempe, Ariz., Feb. 28, 2001.

68. York Clamann, interview with author.

69. Strughold, interview with Thomas, tape 3, side 2, transcript copy DD.

70. Luft, interview with Spidle, p. 5.

71. Affidavit of Joseph Pichotka, in *U.S.A. v. Karl Brandt et al.*, roll 9, p. 8299. Pichotka said that he quickly obtained a gun (how, he did not explain) and rescued the man from the crowd, which was threatening to hang him on the spot. Interestingly, he added that he himself was threatened with "legal proceedings" but that these were quashed. By whose effort, he also did not say.

72. Strughold box, Brooks AFB History Office; photos from the Luft Papers.

73. Strughold, interview with Thomas, tape 3, side 2, transcript DD; Cassidy, *Uncertainty*, p. 526. The British planned to foster a regrowth of German science in Göttingen, which was already well known for physics and aeronautical research.

74. York Clamann, interview with author.

75. Luft, interview with Spidle, p. 5.

CHAPTER 4

1. Michael J. Neufeld, *The Rocket and the Reich: Peenemünde and the Coming of the Ballistic Missile Era*, fig. 98, pp. 221, 230, 327n.13.

2. Tomich, "Air Force Career," p. 11; Armstrong, interview with Bullard and Glasgow, pp. 52–54.

3. Clarence G. Lasby, *Project Paperclip: German Scientists and the Cold War*, pp. 11–14.

4. Cassidy, *Uncertainty*, pp. 128, 132.

5. Lasby, *Project Paperclip*, pp. 51–54.

6. Newell, *Beyond the Atmosphere*, p. 91. For details on the record of the United States, Britain, and Germany in bringing military jets on line, see also Roger E. Bilstein, *Orders of Magnitude: A History of the NACA and NASA, 1915–1990*, pp. 91–93.

7. Lasby, *Project Paperclip*, pp. 17, 19, 20–22.

8. Ibid., pp. 16, 83–84. "Alsos" is the Greek word for "grove." The operation was under the direction of Manhattan Project military leader Gen. Leslie Groves.

9. Luft, interview with Spidle, p. 3.

10. Frank Winter, *Rockets into Space*, pp. 55–56.

11. Robert J. Benford, *Report from Heidelberg: The Story of the Army Air Forces Aero Medical Center in Germany, 1945–1947*, pp. 1–2; U.S. Air Force Surgeon General, *German Aviation Medicine*, vol. 1, p. iv.

12. W. Randolph Lovelace files, folder 1, box 5, Thomas Collection.

13. Leslie E. Simon, *German Research in World War II: An Analysis of the Conduct of Research*, p. viii.

14. Campbell, interview with Hasdorff, pp. 13–17, 35; Armstrong, interview with Bullard and Glasgow, pp. 55, 90. Campbell saw Armstrong as the world's foremost authority on aviation medicine but thought Strughold nearly his peer. Armstrong considered Strughold the luminary and himself someone who "just sort of stumbled through life and accepted things as they came. . . . I never thought of myself as being farsighted in the ordinary sense of the word. I perhaps could flatter myself by simply saying that I was able to see the obvious."

15. Luft to Herbert Hultgren, May 8, 1989, box 1, folder 14, and Luft to K. Kirsch, Feb. 27, 1983, box 5, folder 31, Luft Papers; Luft interview with Spidle, pp. 2–3. He also said that Mayo-educated cardiologist Howard Burchell, then at the Heidelberg CME, was "one of the first Americans to look me up in Berlin. . . . [H]is wise counsel was an important factor in my decision to come to this country in 1947."

16. Armstrong, interview with Bullard and Glasgow, p. 54.

17. Anonymous, interview with author, notes, San Antonio, July 20, 2000. A German master mechanic who came to the United States in the 1950s recalls that Strughold "never actually did anything. But if there was a camera . . ."

18. Armstrong, interview with Bullard and Glasgow, p. 55; Benford, *Report from Heidelberg*, pp. 9, 17–18. Engineer Hans Mauch was Ingeborg Schmidt's brother-in-law and made significant contributions to pressure-suit design at Wright. The other man was Ulrich Henschke.

19. Strughold, interview with Thomas, tape 3, side 2, transcript, pp. 43–44. Strughold said that he had been a POW because of his overnight promotion to colonel.

20. York Clamann, interview with author.

21. FBI FOIA file, Harald von Beckh, U.S. Department of Justice, Washington, D.C. Under the name Harold Juan Widmanstetter, Austrian physician Harald J. von Beckh went to Argentina, as did Heinz von Diringshofen. Von Beckh was invited to Holloman AFB, near Alamogordo, N.Mex., in 1957 to work on issues of weightlessness.

22. Armstrong, interview with Bullard and Glasgow, pp. 55–56.

23. Strughold, interview with Thomas, tape 3, side 2, transcript, p. 44.

24. Benford, *Report from Heidelberg*, p. 1; Strughold, interview with Thomas, tape 3, side 2, transcript, p. 46; U.S. Air Force Surgeon General, *German Aviation Medicine*. Some of the controversy surrounding Strughold's role in the Dachau experiments concerns the fact that he includes some experimental data obtained there but makes no note of the suffering and deaths in this volume. It was likely a conscious decision, but whether it was made by Strughold or an American is not known.

25. James Tent, *Mission on the Rhine: Reeducation and Denazification in American-Occupied Germany*, p. 65. The University of Heidelberg had been a jewel in the Nazi crown, and the party had recruited faculty as active party members. After the war, nearly two-thirds of the professors of medicine and the natural sciences had to be replaced. The school would have known who had cooperated with the Nazis and would have checked and documented every applicant's background. This supports the idea that Strughold had indeed been a known and consistent opponent of the Hitler regime.

26. Strughold, interview with Thomas, tape 3, side 2, transcript, p. 45.

27. Benford, *Report from Heidelberg*, p. 1; "Special Contract for Employment of German Nationals with the War Department in the United States," Dec. 23, 1946, box 1, folder 13, Luft Papers; document I-1, Maj. Gen. Hugh J. Knerr, deputy commanding general of the U.S. Strategic Air Forces in Europe, memorandum for the commanding general of the U.S. Strategic Air Forces in Europe, June 1, 1945. Cited in *Exploring the Unknown: Selected Documents in the History of the U.S. Civilian Space Program*, vol. 4: *Accessing Space*, pp. 32–33. Knerr indicated that a party of Paperclips sent to Wright Field would be assigned a block of houses on base and that "these men should be paid a good salary and in nowise treated as prisoners or slave workers. The scientific mind simply does not produce under duress."

28. Strughold, interview with Thomas, tape 3, side 2, transcript, p. 46; Robert J. Benford to Strughold, Heidelberg, Feb. 4, 1947. However, Benford, an army flight surgeon, urged Strughold to come to the United States, saying, "[W]e feel that the Heidelberg University itself would benefit from your visit to the States because it may prove a valuable link between German and American university circles and may help to reestablish Heidelberg as one of the favorable places for American scientists to go to, a place it has been for such a long time. We also feel that one of the main defects at present is caused by the fact that the Heidelberg University has been cut off from scientific progress in other countries. A visit to the States would bring you up to date in the field of physiology and would be of tremendous importance for your teaching and research in years to come."

29. York Clamann, interview with author.

30. Travel orders, U.S. Army to United States, signed by Capt. Albert Powell by order of Lieutenant Colonel Grieves, May 15, 1947, folder 2, box 1, Luft Papers; Luft, interview with Spidle, p. 7.

31. York Clamann, interview with author; document I-2, memorandum to the director of research and development, DC/S, Material, Attn: General Craigie, "Utilization of German Scientists by the U.S.S.R. and U.S.," Mar. 22, 1948, cited in Logsdon et al., *Exploring the Unknown*, vol. 4, pp. 33–34. The U.S. State Department blocked visas for these scientists, consequently the State-War-Navy Coordination

Committee, which authorized Project Paperclip, decided to bring them in under military custody and legalize their immigration status later.

32. *U.S.A. v. Karl Brandt et al.*, microfilm roll 1, pp. 29, 67; roll 5, pp. 3761–62; roll 7, pp. 6501, 6740–41, 6741–45; roll 8, pp. 7787, 7788, 7792; roll 9, pp. 8313–16, 8328–29, 8398. Clamann provided an affidavit for Romberg and a letter for Becker-Freyseng; Otto Gauer did likewise, and both men were requested as defense witnesses by Ruff. Erich Opitz wrote a letter for Becker-Freyseng, and Luft wrote one for Schaefer and swore an affidavit for Becker-Freyseng. He had been requested as a defense witness but was departing for the United States. Strughold wrote a letter and gave several affidavits on behalf of Schaefer and provided one for Becker-Freyseng, Schröder, and Ruff.

33. Charlotte Becker-Freyseng to Ulrich Luft, Germany, May 30, 1951, and July 13, 1951, in folder 21, box 2; various letters from Bauer in folders 34 and 35, box 3; miscellaneous letters within the correspondence series, all in the Luft Papers.

34. York Clamann, interview with author.

35. Heinz Maier-Leibnitz to Ulrich Luft, Randolph AFB, Nov. 4, 1950, folder 20, box 6, Luft Papers.

36. Armstrong, interview with Bullard and Glasgow, pp. 57–58.

37. York Clamann, interview with author.

38. "Special Contract for Employment of German Nationals with the War Department in the United States," Dec. 23, 1946, folder 13, box 1, and Konrad Büttner to "SAM [School of Aerospace Medicine]—paperclips," Aug. 30, 1957, folder 15, box 3, Luft Papers; Marg, phone interview with author. Hunger had reached such a level that contracts between the United States and individual German scientists guaranteed they would be fed in the mess hall daily and that dependents still in Germany would be provided "2,300 kcal of reasonable variety." Büttner wrote that "Our common problem was for a while to convert a six dollars per diem into CARE parcels."

39. M. H. Fischer to Ulrich Luft, Germany, Mar. 19, 1949, folder 13, box 4; Gertrud Hartmann to Alice and Ulrich Luft, Germany, Jan. 14, 1952, folder 4, box 5; "Herbert and Anneliese" to Ulrich Luft, Germany, Sept. 7, 1948, folder 21, box 2; Annemarie Dieterici to Alice Luft, Germany, July 10, 1948, folder 32, box 3; Charlotte Becker-Freyseng to Ulrich Luft, Germany, May 30, 1951, and July 13, 1951, folder 21, box 2; Inge Erdmann to Ulrich Luft, Germany, Aug. 21, 1946, folder 8, box 4; Paul Bauer to Ulrich Luft, Munich, Oct. 2, 1948, folder 34, box 3; Frank Leberecht to Ulrich Luft, Germany, May 1, 1948, folder 9, box 6; Hans Loeschke to Ulrich Luft, Germany, Aug. 20, 1948, box 6, folder 14; Erich Opitz to Ulrich Luft, Germany, Oct. 9, 1948, folder 11, box 6, Luft Papers.

40. Ulrich Luft to a Prof. Dr. Schäfer, Bad Wildungen, May 13, 1947, folder 2, box 2, Luft Papers.

41. Packing list, July 27, 1950, folder 18, box 1, Luft Papers.

42. Armstrong, interview with Bullard and Glasgow, p. 53.

43. Two good sources on von Braun's career are Neufeld's *Rocket and the Reich* and Frederick I. Ordway III and Mitchell Sharpe's *Rocket Team*, with a foreword by Wernher von Braun.

44. Dempsey, *Fifty Years of Research on Man in Flight*, pp. 57, 61, 62.

45. Ibid., pp. 58, 64; Harry G. Mosely, "U.S. Air Force Experience with Ejection Seat Escape," *Journal of Aviation Medicine* 28, no. 2 (Feb. 1957): 69–73.

46. Edward M. Haight, *Semiannual History: July 1, 1951, to Dec. 31, 1951*, vol. 13 (Montgomery: Maxwell AFB, Air University, 1952), pp. 2, 6, AFHRA. Enlisted medical personnel were trained in Alabama.

47. Peyton, *Fifty Years of Aerospace Medicine*, p. 138.

48. Ordway and Sharpe, *The Rocket Team*, pp. 407–409; Strughold, *The Green and Red Planet*, pp. viii–xi, xv–xvi, 35, 91–97.

49. Peyton, *Fifty Years of Aerospace Medicine*, pp. 139, 141.

50. Ibid., p. 141; Swenson et al., *This New Ocean: A History of Project Mercury*, p. 36. Swenson credits Otto Gauer, who returned to Germany and a distinguished career as a professor of physiology, for the study of the weightless condition and the identification of its seriousness.

51. Peyton, *Fifty Years of Aerospace Medicine*, p. 140.

52. Strughold, interview with Thomas, tape 3, side 2, transcript, p. 46.

53. Peyton, *Fifty Years of Aerospace Medicine*, p. 142.

54. Lasby, *Project Paperclip*, p. 287.

55. Thomas, notes from Strughold interview, p. 9; Strughold, interview with Thomas, tape 3, side 2, transcript, pp. 46–57. Armstrong, Strughold recalled later, "was always open-minded in this respect, and when . . . at a luncheon in Chicago . . . Haber and I gave some talks about the necessity to create a space medicine branch in the . . . medical association, [h]e said in advance that he gave his blessing to everything we should decide about the foundation [of] such a branch."

56. Peyton, *Fifty Years of Aerospace Medicine*, pp. 142–43.

57. Ibid., p. 142; Strughold, interview with Thomas, tape 3, side 2, transcript, p. 48. Fritz Haber is acknowledged as the originator of the piggyback system by which NASA transports the space shuttle from California to Florida.

58. Strughold, interview with Thomas, tape 3, side 2, transcript, p. 48.

59. Campbell, interview with Hasdorff, pp. 21–24.

60. Haight, *Semiannual History: July 1, 1951, to Dec. 31, 1951*, vol. 13, pp. 27–30.

61. Anne M. Platoff, "Eyes on the Red Planet: Human Mars Mission Planning, 1952–1970" (master's thesis, University of Houston, Clear Lake, 1999), p. 14. With the *Collier's* series and his appearances on leading television programs in the early 1950s, von Braun reached around thirty million Americans with his vision of journeys into space.

62. Strughold, interview with Thomas, tape 3, side 2, p. 49.

63. Harry G. Armstrong, foreword to *Physics and Medicine of the Upper Atmosphere*, ed. Clayton S. White and Otis O. Benson Jr., pp. xiii–xv.

64. As a college freshman, Armstrong had even enlisted for a year in the marines as an ordinary infantryman at the tail end of World War I.

65. "Akademischer Alpenverein München," folder 4, box 2, Luft Papers.

66. Copy of Friedrich Luft's birth certificate, Berlin, May 1942, folder 1, box 1, Luft Papers; York Clamann, interview with author; Marg, interview with author.

67. Lasby, *Project Paperclip*, pp. 258–62.

68. Bubel, interview with author.

69. Luft, interview with Spidle, pp. 9–10.

70. Sam White to Ulrich Luft, Albuquerque, June 26, 1953, folder 12, box 9, and Luft to Alfonso del Castillo, Albuquerque, July 6, 1955, folder 17, box 3, Luft Papers. The actual written offer came from White. Handwritten at the bottom of the letter is a postscript: "Randy has asked me to say that should you decide to come to Albuquerque you can count on getting land up by our places on a long-term basis."

71. FBI report, from SAC San Antonio (9-830) to the director of the FBI, Aug. 12, 1958, FBI FOIA file of Hubertus Strughold. The letter was typed in German and sent from Philadelphia. Strughold translated it: "Nazi Pig: I have found you. I shall bring you soon to your court. KZ 34-14587." The alphanumeric entry at the end is likely a *Konzentrationslager*—concentration camp—identification number.

72. "Lenchen" to Konrad Büttner, Ostseebad, Germany, July 1951, English translation by the Federal Bureau of Investigation, FBI file no. 105-HQ-10888, FOIA file on Konrad Büttner, U.S. Department of Justice.

73. York Clamann, interview with author.

CHAPTER 5

1. Peyton, *Fifty Years of Aerospace Medicine*, pp. 133–34, 138.

2. John Paul Stapp, interview with Shirley Thomas, Oct. 14, 1959, tape 1, sides 1 and 2, and tape 2, side 1, Thomas Collection. Wilford Stapp, correspondence with author, July 21, 2003. In her book, Thomas incorrectly has Stapp graduating from high school at age fourteen.

3. Stapp, interview with Thomas, tape 1, side 2; Thomas, *Men of Space*, vol. 1, pp. 69–71; Craig Ryan, *The Pre-Astronauts: Manned Ballooning on the Threshold of Space*, pp. 14–15.

4. Stapp, interview with Thomas, tape 1, side 2; Wilford Stapp and Margaret Stapp, interview with author, notes, San Antonio, July 18, 2000.

5. Stapp, interview with Thomas, tape 1, sides 1 and 2; Stapp and Stapp, interview with author; Wilford Stapp, correspondence with author. The research position still did not fulfill his desire to serve people in need. Consequently, Stapp established "curbside clinics" at both Muroc and Holloman, as he had at an earlier assignment at Davis-Monthan AFB in Tucson, making house calls to people with little or no access to medical care. Throughout his life, he never accepted a penny for his doctoring services.

6. John Paul Stapp, *Reminiscences of Col. John Paul Stapp*, May 1960, interview with Kenneth W. Leish for the Aviation Project, Oral History Research Office, Columbia University, transcript, p. 1.

7. Ryan, *The Pre-Astronauts*, p. 15.

8. Stapp, interview with Thomas, tape 1, side 1.

9. Ryan, *The Pre-Astronauts*, pp. 29–30. The film is titled *On the Threshold of Space*, directed by Robert D. Webb, Twentieth-Century Fox, 1956.

10. Stapp, interview with Thomas, tape 1, side 1.

11. Douglas Martin, "John Paul Stapp, 89, Is Dead: 'The Fastest Man on Earth,'" *New York Times*, Nov. 16, 1999; Robert Murphy, "Murphy's Law," letter to the editor, *Los Angeles Times*, Nov. 29, 1999.

12. Percival Lowell, *Mars* (Boston and New York: Houghton Mifflin, 1895), pp. 3, 7, 35, 48, 75. Lowell had observed the planet between May 24, 1894, and Apr. 3, 1895, and had made 917 drawings and sketches. He took it as quite likely that life existed elsewhere and "simple logic" that there would be an atmosphere on Mars. He concluded that the atmospheric haze he observed was caused by ice crystals and likened portions of the planet's atmosphere to that of the Himalayas.

13. William M. Sinton, interview with author, notes, July 2000, Flagstaff, Ariz.; Sinton, "Further Evidence of Vegetation on Mars," *Science* 130, no. 3384 (Nov. 6, 1959): 1234–37. For a more detailed explanation of research in the 1950s and 1960s on exobiology, see Steven J. Dick, *The Biological Universe: The Twentieth-Century Extraterrestrial Life Debate and the Limits of Science,* and vol. 5 of Shirley Thomas's *Men of Space* series.

14. Sinton, interview with author; Lovelace, interview with Thomas, Jan. 17, 1961, tape 2, side 1; Clyde Tombaugh to Roger Putnam, Las Cruces, N.Mex., July 20, 1953, Tombaugh correspondence file, Lowell Archives. Sinton, who supported the lichen theory, came to Lowell from Harvard in 1957. His specialty was infrared and spectral atmospheric analysis of the inner planets (Mercury, Venus, and Mars). Lovelace also thought life might exist on Mars. Tombaugh, the discoverer of Pluto and an astronomy professor at New Mexico State University, was enthusiastic about the possibility of plant life, believing that Syrtis Major was "the richest vegetational region on the planet." Also, program of the Astronomical Society of the Pacific in conjunction with the International Mars Committee, Arizona State College, Flagstaff, Ariz., June 16–19, 1957, Putnam in E. C. Slipher correspondence file, Lowell Archives. Astronomers from Athens, the Meudon Observatory in Paris, and the Pic du Midi Observatory in France gave talks upholding the theory.

15. Strughold, *The Green and Red Planet,* p. xvi.

16. Strughold, interview with Thomas, folder 1, box 8; "An Intro to Astrobiology," *Astronautics* (Dec. 1960): 85–90.

17. V. M. Slipher to Lyman J. Briggs, National Geographic Society, May 14, 1953, V. M. Slipher correspondence file, "Briggs, Dr. Lyman J., Correspondence" folder, Lowell Observatory Archives; Sinton, interview with author; E. C. Slipher, *Mars 1956: Report of the International Mars Committee* (Dec. 1964), IMC file, Lowell Archives.

18. Peyton, *Fifty Years of Aerospace Medicine,* pp. 183–84; Haight, *Semiannual History: July 1, 1957, to Dec. 31, 1957,* vol. 25, pp. 31–32, AFHRA; samples came from three hot, arid sites: the Grand Canyon, the Petrified Forest, and the Painted Desert in Arizona, and one arctic region, McGonagel Pass in Alaska.

19. Newell, *Beyond the Atmosphere,* pp. 33–35; Roger D. Launius, "Early U.S. Civil Space Policy, NASA, and the Aspiration of Space Exploration," in *Organizing for the Use of Space: Historical Perspectives on a Persistent Issue,* ed. Launius (San Diego: Univelt, 1995), p. 69; John E. Naugle, *First among Equals: The Selection of NASA Space Science Experiments* (Washington, D.C.: NASA, 1991), pp. 1–4.

20. Ordway and Sharpe, *The Rocket Team,* p. 400; Ray A. Williamson, "Access to Space: Steps to the Saturn V," in *Exploring the Unknown,* vol. 4: *Accessing Space,* ed. Logsdon et al., p. 5; Swenson et al., *This New Ocean,* p. 19. Williamson places the number at 67 between 1946 and 1951, Swenson at 66 from April 1946 to October 1951, citing a joint report by the army and General Electric.

21. Newell, *Beyond the Atmosphere*, pp. 35–36, 75–81.

22. Peyton, *Fifty Years of Aerospace Medicine*, p. 147.

23. "Medical Research in Rockets," memo dated Sept. 7, 1949, and "Request for Consultation," Aug. 18, 1949, Col. Otis O. Benson Jr., USAF (MC), commandant of the SAM to the officer-in-charge, Ordnance Research and Development Division (Rocket), Fort Bliss, Tex., Strughold Papers. The term "warhead" was Benson's choice of words.

24. Newell, *Beyond the Atmosphere*, p. 37.

25. Ibid., p. 36; Swenson et al., *This New Ocean*, p. 19; Peyton, *Fifty Years of Aerospace Medicine*, pp. 148–49. Four monkeys died.

26. Swenson et al., *This New Ocean*, p. 50.

27. E. O. Hurlburt, "Physical Characteristics of the Upper Atmosphere of the Earth," in *Physics and Medicine of the Upper Atmosphere*, ed. White and Benson, pp. 39–40.

28. DeVorkin, *Science with a Vengeance: How the Military Created the U.S. Space Sciences after World War II*, pp. 11–12.

29. William W. Kellogg, "Temperatures and Motions of the Upper Atmosphere," *Physics and Medicine of the Upper Atmosphere*, ed. White and Benson, pp. 57, 59; James A. Van Allen, "The Nature and Intensity of the Cosmic Radiation," pp. 239–66, in the same volume; Ryan, *The Pre-Astronauts*, pp. 22–23.

30. Kellogg, "Temperatures and Motions," pp. 56–57, 63–64; Van Allen, "The Nature and Intensity of the Cosmic Radiation," p. 253; DeVorkin, *Science with a Vengeance*, pp. 273, 289–94; Sydney Chapman, *IGY: Year of Discovery*, pp. 58–59, 55, 63–64.

31. Newell, *Beyond the Atmosphere*, p. 35; cited in Walter Sullivan, *Assault on the Unknown*, pp. 20–22, 31.

32. Paul Dickson, *Sputnik: The Shock of the Century*, pp. 76–77, 136–37; Arthur C. Clarke, *The Making of a Moon: The Story of the Earth Satellite Program* (New York: Harper, 1957), pp. 32–33.

33. Newell, *Beyond the Atmosphere*, pp. xiii, 40, 42, 46–49, 429, 431–32. The group was active until 1960. The Space Science Board, which the National Academy of Sciences had created in 1958, then picked up the reins.

34. Chapman, *IGY: Year of Discovery*, pp. 57–59, 66–67.

35. DeVorkin, *Science with a Vengeance*, pp. 15–16, 250–52, 261; Swenson et al., *This New Ocean*, p. 49.

36. Benford, *Doctors in the Sky*, pp. 202–212.

37. Campbell, interview with Hasdorff, pp. 5, 25–26, 50. Campbell credits Andrew Ivy with the idea for the group. Ivy was a renowned medical researcher who had been a key prosecution witness at the Nuremberg trials of Strughold's colleagues. He was considered an expert on medical ethics and practices.

38. "Meeting of Informal Committee on Space Medicine," *Journal of Aviation Medicine* 22, no. 2 (Apr. 1951): 163–64; Heinz Haber, "Space Medicine Association of the Aero Medical Association," *Journal of Aviation Medicine* 25, no. 4 (Aug. 1954): 425.

39. Campbell, interview with Hasdorff, pp. 26–27.

40. Hermann J. Schaefer, "Cosmic Radiation," *Journal of Aviation Medicine* 21, no. 5 (Oct. 1950), and Fritz Haber and Heinz Haber, "Possible Methods of Producing the

Gravity-Free State for Medical Research," pp. 395–400 in the same volume; Strughold et al., "Where Does Space Begin? Functional Concept of the Boundaries between Atmosphere and Space," *Journal of Aviation Medicine* 22, no. 5 (Oct. 1951): 342–49, 357; H. Haber and S. J. Gerathewohl, "Physics and Psychophysics of Weightlessness," *Journal of Aviation Medicine* 22, no. 3 (June 1951): 180–89.

41. Hermann J. Schaefer, "New Knowledge of the Extra-Atmospheric Radiation Field," *Journal of Aviation Medicine* 29, no. 7 (July 1958): 492–500. Another reason was the nuclear-powered aircraft the USAF had contemplated since 1947. Although the project was canceled, a nuclear ramjet and a nuclear reactor for a rocket engine evolved from the studies, and interest in nuclear propulsion for aircraft and rockets continued at least until the 1990s.

42. Peyton, *Fifty Years of Aerospace Medicine*, p. 128; FBI FOIA file of Siegfried Gerathewohl.

43. Siegfried J. Gerathewohl and Herbert D. Stallings, "The Labyrinthine Posture Reflex (Righting Reflex) in the Cat during Weightlessness," *Journal of Aviation Medicine* 28, no. 8 (Aug. 1957): 345–55. During the takeoffs and landings, Gerathewohl held the presumably sedated cat in his lap.

44. Siegfried J. Gerathewohl et al., "Sensomotor Performance during Weightlessness: Eye-Hand Coordination," *Journal of Aviation Medicine* 28, no. 2 (Feb. 1957): 7–12; Siegfried J. Gerathewohl and Herbert D. Stallings, "Experiments during Weightlessness: A Study of the Oculo-Agravic Illusion," *Journal of Aviation Medicine* 29, no. 7 (July 1958): 504–516; Swenson et al., *This New Ocean*, p. 38.

45. Stapp, *Reminiscences of John Paul Stapp*, p. 3. Stapp estimated that, at ejection, a pilot would pull thirty-six Gs over a period of two seconds.

46. George F. Meeter, *The Holloman Story: Eyewitness Accounts of Space Age Research*, p. 53. Scant history exists on twentieth-century animal experimentation in America. Most of the available information deals with current activities of animal-rights groups. One writer who gave a few pages in answer to the question of military laboratories is Amy Blount Achor, whose *Animal Rights: A Beginner's Guide* (Yellow Springs, Ohio: WriteWare, 1996) describes the military's treatment of animals as "notoriously horrific."

47. Ryan, *The Pre-Astronauts*, p. 14.

48. Engle and Lott, *Man in Flight*, pp. 101–102.

49. Ibid., pp. 102–103; Jon Franklin and John Sutherland, *Guinea Pig Doctors: The Drama of Medical Research through Self-Experimentation*, pp. 297–98.

50. Franklin and Sutherland, *Guinea Pig Doctors*, pp. 298–300.

51. Shirley Thomas, "John Paul Stapp," in *Men of Space*, vol. 1, pp. 75, 77; Ryan, *The Pre-Astronauts*, pp. 17–18.

52. Quote in "The Fastest Man on Earth," *Time*, Sept. 12, 1955, p. 86.

53. Ryan, *The Pre-Astronauts*, p. 17.

54. John Paul Stapp, "Effects of Mechanical Forces on Living Tissues: Abrupt Deceleration and Windblast," *Journal of Aviation Medicine* 25, no. 4 (Aug. 1955): 268–88; Stapp, interview with Thomas, tape 1, side 2.

55. Thomas, "John Paul Stapp," in *Men of Space*, vol. 1, p. 81.

56. Engle and Lott, *Man in Flight,* p. 103.

57. Meeter, *The Holloman Story,* pp. 103–109.

58. John Paul Stapp, "Human Tolerance Factors in Supersonic Escape," *Journal of Aviation Medicine* 28, no. 1 (Feb. 1957): 77–82.

59. Ryan's *Pre-Astronauts* is the best source on military balloon programs from 1956 to 1966 and on their long-term results, providing much detailed information and participant commentary. Another excellent source is DeVorkin's *Race to the Stratosphere: Manned Scientific Ballooning in America,* which sets the Holloman work in the larger context of twentieth-century atmospheric physics. David Simons's *Man High* covers his own flight in fair detail and describes his relationship with Stapp and the lab's struggle for air force support. See also his "Pilot Reactions during 'Man High II' Balloon Flight," *Journal of Aviation Medicine* 29, no. 1 (Jan. 1958): 1–14.

60. Swenson et al., *This New Ocean,* p. 38.

61. "In Memoriam: Harald J. von Beckh, Space Scientist, Dies at 73," *Aviation, Space, and Environmental Medicine* 62, no. 2 (Feb. 1991): 200; FBI FOIA file on Harald von Beckh; Heinz von Diringshofen, "'Long Chair' Position for Fighter Pilots," *Journal of Aviation Medicine* 26, no. 12 (Dec. 1955): 467ff; Meeter, *The Holloman Story,* p. 113. Meeter hints that it was Stapp who extended the invitation. Government documents created in 1963 show him as having changed his name from "Harald Juan Albrecht von Beckh Widmanstetter" to "Harald John von Beckh" at some point. Since his parents were listed as Johannes A. von Beckh and Elizabeth Flach-Mille, it is possible that he had actually added the "Widmanstetter" to make leaving Austria and entering Argentina a bit easier.

62. Siegfried Gerathewohl, "The Peculiar State of Weightlessness," *Epitome of Space Medicine* (Randolph AFB, SAM, ca. 1957), pp. 16–20; Meeter, *The Holloman Story,* pp. 112–13; Engle and Lott, *Man in Flight,* p. 272. The turtles were on a seat next to von Beckh. During weightlessness, the tank would stay on the seat while the turtles, still in their water, would rise. While flying the plane, von Beckh had to reach over each time, lift the tank, fit it back around the water again, hold it in place until gravity in the aircraft returned to normal, and then lower it gently back down to the seat.

63. Meeter, *The Holloman Story,* p. 114.

64. Harald von Beckh, "Flight Experiments about Human Reactions to Accelerations Which Are Followed or Preceded by the Weightless State," technical report AFMDC-TN-58-15, ASTIA document no. 154108, AFHRA.

65. Swenson et al., *This New Ocean,* p. 42; Meeter, *The Holloman Story,* p . 104.

66. Harald J. von Beckh, "Multi-Directional G Protection in Space Flight and during Escape, a Theoretical Approach," *Journal of Aviation Medicine* 29, no. 5 (May 1958): 335–42; von Diringshofen, "'Long Chair' Position for Fighter Pilots," pp. 467–70.

67. Harry G. Moseley, "U.S. Air Force Experience with Ejection Seat Escape," *Journal of Aviation Medicine* 28, no. 1 (Feb. 1957): 69–73; Stapp, "Human Tolerance Factors in Supersonic Escape," pp. 77–82. Another fourteen percent of those who ejected experienced "major" injuries.

68. Moseley, "U.S. Air Force Experience with Ejection Seat Escape," pp. 69–73.

69. Stapp, "Human Tolerance Factors in Supersonic Escape," pp. 77–82.

70. Stapp, interview with Thomas, tape 3, side 1; Ryan, *The Pre-Astronauts*, pp. 154, 160–62, 168–76, 193–98, 201–218.

71. Stapp, interview with Thomas, tape 1, side 2; Ryan, *The Pre-Astronauts*, p. 287.

72. Ryan, *The Pre-Astronauts*, p. 65.

73. Ibid., pp. 87, 162.

74. Ibid., p. 19; Thomas, *Men of Space*, vol. 1, pp. 85–86; Stapp, interview with Thomas, tape 1, side 2, and tape 2, side 1.

75. Ryan, *The Pre-Astronauts*, pp. 123, 162; Stapp and Stapp, interview with author.

76. Henry Fountain, "Dr. Donald [*sic*] D. Flickinger, 89, a Pioneer in Space Medicine," obituary, *New York Times*, Mar. 9, 1997, p. 42; Eric Sevareid, *Not So Wild a Dream* (New York: Knopf, 1946), pp. 265–72, 276–81, 289–95, 297–300, 308–309; Eloise Engle, *Pararescue: What Men Dare Do* (New York: John Day, 1964), pp. 55–56; Shirley Thomas, "Don D. Flickinger," in *Men of Space*, vol. 3, pp. 83–87, 89. The Air Rescue Service initiated the Don Flickinger Trophy for pararescue teams in 1954.

77. Ryan, *The Pre-Astronauts*, p. 65.

78. Don D. Flickinger, "Interview of Brig. Gen. Donald [*sic*] D. Flickinger," by Max Rosenberg, H. L. Brown, and Mae Mills Link (uncredited), Washington, D.C., May 25, 1961, for the USAF Oral History Program, transcript, pp. 18, 22–25, AFHRA. Flickinger was given the choice of a transfer to a nonspace job in Hawaii or retirement. In the interview he implies that this was because of his outspokenness over NASA's growing control of the nation's manned space program and the diminution of the military's program.

79. Don Flickinger, "Sky Unlimited: A Panel Discussion on Extreme Speed and Altitude," reprinted in *Journal of Aviation Medicine* 26, no. 4 (Dec. 1955): 503–12.

80. David H. Beyer and Saul B. Sells, "Selection and Training of Personnel for Space Flight," *Journal of Aviation Medicine* 28, no. 1 (Feb. 1957): 1–6.

81. Ibid., pp. 2, 3, 5. The von Braun publication referred to is a translation of *The Mars Project* (Urbana: University of Illinois, 1953).

82. Robert T. Clark, memo, "Ad Hoc Work Committee," Feb. 11, 1958, Hans-Georg Clamann Papers, uncatalogued.

83. Bruno Balke and J. Gordon Wells, memo to R. T. Clark, "Report of Committee Meeting on Requirements for Crew Members in Extra-Terrestrial Flights," Feb. 19, 1958, Hans-Georg Clamann Papers, uncatalogued. The final requirements did not mandate that a candidate be a nonsmoker, and a height restriction of under six feet was imposed because of capsule-size constraints.

84. Bruno Balke, "Ceiling Altitude Tolerance following Physical Training and Acclimatization," *Journal of Aviation Medicine* 29, no. 1 (Jan. 1958): 40–47. Balke estimated that the altitudes achievable by mountaintop conditioning were equivalent to what explorers on Mars would experience in terms of barometric pressure. He concluded that once on the red planet, "man could spend some time with only the relatively simple protection of pressure breathing."

85. Balke and Wells, "Report of Committee Meeting on Requirements," pp. 80, 176.

86. Jay Miller, *The X-Planes: X-1 to X-29* (Marine on St. Croix, Minn.: Specialty Press, 1983), p. 101.

87. Myron B. Gubitz, *Rocketship X-15: A Bold New Step in Aviation*, pp. 80, 176.

88. Ibid., pp. 61–64, 72–73, 155–56; Dennis R. Jenkins, *Hypersonics before the Shuttle: A Concise History of the X-15 Research Airplane* (Washington, D.C.: NASA, 2000), p. 70; Ryan, *The Pre-Astronauts*, p. 218. Kittinger's jump from 102,800 feet, still the world's record, took thirteen minutes and forty-five seconds.

89. Gubitz, *Rocketship X-15*, pp. 154–55, 159, 160, 161, 166; Frederick R. Ritzinger Jr. and Ellis G. Aboud, "Pressure Suits: Their Evolution and Development," *Air University Review*, ca. 1962, pp. 23–32, box 13, Thomas Collection.

90. Gubitz, *Rocketship X-15*, pp. 160, 161, 166.

91. Ibid., pp. 161, 162, 163, 166.

92. Ibid., pp. 175, 176; Guenther et al., *North American X-15/X-15 A-2*, p. 11; Jenkins, *Hypersonics before the Shuttle*, p. 69.

93. Gubitz, *Rocketship X-15*, pp. 165, 170, 171, 173–75; W. D. Kay, "The X-15 Hypersonic Flight Research Program: Politics and Permutations at NASA," in *From Engineering Science to Big Science: The NACA and NASA Collier Trophy Research Project Winners*, ed. Pamela Mack (Washington, D.C.: NASA, 1998), pp. 155–56; Miller, *The X-Planes*, p. 107; Chris Pocock, "From the Shadows: Early History of the U-2," in *Code One* 17, no. 1 (first quarter, 2002): 14. Actually, the U-2 spyplane, whose pilots Lovelace also screened, had already surreptitiously broken what was then the world altitude record, flying higher than 66,000 feet five times in their first week of operation in late 1955.

Chapter 6

1. Haight, *Semiannual History: Jan. 1, 1952, to June 30, 1952*, vol. 14, p. 67.

2. Haight, *Semiannual History: July 1, 1954, to Dec. 31, 1954*, vol. 19, p. 5.

3. Haight, *Semiannual History: July 1, 1957, to Dec. 31, 1957*, vol. 25, p. 54.

4. Cited in Roger D. Launius, "Prelude to the Space Age," in *Exploring the Unknown: Selected Documents in the History of the U.S. Civilian Space Program*, vol. 1: *Organizing for Exploration*, ed. John M. Logsdon et al., p. 16.

5. David Callahan and Fred I. Greenstein, "The Reluctant Racer: Eisenhower and U.S. Space Policy," in *Spaceflight and the Myth of Presidential Leadership*, ed. Roger D. Launius and Howard E. McCurdy, p. 21.

6. Robert Dallek, "Johnson, Project Apollo, and the Politics of Space Program Planning," in *Spaceflight and the Myth*, pp. 69–70; Eilene Galloway, "Organizing the United States Government for Outer Space, 1957–1958," in *Reconsidering Sputnik*, pp. 309–10.

7. *History of the USAF Aerospace Medical Center Air Training Command*, vol. 2: *July 1, 1960–Dec. 31, 1960* (San Antonio: Brooks AFB, USAF Aerospace Medical Center, 1961), pp. 11–12, AFHRA.

8. *School of Aviation Medicine, USAF: Semiannual History*, vol. 23: *July 1–Dec. 31, 1956* (San Antonio: Randolph AFB, USAF School of Aviation Medicine, 1957), p. 14.

9. Bubel, Dornes, York Clamann, and anonymous, interviews with author.

10. Peyton, *Fifty Years of Aerospace Medicine*, pp. 192–94; Constance McLaughlin Green and Milton Lomask, *Vanguard: A History* (Washington, D.C.: NASA, 1970), pp.

240, 288–93. This small satellite, just one-fiftieth the size of *Sputnik*, had been boosted by a Jupiter C missile based on von Braun's V-2s. It carried a cargo of miniaturized scientific equipment to study the environment of Earth's orbit. In contrast to the Soviets' first effort, which merely broadcast a signal to let observers know that it was in orbit, the American satellite collected data for four months and transmitted that information to scientists in the United States. This allowed physicist James Van Allen of the University of Iowa to verify his theory that electromagnetic radiation surrounded the earth near the poles.

The National Institutes of Health had proposed a biology experiment, but the selection panel turned it down. No other life-science experiment was ever flown on Vanguard or, for that matter, on the other IGY satellite series, Explorer. See John E. Naugle, *First among Equals: The Selection of NASA Space Science Experiments* (Washington, D.C.: NASA, 1991), pp. 7–11, for an explanation of the selection process.

11. George R. Steinkamp and Willard R. Hawkins, "Medical Experimentation in a Sealed Cabin Simulator," in *Physics and Medicine of the Atmosphere and Space*, ed. Otis O. Benson and Hubertus Strughold, pp. 371–73.

12. Peyton, *Fifty Years of Aerospace Medicine*, pp. 193–94.

13. Strughold, interview with Thomas, tape 4, side 1, transcript, pp. 53–54; tape 3, side 2.

14. Ibid., tape 4, side 1, transcript, p. 54; "Record of Organizational Meeting of Special Senate Committee on Space and Astronautics, Feb. 20, 1958," p. 2; envelope marked " 'Outer Space Committee' organizational meeting," U.S. Senate, 1949–1961, Special Committee on Space and Astronautics Collection, Johnson Library.

15. Since the fortieth anniversary of the *Sputnik* launch, the literature on that event has increased significantly. Earlier works include Roger D. Launius, *NASA: A History of the U.S. Civil Space Program*; Alan J. Levine, *The Missile and Space Race*; Dwight D. Eisenhower, *Waging Peace, 1956–1961* (Garden City, N.Y.: Doubleday, 1965); Walter A. McDougall, *The Heavens and the Earth: A Political History of the Space Age*; as well as Ordway and Sharpe, *The Rocket Team*; Winter, *Rockets into Space*; and Swenson et al., *This New Ocean*.

16. James J. Harford, "Korolev's Triple Play: Sputniks *1, 2*, and *3*" in *Reconsidering Sputnik*, pp. 75, 77.

17. Divine, *The Sputnik Challenge*, p. 11.

18. Document I-4, Homer J. Stewart, chair, Ad Hoc Advisory Group on Special Capabilities, report to Donald A. Quarles, assistant secretary of defense (research and development), Aug. 4, 1955, pp. iii, 1, 3–8, cited in *Exploring the Unknown*, vol. 4: *Accessing Space*, ed. Logsdon et al., pp. 38–43.

19. Ray A. Williamson, "Access to Space: Steps to the Saturn V," p. 6 fn. Williamson states that the von Braun team "did not accept gracefully" the decision to go with the Vanguard, and there was concern that the team might try to orbit a satellite without approval. Consequently, when the Army Ballistic Missile Agency made a test launch in early 1957, the upper stage of the vehicle was reportedly ordered filled with sand so that it could not reach orbit.

20. Harford, "Korolev's Triple Play," pp. 75, 77.

21. Chapman, *IGY: Year of Discovery*, p. 105.

22. "Soviet Engineers Constructing Two Rockets," *Bulletin of the American Interplanetary Society* (Jan. 1952): 1, Strughold Papers, uncatalogued.

23. Sullivan, *Assault on the Unknown*, p. 56.

24. Harford, "Korolev's Triple Play," pp. 77–78.

25. Sullivan, *Assault on the Unknown*, pp. 49, 58–60.

26. Ingeborg Schmidt, "Visibility of Artificial Satellites of the Planet Earth," *Journal of Aviation Medicine* 28, no. 5 (Oct. 1957): 435–46. In her acknowledgements, Schmidt expresses gratitude to Hubertus Strughold for suggesting the idea.

27. Recent historiography on the Soviet view of *Sputnik*, based on newly opened archives there, is that their program, like the American one, was fragmented into factions: scientific goals vs. military payloads, big rockets vs. smaller rockets, and manned flight vs. unmanned flight. See William P. Barry, "How the Space Race Began," Society for History in the Federal Government, *Occasional Papers* 1 (1997): 1–12, and Asif A. Siddiqi, *Challenge to Apollo: The Soviet Union and the Space Race, 1945–1974*, pp. 119–203.

28. Ryan, *The Pre-Astronauts*, pp. 293–94. Right up until Yuri Gagarin's launch on Apr. 12, 1961, the United States thought it had a chance to be first to put a human into space. One USAF plan, hatched in 1960, would have launched a test pilot toward space in the nose cone of a Redstone rocket, then, using an explosive ejection seat, sent him on a further upward/forward trajectory that would briefly put his spacesuit-clad body into space before he began falling, hopefully to parachute to a safe landing. Joseph Kittinger volunteered for the mission, but somewhere in the chain of command the idea was squelched, presumably for safety and publicity reasons.

29. Swenson et al., *This New Ocean*, pp. 69, 70, 73, 74, 80, 81–83, 99–100, 101–102, 171. At the same time, the von Braun group wanted to grab the headlines with a manned ballistic shot the following year, in 1959, using a modified Redstone and a steep trajectory. Called "Man Very High," the project called for a volunteer to ride in a redesigned Man-High balloon gondola and function only as a passenger. Joachim Kuettner, a former Messerschmitt test pilot with doctorates in law, physics, and astronomy and one of a tiny elite who had test-flown a manned V-1 rocket—and lived—was asked to lead the project. Hugh Dryden referred to it in House hearings as being of "about the same technical value as the circus stunt of shooting a young lady from a cannon."

30. Ibid., p. 2.

31. "Press Release: Opening Statement by Chairman Lyndon B. Johnson before the Senate Special Committee on Space and Astronautics, May 6, 1958," p. 1, Sen. Mundt folder, Senate Committee on Space and Astronautics; Committee on Aeronautics and Space Science, container no. 358, Johnson Library.

32. "Statement of Loftus E. Becker, the Legal Adviser, Department of State, for Delivery on Wednesday, May 13, 1958, before the Special Senate Committee on Space and Astronautics," pp. 8–9, Sen. Mundt folder.

33. A. Scott Crossfield with Clay Blair Jr., *Always Another Dawn: The Story of a Rocket Test Pilot*, p. 27.

34. Naugle, *First among Equals*, p. 23.

35. Newell, *Beyond the Atmosphere*, pp. 106–107.

36. Divine, *The Sputnik Challenge*, p. 103.

37. Callahan and Greenstein, "The Reluctant Racer: Eisenhower and U.S. Space Policy," p. 38.

38. Henry C. Dethloff, *Suddenly Tomorrow Came: A History of the Johnson Space Center*, p. 14.

39. A good example of such beliefs is contained in Hugh L. Dryden, "Spiritual Leadership in the Space Age," commencement address, Drew University, Madison, N.J., June 6, 1960, folder 1, box 5, Thomas Collection.

40. "Statement of Dr. Hugh L. Dryden, director, National Advisory Committee for Aeronautics, before the Special Committee on Space and Astronautics United States Senate, May 13, 1958," p. 3; "Statement by the Honorable Wilber M. Brucker, Secretary of the Army, before Senate Special Committee on Astronautics and Space Exploration," May 8, 1958; "Statement of Roy W. Johnson, director, Advanced Research Projects Agency before the Senate Special Committee on Space and Astronautics," n.d.; "Statement of Donald A. Quarles, Deputy Secretary of Defense before the Senate Select Committee on Space and Astronautics," May 7, 1958; "Statement of Alan T. Waterman, Director, National Science Foundation, before the Senate Special Committee on Space and Astronautics," May 7, 1958, all in Sen. Mundt folder; and "Statement of Maurice H. Stans, Director of the Bureau of the Budget, before the Special Committee on Space and Astronautics of the Senate on S. 3609, the 'National Aeronautics and Space Act of 1958,' May 13, 1958, 3–5," Sen. Magnuson folder, Senate Committee on Space and Astronautics; Committee on Aeronautics and Space Science, container no. 358.

41. "Statement of Dr. Hugh L. Dryden," pp. 7–8; "Statement of Donald A. Quarles," pp. 1–2.

42. "Statement by the Honorable Wilber M. Brucker," p. 2.

43. Callahan and Greenstein, "The Reluctant Racer: Eisenhower and U.S. Space Policy," p. 40.

44. James R. Killian, *Sputnik, Scientists, and Eisenhower: A Memoir of the First Special Assistant to the President for Science and Technology* (Cambridge: MIT Press, 1977), p. 286.

45. "Statement of Roy W. Johnson," p. 5.

46. "Statement of Alan T. Waterman," p. 6.

47. Launius, *NASA: A History of the U.S. Civil Space Program*, pp. 30–32.

48. Divine, *The Sputnik Challenge*, p. 191.

49. Dethloff, *Suddenly Tomorrow Came*, p. 19.

50. Elliott, "'On a Comet, Always,'" pp. 369, 372–73.

51. Spidle, *The Lovelace Medical Center*, pp. 106, 116–17, 133; Michael R. Beschloss, *Mayday: Eisenhower, Khrushchev, and the U-2 Affair*, p. 109.

52. McDougall, *The Heavens and the Earth*, p. 165.

53. Andrei G. Kousnetzov, "Some Results of Biological Experiments in Rockets and *Sputnik 2*," a speech at the Third European Congress of Aviation Medicine, Louvain, Belgium, Sept. 1958, reprinted in *Journal of Aviation Medicine* 29, no. 11 (Nov. 1958): 781–84. Kousnetzov stated that the USSR had been carrying out biological research in space flight since 1949, first using rockets of an unnamed type that carried unspecified animals to a height of approximately two hundred kilometers (110 miles). Catapult experiments had come later. Then Laika was placed in orbit aboard *Sputnik 2* in a custom-built

cabin that exposed her to transverse acceleration. Thanks to automatic recording and transmission of her vital signs, researchers could see that her heartbeat and respiration were three times what they had been on Earth. Beyond that terse report, the Soviets shared nothing.

54. Shirley Thomas, *Men of Space*, vol. 2, pp. 107–108; Lovelace, interview with Thomas, tape 1, side 1.

55. Swenson et al., *This New Ocean*, pp. 75–76, 120.

56. John Pitts, *The Human Factor: Biomedicine in the Manned Space Program to 1980*, pp. 15–16.

57. Swenson et al., *This New Ocean*, pp. 114–15, 129–30, 131.

58. Ryan, *The Pre-Astronauts*, p. 249, 249 fn.

59. Link, *Space Medicine and Project Mercury*, chap. five, "Medical Aspects of Astronaut Selection and Training," electronic version, n.p.

60. Memorandum from Robert B. Voas, human-factors assistant to the director to Robert Everline, Mercury Project Office, Aug. 28, 1963, "Preliminary Draft of Astronaut Selection Section," *Mercury Technical History*, p. 14, Mercury astronaut selection file, NASA History Office.

61. Swenson et al., *This New Ocean*, pp. 131, 160–61; Spidle, *The Lovelace Medical Center*, p. 134; Link, *Space Medicine in Project Mercury*, chap. five; Voas, "Preliminary Draft of Astronaut Selection Section," pp. 19–22.

62. Spidle, *The Lovelace Medical Center*, pp. 133–34; Link, *Space Medicine in Project Mercury*, chap. five.

63. W. Randolph Lovelace II et al., "Selection Program for Astronauts for the National Aeronautics and Space Administration," hand-dated Nov. 5, 1959, p. 2, Mercury astronaut selection file, NASA History Office.

64. Ibid., p. 4; Spidle, *The Lovelace Medical Center*, pp. 134–37; Link, *Space Medicine in Project Mercury*, chap. five.

65. Link, *Space Medicine in Project Mercury*, chap. five; Lovelace et al., "Selection Program for Astronauts," p. 4.

66. Lovelace et al., "Selection Program for Astronauts," p. 3.

67. Voas, "Preliminary Draft of Astronaut Selection Section," p. 26; Charles L. Wilson, ed., *Project Mercury Candidate Evaluation Program*, Dec. 1959, p. 1, WADC technical report 59-505, project no. 7164, task no. 71832. Mercury astronaut selection file, NASA History Office. Scuba divers may have been used because of their unusually well-developed lung capacity. Scott Carpenter was a diver and went on to participate in navy studies of undersea habitats in the mid- and late 1960s.

68. Charles L. Wilson, "Physical Fitness Tests," in *Project Mercury Candidate Evaluation Program*, ed. Wilson, p. 49. The treadmill test was recommended by Bruno Balke.

69. C. E. Clauser, "Anthropometric Studies," in *Project Mercury Candidate Evaluation Program*, ed. Wilson, p. 23.

70. Swenson et al., *This New Ocean*, p. 162.

71. Link, *Space Medicine in Project Mercury*, chap. five; J. Gold, "Heat Tests," in *Project Mercury Candidate Evaluation Program*, ed. Wilson, pp. 27–30, 41, 43.

72. Swenson et al., *This New Ocean*, p. 239.

73. D. J. Baker and R. G. Hansen, "Biological Acoustical Tests, Part One: Intelligibility Measure," pp. 27–30; C. L. Wilson, "Physical Fitness Tests," p. 69; J. E. Steele, "Biological Acoustical Tests: Part Two, Effect of Noise on the Ability to Perform Addition," pp. 31–32; R. R. Coermann et al., "Biological Acoustical Tests, Part Three: The Influence of Vibration on Holding the Horizontal Position Utilizing the Equilibrium Chair," pp. 33, 38, all in *Project Mercury Candidate Evaluation Program*, ed. Wilson. The seven Mercury finalists received only average ratings on the audibility tests.

74. E. L. Lindberg, "Acceleration Tests," in *Project Mercury Candidate Evaluation Program*, ed. Wilson, pp. 11–12, 15. The average adult on a roller coaster can handle five Gs before blacking out.

75. C. L. Wilson, "Physical Fitness Tests," pp. 63–72.

76. Lovelace, interview with Thomas, tape 1, side 1.

77. Swenson et al., *This New Ocean*, pp. 162–63; Voas, "Preliminary Draft of Astronaut Selection Section," p. 27.

78. Patricia A. Santy, *Choosing the Right Stuff: The Psychological Selection of Astronauts and Cosmonauts*. Former NASA psychiatrist and flight surgeon Santy gave a very critical analysis and review of the agency's early efforts in using psychological evaluations for astronaut selection. Not only did their methodology antagonize the pilots, she said, but the agency also compounded its errors by dropping their postflight follow-up analysis before the end of the Mercury program and losing much of the information.

79. C. L. Wilson, "Physical Fitness Tests," in *Project Mercury Candidate Evaluation Program*, ed. Wilson, pp. 52, 53, 63, 77.

80. "The Candidate Evaluation Committee," in *Project Mercury Candidate Evaluation Program*, ed. Wilson, p. 89. In "Discussion and Recommendations," p. 99 in the same volume, Wilson notes that "The main value of a severely stressful physiological test was the interpretation of the psychological response to that stress test. Whenever a subject terminated a severe test for psychological reasons, he was not recommended by the Committee."

81. Wilson, ed., *Project Mercury Candidate Evaluation Program*, pp. 41–47. Of the seven, only three of the Mercury astronauts scored the highest in any particular medical category: one for resistance to heat, another for physical fitness, and a third for psychological fitness. This tends to support the statements that the committee was attempting to match specific skills with the program's needs more than it was looking for physiological perfection and that the medical personnel were the Mercury astronauts' allies in the fight to be pilots rather than mere passengers.

82. "The Candidate Evaluation Committee," in *Project Mercury Candidate Evaluation Program*, ed. Wilson, p. 89. Six of the Mercury astronauts were "outstanding," with no medical reservations.

83. Swenson et al., *This New Ocean*, pp. 163–64; Voas, "Preliminary Draft of Astronaut Selection Section," p. 30.

84. Dwayne Day, "Invitation to Struggle: The History of Civilian-Military Relations in Space," in *Exploring the Unknown: Selected Documents in the History of the U.S. Civilian Space Program*, vol. 2: *External Relationships*, ed. John M. Logsdon et al., p. 233.

85. Cited in McDougall, *The Heavens and the Earth*, p. 114.

86. Ibid., p. 158.

87. "Memorandum for the Secretary of Defense; Chairman, the National Advisory Committee for Aeronautics from the White House, Apr. 2, 1958," p. 1, Sen. Mundt folder.

88. Launius, *NASA: A History of the U.S. Civil Space Program*, pp. 34–35. "Reconnaissance" in this sense refers to spy satellites.

89. "Statement by the Honorable Wilber M. Brucker, Secretary of the Army, before Senate Special Committee on Astronautics and Space Exploration," May 8, 1958, p. 5, Sen. Mundt folder.

90. Howard McCurdy, "Organizing for Space: The Popular Culture of Cold-War America," p. 38; Sylvia K. Kraemer, "NASA and the Challenge of Organizing for Exploration," pp. 94–96, both in *Organizing for the Use of Space: Historical Perspectives on a Persistent Issue*, ed. Roger D. Launius (San Diego: Univelt, 1995).

91. Launius, *Organizing for the Use of Space*, p. 5; "Statement of Donald A. Quarles," pp. 1–2.

92. Rick Sturdevant, "The United States Air Force Organizes for Space: The Operational Quest," in *Organizing for the Use of Space*, ed. Launius, pp. 165–69; McDougall, *The Heavens and the Earth*, p. 107.

93. Sturdevant, "The United States Air Force Organizes for Space: The Operational Quest," in *Organizing for the Use of Space*, ed. Launius, pp. 169–70.

94. Otis O. Benson Jr., preface to *Physics and Medicine of the Atmosphere and Space*, ed. Benson and Strughold, p. xii.

95. Strughold, "The Ecosphere of the Sun," *Journal of Aviation Medicine* 26, no. 8 (Aug. 1955): 323–38; Strughold, "Gravitational Environment of Space," a talk presented at the Second International Symposium on the Physics and Medicine of the Upper Atmosphere and Space, Sept. 10–12, 1958, San Antonio.

96. Dietrich E. Beischer, "Potentialities and Ramifications of Life under Extreme Environmental Conditions," *Journal of Aviation Medicine* 29, no. 7 (July 1958): 500–503. The Naval School of Aviation Medicine scientist enjoyed the esoteric. One of his weightlessness adaptation studies included tiny magnetic shoes for kittens and mice.

97. John D. Fulton, "Survival of Terrestrial Microorganisms under Simulated Martian Conditions" in *Physics and Medicine of the Atmosphere and Space*, pp. 606–13.

98. Gerard Kuiper, "The Environments of the Moon and the Planets," in *Physics and Medicine of the Atmosphere and Space*, pp. 577–83.

CHAPTER 7

1. "Should a Girl Be First in Space?" *Look* 24, no. 3 (Feb. 2, 1960): 112ff; Weitekamp, *The Right Stuff, the Wrong Sex*, pp. 142–43, 150–51, 154–55, 163–67.

2. Spidle, *The Lovelace Medical Center*, p. 138; Lillian Kozloski and Maura J. Mackowski, "The Wrong Stuff," *Final Frontier* 3, no. 3 (May/June 1990): 20–23, 52–55; Jerrie Cobb, "Summary," June 15, 1961, Jerrie Cobb file, NASA History Office. The Soviets had selected Valentina Tereshkova and other female cosmonaut candidates in 1961.

3. Deborah G. Douglas, *United States Women in Aviation 1940–1985*, p. 51. Of the 25,000 young women who applied for admission to the WASP training program, 1,800 were accepted. Of these, 1,074 earned their wings. Thirty-eight were killed in the line of duty.

4. "Three Yanks, Two Britons Top Flyers," *Dayton Daily News*, Oct. 15, 1972, p. 25-A, Jerrie Cobb file, International Women's Air and Space Museum.

5. Kozloski and Mackowski, "The Wrong Stuff," pp. 20–23, 52–55.

6. In the late 1960s, Cobb gave up her battle with Washington and became a freelance flying missionary in the Amazon, relying solely on sporadic donations to finance her solo work. Nominated in 1980 for the Nobel peace prize, she scrupulously avoided public attention but was still the subject of a fair amount of media coverage. An interesting but unflattering portrait of Cobb and her work appeared as "The Discarded Astronaut," by Meg Laughlin, in *Tropic Magazine*, the *Miami Herald*, June 12, 1983.

7. Jerrie Cobb with Jane Rieker, *Woman into Space*, pp. 131–33.

8. Kozloski and Mackowski, "The Wrong Stuff," pp. 20–23, 52–55.

9. Weitekamp, *The Right Stuff, the Wrong Sex*, p. 201. These connections were likely made through Lovelace's Aero Medical Association membership and his position within NASA.

10. Television interview with the "future lady astronaut trainees" (FLATs) at the National Air and Space Museum for *NBC DATELINE* in December 1994.

11. Cobb and Rieker, *Woman into Space*, pp. 151–52. After her Albuquerque tests but before the Time, Inc., press conference, Cobb was sent to NASA's Lewis Research Center in Cleveland (now the John Glenn Research Center) to "fly" the MASTIF (Multi-Axis Spin-Test Inertia Facility). This device operated as an enormous gyroscope in which a pilot occupied a small space in the center, outfitted with controls. The pilot's job was to maintain stability on all three axes as the MASTIF gyrated. The only written record of this experience that I have uncovered is Cobb's autobiographical account, which does not specify how she received clearance to use this vehicle. It is reasonable to assume that Lovelace made that arrangement, further validating her belief that he was acting on behalf of the space agency.

12. Jacqueline Cochran to Eloise Engle, Jan. 19, 1962, correspondence file, manuscript materials, Cochran Papers; Cobb and Rieker, *Woman into Space*, p. 154. A good source of information about the arrangement is a book by former *Life* reporter Loudon Wainwright, titled *Great American Magazine: An Inside History of* Life (New York: Knopf, 1986).

13. "A Lady Proves She's Fit for Space Flight," *Life*, Aug. 29, 1960, pp. 73–77. See Cobb and Rieker, p. 156, for the Rome Olympics incident.

14. Program for the Second International Symposium on Submarine and Space Medicine, Karolinska Institutet, Stockholm, Aug. 18–19, 1960, Yuri Gagarin file, folder 1, Thomas Collection.

15. "From Aviatrix to Astronautrix," *Time*, Aug. 29, 1960, p. 41.

16. Cobb and Rieker, *Woman into Space*, pp. 154–64.

17. Cited in Kozloski and Mackowski, "The Wrong Stuff," pp. 20–23, 52–55.

18. "NASA Refutes Space Girl's Story," *New York World Telegram*, Sept. 29, 1960, p. 30; "No Women in Space," *Science News Letter*, Oct. 8, 1960, p. 230.

19. Donald Cox, "Women Astronauts," *Space World* (Sept. 1961): 37, 58–60.

20. Weitekamp, *The Right Stuff, the Wrong Sex*, pp. 157–58, 167. Weitekamp cites a letter from Flickinger to Lovelace dated Dec. 20, 1959, in which he says that he will turn over the names to Lovelace. It is not known whether he received or used Flickinger's list and which names were on it. In Cobb's autobiography, *she* claims to have come up with most or all of the candidates, and Cochran makes a similar claim in *her* book.

21. Cobb and Rieker, *Woman into Space*, p. 191. Cobb does not specify what records she checked but writes that she ultimately recommended seven of the twelve women who passed the exams.

22. Bill Robie, *For the Greatest Achievement: A History of the Aero Club of America and the National Aeronautic Association*, pp. 183–84, 186. Cochran was known within the NAA for letting nothing get in the way of American aerospace preeminence. She wanted the public to be aware of the relationship of aviation and space to national security and encouraged NAA members to set records that would keep American names at the top of the FAI lists.

23. Cochran and Brinley, *Jackie Cochran*, p. 353.

24. Donald R. Baucom, "Floyd Bostwick Odlum: 1892–1976," n.d., folder 17, box 3, MSS 4/5, Cochran Papers; Spidle, *The Lovelace Medical Center*, pp. 62–63, 78–81, 123.

25. Cochran to Alice and Ulrich Luft, New York, May 13, 1959, C-miscellaneous folder, box 3, Luft Papers.

26. Cochran and Brinley, *Jackie Cochran*, pp. 7–11, 15–16, 316–18. Reared by a poor white family in rural Florida that labored for various sawmills in the Panhandle region, Cochran never knew her exact age but estimated that she had been born about 1908. She was a foster child and, given the poverty and migratory status of her childhood, had only two years of schooling, enough to achieve a very basic literacy.

27. Ibid., p. 317.

28. NAA interoffice communication, Dec. 6, 1960; NAA interoffice communication, Cochran to Ralph V. Whitener, Dec. 24, 1960; letter, Whitener to Cochran, Washington, D.C., Dec. 29, 1960, Cochran Papers.

29. Letter, Jacqueline Cochran to Randolph Lovelace, Jan. 14, 1961; letter, Floyd B. Odlum to Lovelace, Feb. 6, 1961; letter, Odlum to Lovelace, July 19, 1961; letter, Odlum to Lovelace, Nov. 17, 1961, all in the Lovelace Foundation file, Cochran Papers. Cochran sent a check for $500, and Odlum made two stock transfers totaling $18,700. Lovelace also noted that Jerrie Cobb donated $300.

30. The Jacqueline Cochran Papers contain numerous thank-you letters from the women acknowledging her role.

31. The twelve who passed were Gene Nora Stumbough, twins Jan Dietrich and Marion Dietrich, Irene Leverton, Mary Wallace Funk, Rhea Hurrle, Jerri Sloan, Sarah Gorelick, Jane Hart, Bernice Steadman, Jean Hixson, and Myrtle Cagle.

32. "A Mrs. in the Missile," *Los Angeles Times*, n.d.; "Twelve Women Test for Space," *Washington Post*, Jan. 27, 1961; "Woman Astronaut, Scientist Probe Secrets of Outer Space," *Dallas Times Herald*, n.d.; "Women to Take Astronaut Tests," *New York Times*, June 26, 1961. Clippings file, manuscript materials, Cochran Papers.

33. Jerrie Cobb, "Space for Women?" Speech in Feb. 1962 at the First International

Women's Space Symposium in Los Angeles, reprinted in the *Congressional Record*, 87th Cong., 2d sess., Mar. 15, 1962, Cochran Papers; Jackson, "Bruno Balke Welcomes—and Creates—Avalanches," p. 98. Balke had left the school and gone to work at the Oklahoma FAA facility by then.

34. "A Damp Prelude to Space," *Life*, Oct. 24, 1960.

35. Cobb and Rieker, *Woman into Space*, p. 173.

36. The navy had sent its flight surgeons to the San Antonio school for many years until opening a naval flight-surgeon's training program in 1939. There were only a few navy aerospace-medicine specialists active nationally, most notably Ashton Graybiel, but Lovelace would have had many opportunities for contact with them and likely thought of Pensacola as the place to test the women for overwater flights.

37. Cobb and Rieker, *Woman into Space*, pp. 193–201.

38. Letter, Lovelace to Webb, Washington, D.C., Apr. 20, 1961; appointments calendar, May 1961, both in Webb Papers. As of April 20, Webb and Lovelace had never met but anticipated doing so in Tulsa. Lovelace came to Washington, D.C., in May, however.

39. W. Henry Lambright, *Powering Apollo: James E. Webb of NASA*, pp. 72, 74; Swenson et al., *This New Ocean*, p. 131; letters from Thomas J. Harris to James Webb, Oklahoma City, May 1, 1961; May 9, 1961; May 27, 1961; and May 25, 1964, all in general correspondence in the H folder, box 70, NASA correspondence file Alpha; letter, Harris to Webb, Feb. 15, 1961, folder, box 30, NASA chronological file, both in Webb Papers. The best discussion of Webb as a manager is found in Lambright's book. While historians consistently cite Webb's reluctance to take the NASA job because he was not an engineer, he was familiar with the aerospace manufacturing industry. He had also sat on the McDonnell Aircraft board of directors when the St. Louis firm was designing and fabricating the Mercury space capsules.

40. Copy of Webb's Tulsa speech, hand-edited, June 16, 1961, for the "First Conference on the Peaceful Uses of Space," box 198, Webb Papers; Cobb and Rieker, *Woman into Space*, p. 201. Cobb adds that, seated at the head table before an audience of two thousand, she had one NASA official on her left and Webb on her right. He was "adding last-minute notes to his speech all during dinner." Interestingly, Weitekamp says that Cobb was not at the dinner at all.

Weitekamp (pp. 255, 267–68) concludes that Webb decided to appoint Cobb to shut her up since Kennedy had just committed NASA to a ten-year, Cold-War space race. This is certainly a plausible notion; however, Webb had been named administrator of NASA just four months previously, and news coverage of the study had been sporadic. He might have been hoping the Cobb announcement would generate favorable publicity. In either case, it appears to have been a spur-of-the-moment decision, and Webb might well have had both goals in mind.

41. Cobb and Rieker, *Woman into Space*, p. 201.

42. Jerrie Cobb, paper presented at the annual meeting of the Aviation and Space Writers Association, May 1, 1961, Jerrie Cobb file, NASA History Office. Cobb argued that military pilots should be reassigned to the military's manned space program and that civilians, including women, should be hired for NASA's flights.

43. Cobb and Rieker, *Woman into Space,* pp. 203, 207.

44. Lovelace, interview with Thomas, tape 2, side 1. In 1960, two and a half years before the congressional hearings, Lovelace told Thomas that women belonged in space but only in support jobs, such as scientist and technician, most likely when the United States had a space station in orbit.

45. Jerrie Cobb to Charles H. Roadman, Office of Life Sciences Programs, NASA, June 16, 1961; Roadman to Cobb, June 29, 1961; and James Webb to Cobb, Sept. 20, 1961, Jerrie Cobb correspondence file, NASA History Office Archives.

46. Cobb to Roadman, June 16, 1961; Roadman to Cobb, June 29, 1961; Roadman to Cobb, Sept. 20, 1961, all in the Jerrie Cobb file, NASA History Office.

47. Jerrie Cobb to James Webb, Mar. 30, 1962, Jerrie Cobb correspondence file, NASA History Office Archives.

48. Cobb and Rieker, *Woman into Space,* p. 6. Cobb's maternal grandfather was Rep. Ulysses Stevens Stone.

49. Lyndon Johnson to James Webb, Mar. 15, 1962; Jerrie Cobb to Lyndon Johnson, Apr. 17, 1962. Science: Space and Aeronautics (Women in Space) folder, container no. 183, vice presidential 1962 subject file, Johnson Presidential Library.

50. Jane Hart to Jacqueline Cochran, June 22, 1962, correspondence file, manuscript materials, Cochran Papers. Hart was politician enough to also advise Cochran of the goings-on, apparently without Cobb's knowledge, and to state that she had concerns about the motives of the congressmen involved. She expressed disappointment to Cochran that Miller had appointed New York Rep. Victor Anfuso as chair of the special subcommittee, noting that "Miller's views rather favored the broad approach; the research program rather than the 'crash' program. I am not sure what Mr. Anfuso thinks about this. The circumstances of the redistricting in New York State which puts Anfuso in a primary contest with the venerable Mr. Rooney causes me some concern. I do not want this hearing to become an attention-getting device for Mr. Anfuso."

51. Letter, Webb to Cochran, Washington, D.C., July 12, 1962, Astronauts: file on women, Webb Papers.

52. House Committee on Science and Astronautics, hearings before the Special Subcommittee on the Selection of Astronauts, 87th Cong., pp. 23–28, 40, 44–75.

Many first-person accounts have been written by WASPs, particularly in the past decade, but little on the program as a whole. *Clipped Wings: The Rise and Fall of the Women Airforce Service Pilots (WASPs) of World War II,* by American studies professor Molly Merryman, is useful because it places the WASPs in the context of the overall air-war effort. In particular, it shows the lack of political clout they had in comparison with the men's, civilian ferry pilots, instructors, and military fliers returning from Europe and facing redeployment in the Pacific. A good first-person work is the two-volume *Sisters in the Sky,* by Adela Riek Scharr, who also served in a predecessor group, the WAF (Women's Air Force), and remained in the U.S. Air Force Reserve until her retirement.

53. For example, "Of Sex and Spaceniks: Cochran Briefs Congress" with photo of Cobb and Hart, *New York Daily News,* July 18, 1962, n.p., Jerrie Cobb file, NASA History Office.

54. Phyllis Battelle, "Assignment: America Blasts Astronette Blaster," *New York Journal-American,* July 25, 1962, p. 27; Bill Moore, "It Says Here: Still Struggling to Get a

Chance at Space," *Kansas City Star*, Sept. 28, 1962; "In the Same Boat," *Ebony*, Oct. 1962, pp. 72–73; Clare Booth Luce, "Without Portfolio," *McCall's*, May 1963, p. 16; "Women Astronauts Needed," in (Newport News) *Times Herald*, June 17, 1963; Richard Starnes, "Give the Girls a Lift," *New York World-Telegram*, July 5, 1963; Robert C. Ruark, "Why Not Put a Lady in Space?" *Telegram*, Aug. 7, 1962; Phyllis Battelle, "Why Not Women in Outer Space?" *San Francisco News Call Bulletin*, July 24, 1962. A few editorials were negative; see "Space Women Expensive," *Science News Letter* 82, no. 70 (Aug. 4, 1962). Even the syndicated comics offered commentary on the women's quest. See *Smilin' Jack*, Oct. 21, 1962; *Glamour Girls*, Oct. 21, 1962; *Grin 'n' Bear It*, Oct. 1, 1962, Jerrie Cobb files, NASA History Office.

55. Neal Stanford, "Washington Report: High G."

56. Appointment affidavit, Jacqueline Cochran, June 11, 1963; memo, R. P. Young to James Webb, June 10, 1963, both in NASA consultant file, manuscript materials, Cochran Papers; memo, Clare F. Farley, executive officer of NASA to Banks, cc: Homer Newell, June 22, 1971, Jacqueline Cochran file, NASA History Office Archives.

57. James Webb to Jerrie Cobb, Apr. 5, 1963, Jerrie Cobb correspondence file, NASA History Office Archives.

EPILOGUE

1. Luft, interview with Spidle, p. 34; photos dated 1976 of Luft and Balke at the crash site, the wreckage still visible, in the Luft Papers.

2. Luft, interview with Spidle, pp. 34–35.

3. Ibid., pp. 35–36.

4. Ibid., pp. 34–35.

5. Luft to Michael Penford, Dec. 22, 1965, folder 24, box 9, Luft Papers.

6. It is difficult to determine how correct this opinion might be. One former SAM employee related an incident in which Flickinger publicly rebuked Benson—in front of his peers—from the podium at an aeromedical conference at the school in 1960 or 1961, accusing him of failing to support space exploration. The employee also said that the team that Armstrong had put together, Benson tried to pull apart, citing Luft's departure as having been caused by Benson's lack of support of the Paperclips. This contradicts what Benson wrote in various books and papers, and, after retirement, he took the job of staff director of bioscience and biomedical engineering for the Southwest Research Institute in San Antonio. Essentially an air force spin-off, Southwest contracted life-sciences studies related to the space program.

7. York Clamann, interview with author; Bubel, interview with the author.

8. York Clamann, interview with author.

9. Spidle, *The Lovelace Medical Center*, pp. 139–42.

NOMENCLATURE
AND SOURCES

NOMENCLATURE

The School of Aviation Medicine was always referred to as such from conception until 1961, when its name was changed to the School of Aerospace Medicine. However, the main human-factors laboratory in Ohio changed its name as the political winds blew. In 1934, Harry Armstrong was initially assigned to the Materiel Division, Engineering Section, Equipment Branch, at what was then called Wright Field. In 1935, this became the Physiological Research Laboratory within the Equipment Branch. In 1939, its name became the Aero Medical Research Unit, part of the newly named Equipment Laboratory until July 1, 1942, when it became the Aero Medical Research Laboratory (AMRL) for five entire months. It was then renamed the Aero Medical Laboratory (AML) and, in the 1980s, became the Aerospace Medical Research Laboratories (AMRL). At some later point, the entire set of human-factors facilities nationwide was renamed the Armstrong Laboratories. Additionally, Wright Field became Wright-Patterson Air Force Base after World War II. To avoid confusion, I refer to the lab that Armstrong founded in Ohio as "the Wright Lab" or a similar descriptive term. Later field units of the Wright Lab are referred to by their geographic locations.

Sources

This book attempts to clear up misinformation about aviation medicine's history, particularly in Hitler-era Germany, that has been published in popular histories. Errors in such books have unfortunately been reprinted in magazines, newspapers, on the Internet, and in other books by authors who have failed to do any primary-source research themselves. What little scrutiny of sources that anyone has done has been narrowly focused, and evidence has been taken out of context, misinterpreted, or mistranslated. This book makes extensive use of a variety of primary historical sources. However, some readers may be unwilling to accept evidence that comes from an individual or organization they believe to be untruthful. Therefore, I am including an explanation of these sources and how I evaluated, chose, and used them.

German

Finding and evaluating sources on the lives and activities of the German scientists before they came to the United States was a challenge. It is a hurdle faced by researchers who study emigrants of any place or era because the written evidence of their actions is usually left behind. In this case, the matter was complicated by the fact that these subjects had lost a war that reached global proportions. Records of ordinary activities and relationships, such as clubs, friendships, marriages, trips, and university studies were preserved only if the site where they were stored remained intact and someone had the time and opportunity to salvage them and bring them to the new country. Bombs might destroy an institution; plunderers might remove objects, papers, photos, or books from a university; and politics might declare that some memories—and therefore some records—were better off left unexamined and unremembered.

Such was the case with the Luftwaffe scientists. When the Allies entered the vanquished Germany in 1945, they immediately began looking both for those whom they could charge with what they termed "crimes against humanity" and for the evidence needed to indict and convict those people. This was a new legal strategy, developed during the war as a means to force an accounting for the genocidal scope and nature of the Nazis' actions. In studying the records left behind or captured soon after VE Day and in querying former concentration-camp inmates, the Allies discovered that these prisons and their inhabitants had been used by German physicians and scientists, who until then were considered the best in the world, for medical experiments that in many cases were nothing but torture or murder. Several aviation-medicine researchers, including some already employed by the United States, were arrested and tried at Nuremberg for their role in experiments in high altitude and in cold-weather environments conducted at Dachau. Most of them were exonerated. However, suspicion dogged these people—and, by association, their colleagues—throughout their lives.

The Germans who came to the United States worked and lived under surveillance by the FBI for years. One reason was the fear that a Nazi might have slipped through the screening process; another was that links to what was then East Germany might make them subject to Soviet control and therefore spies for Communism. Some of the emigrants eschewed further contact with their former associates in Germany. All of them were subject to renewed questioning by the Immigration and Naturalization Service, and at least one (and later his widow) was the object of pursuit by inquisitive reporters and the Anti-Defamation League.

Historians must question whether a particular German might have hidden or destroyed incriminating documents, lied to the Nuremberg tribunal, or colluded with another person to avoid imprisonment or execution. Fortunately, there are primary and secondary sources that can shed light on questions of guilt regarding the human-experimentation charges and the likelihood of deceit or collusion after the event. Such deceit, it should be noted, is of interest not only in dealing with the question of Nazism but also in evaluating the veracity of everything else the person "recalled" in later years.

The primary document of use is the transcript of the first of a series of trials at Nuremberg, *U.S.A. v. Karl Brandt et al.*, also known as the "Physicians' Trial" or the "Doctors' Trial." It is available on microfilm from the National Archives and Records Administration in College Park, Maryland. It is important here to differentiate between the microfilmed, unabridged version of the transcripts and the bound, abridged copies that many libraries hold. Much of the material relating to the aviation-medicine researchers who were acquitted was removed in the editing process. This is also the case for *U.S.A. v. Erhard Milch,* the second Nuremberg trial, in which the charges of human experimentation were brought against the number-two man in the Luftwaffe. Because Milch was also acquitted of those specific charges, much of the testimony pertinent to this study was omitted from the abridged-text version.

Brandt offers as many of the facts related to the events at Dachau as we are ever likely to have, but it also contains excellent portrait sketches of key people who were engaged in aviation-medicine research. Moreover, it offers information about the relationship among the various Luftwaffe-sponsored labs, the German medical-education system, attitudes toward human experimentation and self-experimentation, research protocols, and the mechanics of working within the National Socialist system. Each person on trial had to produce a detailed biography, which was read into the record, and each person testified at length about his training, experience, and activities during the war. Cross-examination usually involved additional questions about beliefs and motivations, standard practices within the profession, and corroboration of the activities, beliefs, and backgrounds of the other defendants. Colleagues and longtime friends (including some Germans who were already packing for the United States) submitted affidavits regarding the professional and personal demeanor and actions of the men on trial, including their political beliefs. Government documents, diaries, paperwork, lab notebooks, and correspondence were read aloud or referred to during the trial, and copies were included as part of the permanent record. Finally, a surprising number of former inmates were located and summoned to testify about their own experiences. In doing so (regardless of whether all of their testimony was accurate or complete), they also provided a glimpse into conditions at the camps: the ethnic, religious, and political makeup of the inmate population; the layout of the sites; the motivations, actions, and demeanor of the physicians; the operation of the medical equipment; and the sub rosa means by which inmates survived their experience.

Because of the richness of the detail provided on these tapes and the corroboration given by multiple sworn testimonies, expert witnesses, and documents, I have used the microfilms in relevant chapters. Wherever possible, I also provide additional citations. These bear out the court evidence.

I believe the likelihood that the aviation-medicine defendants and those who gave affidavits on their behalf are lying is slim, for several reasons. One, torture was carried out at Dachau, but it was proven to have been done by other people who reported directly to Heinrich Himmler and who used established, reputable medical researchers as a screen. Two, a decade earlier these scientists had been publishing their experiments in recognized, widely cited scientific journals. Comparison with these earlier articles affirms the consistency between their actions at Dachau and longtime accepted practices in their field. Three, testimonies from the acquitted, those defendants who were found guilty, and former inmates largely corroborated each other and were supported by the documentary evidence that the Allied prosecutor used.

A second source for recreating the medicine and science of prewar and wartime Germany is *German Aviation Medicine, World War II* (Washington, D.C.: Government Printing Office, 1950). It is a compilation of research papers, introduced by new material written by Hubertus Strughold. It is also a second source of information on the organization of aeromedical research in Germany, activities in the laboratories, research practices, and the results obtained. It is possible to compare some of the articles in the book with earlier versions published in German medical journals and to see that they were faithfully reproduced. The veracity of the book, though, has been questioned by people who have been concerned about the fact that Strughold did not specify that some of the authors and other people cited had been tried at Nuremberg. They have also claimed that some of the research results were obtained from inmate test subjects. These charges are true.

Hubertus Strughold, who plays a key role in the history of German aviation medicine, served as editor for the project and wrote the historical and explanatory chapters. He attributes some of the information in that section to "the last chief of the aeromedical section attached to the *Chef des Sanitätswesen der Luftwaffe*" but does not state outright that this was his former part-time employee, Hermann Becker-Freyseng, who was tried and convicted at Nuremberg. Similarly, he includes a chapter titled "Development, Organization, and Experiences of Aviation Medicine in Germany during World War II," which describes research by the Luftwaffe and university scientists on frostbite and the warming of hypothermia victims, but he does not mention that their activities were part of the deadly cold experiments at Dachau and Auschwitz. Similarly, he says nothing about the poisoning of Gypsy inmates by the forced intake of seawater (and the withholding of fresh water) in his discussion of wartime seawater desalinization research.

The concerns expressed by writers such as journalist Linda Hunt are that these deletions allowed unscrupulous people (and here she includes Strughold) to enter the United States under false pretenses, that is, they lied during questioning about their wartime activities. Ethicists object because they feel that data wrongly obtained (in other words, from experimental subjects not truly at liberty to volunteer or decline) should not be used or even cited for others to use.

From a historian's perspective, the matter of using the actual chapters is somewhat moot because most of them are reprints of papers already published in defunct German journals. In the first two chapters, Strughold's introductory and historical essays, I have found no evidence that he actually lied about any of the facts; everything he says is supported by several other sources. However, as already noted, he leaves things out. The reader must guess whether this is due to a belief that it was simply irrelevant, an embarrassment to Germans who did not engage in such practices or to their new employer (the U.S. Army Air Corps), or a determined, prevaricating effort (apparently unsuccessful) to allow unethical researchers to enter the United States. We may never know which (if any) of these motives were Strughold's and whether anyone in the American military knew the about these oversights and chose to look the other way.

American

The chief caution regarding U.S. military sources is that official unit histories published during this period not only reflect the culture of the time but also are rather blatantly biased in favor of the organizations they chronicle. The authors were typically civilian public-relations writers or secretaries assigned to that unit, and their point of view is evident on every page. Not only is this particular air force base the best base in the world, the author implies, but its commander is the finest officer in the military, its employees are the hardest working, and its buildings the most attractive. On the other hand, it has had the most miserly budget and the most demanding projects to work on and all the while has been dreadfully understaffed. Aside from that, these official histories are usually good sources of detail (including photos) not found in publications that address activities at higher organizational levels.

Anniversary or project histories that commemorate specific labs, wars, or research programs are likewise factual but larded with laudatory prose. In the case of medicine, the aim is usually to prove that one person or another was the first to do or discover something. For example, the authors who were charged with writing fifty-year anniversary books for the School of Aviation Medicine and the Wright Lab both argue that Harry Armstrong, another key figure in this book, was fully responsible for the resurgence of aviation medicine in the United States. All the evidence strongly supports their claim, thus the basis for the name "Armstrong Laboratories." However, the authors of the nine-hundred-plus-page *Medical Support of the Army Air Forces in World War II*, an official history published ten years after the war's end, credit someone higher up, Gen. Malcolm Grow, with being the brains and driving force behind practically everything the medical corps ever accomplished. In reality, Grow spent almost no time in a laboratory and published little in scientific journals during his military career.

Both sorts of official histories are replete with useful statistics, names, charts, and photographs, and they do a good job of explaining the problems that flight surgeons and air surgeons were up against and the military and humanitarian significance of their work. However, the base histories were typically written by someone on the scene and reflect the current objectives of the author, that is, establishing someone's preeminence for posterity, while the anniversary books have the additional challenge of interpreting events of longer ago. I suspect that the authors of *Medical Support of the Army Air Forces in World War II* relied too much on the memories of high-ranking officers and did not double- and triple-check the character evaluations they were offered. There is ample evidence to prove Harry Armstrong's preeminence in and contributions to the field, but he was also well known to eschew praise for himself and instead give credit to everyone else. As USAF surgeon general at the time, Armstrong was most likely interviewed but did not change his self-deprecating tendencies. The result is that credit for his accomplishments has been distributed unevenly, and these misstatements have been repeated in some secondary histories. I chose to cite only the hard data and chronologies from this source. With base histories, I used nearly everything but verified details of character with personal interviews and other research.

Archives

The Aeromedical Library at Brooks Air Force Base has a collection of old aviation-medicine books, many of which appear to have belonged to the Germans who came to the School of Aviation Medicine. Up against one wall are several cardboard boxes labeled with Hubertus Strughold's name and several file cabinets that are said to contain the records of Strughold and Col. John Paul Stapp. Searching through these files revealed that many of them must have been the property of Hans-Georg Clamann, Strughold's longtime friend and chief assistant in Germany, who also came to Texas after the war. In citing the documents found in this box, I have distinguished between the two Germans by saying that the citations are from "the Uncatalogued Papers of Hans-Georg Clamann" or "the Uncatalogued Papers of Hubertus Strughold." These papers may never be cataloged and are not listed in the National Union Catalog of Manuscript Collections (NUCMC) or in online sources. One reason for this disorganization is lack of money and staff at the library, but another may be the controversy over Strughold's activities in wartime Germany. The library was named the Strughold Aeromedical Library after his retirement, but opposition by the Anti-Defamation League after his death forced the removal of the name "Strughold." The holes in the side of the building can still be seen.

Oral Histories

The archived oral histories I have used presented few problems in terms of consistency with other sources, with the exception of the informants' ability to remember exact dates. An example is the first meeting between Hubertus Strughold and Harry Armstrong. In a 1981 journalistic interview, Armstrong remembered it as having taken place in 1934. However, he also said that Strughold was a research fellow in Cleveland that year (he had actually been there in 1929), that both were publishing a book on aviation medicine (both wrote their books in 1939), and that both held the same job (which Strughold did not get until 1935). In 1959, Strughold told an interviewer first that the meeting took place in Washington, D.C., in 1938, but a year later he said that it had been in The Hague in 1929. Thankfully, Strughold also remembered that the occasion was a conference in the United States at which he had been made an honorary member of the Aero Medical Association. An issue of the *Journal of Aviation Medicine* describes that event, including Strughold's introduction, and notes that Armstrong was presenting a paper, his first, at the meeting. The location was New York City; the year, 1937.

Neither man had any reason to make up these dates and cities; I believe the dates they gave are simply the result of faulty memories after a lifetime of conventions and professional acquaintances. Armstrong recalled that he and Strughold became "quite good friends" for the two or three days of the conference, based on their mutual interests and the fact that they were the same age. This is probably true. This is not the most blatant such error, but I have attempted to verify all of the dates and events related in oral histories with other sources.

One excellent and little-used source is the collection of oral-history interviews, notes, and transcriptions by journalist Shirley Thomas in the Lilly Library of Indiana University in Bloomington. A nice surprise was that every word of the interviews was not transcribed. Listening to the tapes, one hears the entire conversation, plus the expression in their voices, laughter, accents, interruptions, and background color. Don Flickinger, for example, who was a gourmet cook, was taped while fixing something for himself and Thomas to eat. One can catch misinterpretations made by the transcriptionist and occasionally find a short interview with a colleague that did not make it into the transcription at all.

These tapes and notes are treasures, but footnoting became rather cumbersome because of the multiple transcripts and the tapes. To be as complete as possible, the transcription number, page, and tape are all included in each citation.

Scientific Journals

Scientific and medical publications were a significant source, not only because of the data in the articles but also because American publishers sometimes included a verbatim account of an annual convention. Especially in the prewar years, this includes opening remarks, banquet speeches, meetings of specialty subgroups, discussions after a paper, and the business meetings. They are quite useful as aids to understanding the social culture of the medical profession during that era. In two cases, for example, prominent dinner speakers from government and medicine opened their remarks with jokes about minorities. In Germany and in Italy, however, no spontaneous give-and-take, discussions, editorials, or business are included because the journals did not accompany membership in an organization. In a rare few instances, though, a speech by a speaker from an outside agency was reprinted. These invariably extol the virtues of fascism or the Nazi system and, in Germany, praise Hermann Göring, whose photograph—in a flattering, heroic pose—is usually included. Above all, the speeches give credit for everything good that happened in Germany to *der Führer*, Adolf Hitler.

BIBLIOGRAPHY

COLLECTIONS AND ARCHIVES

Aerospace Medicine and Human Factors Engineering Collection. Fordham Health Sciences Library, Wright State University School of Medicine, Dayton, Ohio.

Air Force Historical Research Agency. Maxwell AFB, Montgomery, Ala.

Brooks Air Force Base Office of History archives, Aeromedical Library archives, and Museum of Aerospace Medicine (Hangar Nine). Brooks AFB, San Antonio, Tex.

Cochran, Jacqueline, Papers. Dwight D. Eisenhower Presidential Library, Abilene, Kans.

Columbia University Oral History Collection, New York.

Federal Bureau of Investigation. Records. Department of Justice, Washington, D.C.

High-Altitude Medicine Collection. Mandeville Special Collections Library, University of California at San Diego.

International Women's Air and Space Museum archives, Cleveland, Ohio.

Johnson, Lyndon B. U.S. Senate Papers and Vice Presidential Papers. Lyndon B. Johnson Presidential Library, Austin, Tex.

Lowell Observatory archives. Flagstaff, Ariz.

NASA Headquarters History Office archives. Washington, D.C.

New Mexico Medical History Program, University of New Mexico Health Sciences Center Library, University of New Mexico, Albuquerque.

Nuremberg War Crimes Trials. Records. *United States of America v. Karl Brandt et al.* (case 1), November 21, 1946, to August 20, 1947 (microfilm 887), and *United States of America v. Erhard Milch* (case 2), October 1946 to April 1949 (microfilm M888). National Archives and Records Administration, College Park, Md.

Rockefeller Archive Center, Rockefeller University, Sleepy Hollow, N.Y.

Central Periodicals Holdings. San Antonio Public Library, San Antonio, Tex.

Thomas, Shirley. Collection. Lilly Library, Indiana University, Bloomington, Ind.

Webb, James E., Papers. Harry S. Truman Presidential Library, Independence, Mo.

Books

Altman, Lawrence K. *Who Goes First? The Story of Self-Experimentation in Medicine.* New York: Random House, 1987.

Annas, George G., and Michael A. Grodin. *The Nazi Doctors and the Nuremberg Code: Human Rights in Human Experimentation.* New York: Oxford University Press, 1992.

Armstrong, Harry G., ed. *Aerospace Medicine.* Baltimore: Williams and Wilkins, 1961.

———. *Principles and Practices of Aviation Medicine.* Baltimore: Williams and Wilkins, 1939, 1943, 1952.

Atkinson, Joseph D., and Jay M. Shafritz. *The Real Stuff: A History of NASA's Astronaut Recruitment Program.* New York: Praeger, 1985.

Bainbridge, William Sims. *The Spaceflight Revolution: A Sociological Study.* Malabar, Fla.: Krieger, 1983.

Baker, Robert B., Arthur L. Caplan, Linda L. Emanuel, and Stephen R. Latham. *The American Medical Ethics Revolution: How the AMA's Code of Ethics Has Transformed Physicians' Relationships to Patients, Professionals, and Society.* Baltimore: Johns Hopkins University Press, 1999.

Benford, Robert J. *Doctors in the Sky: The Story of the Aero Medical Association.* Springfield, Ill.: Charles C. Thomas, 1955.

———. *The Heritage of Aviation Medicine: An Annotated Directory of Early Artifacts.* Washington, D.C.: Aerospace Medical Association, 1979.

———. *Report from Heidelberg: The Story of the Army Air Force's Aero Medical Center in Germany, 1945–1947.* Germany: Graf, 1947.

Benson, Otis O., Jr., and Hubertus Strughold. *Physics and Medicine of the Atmosphere and Space.* New York: John Wiley and Sons, 1960.

Beschloss, Michael R. *Mayday: Eisenhower, Khrushchev, and the U-2 Affair.* New York: Harper and Row, 1986.

Bilstein, Roger E. *Orders of Magnitude: A History of the NACA and NASA, 1915–1990.* Washington, D.C.: NASA, 1989.

Bulkeley, Rip. *The Sputniks Crisis and Early United States Space Policy: A Critique of the Historiography of Space.* Bloomington: Indiana University Press, 1991.

Campbell, Paul A. *History of the Space Medicine Branch of the Aerospace Medical Association.* Houston: Johnson Space Center, 1979.

Caplan, Arthur L., ed. *When Medicine Went Mad: Bioethics and the Holocaust.* Totowa, N.J.: Humana Press, 1992.

Cassidy, David C. *Uncertainty: The Life and Science of Werner Heisenberg.* New York: Freeman, 1992.

Chapman, Sidney. *IGY: Year of Discovery.* Ann Arbor: University of Michigan Press, 1959.

Clark, Burton R., ed. *The Research Foundations of Graduate Education: Germany, Britain, France, United States, Japan.* Berkeley: University of California Press, 1993.

Cobb, Jerrie, with Jane Rieker. *Woman into Space.* Englewood Cliffs, N.J.: Prentice-Hall, 1963.

Cochran, Jacqueline. *The Stars at Noon.* Boston: Little, Brown, 1954.

————, with Maryann Bucknam Brinley. *Jacqueline Cochran: An Autobiography*. New York: Bantam, 1987.

Cooper, Henry S. F., Jr. *The Search for Life on Mars: Evolution of an Idea*. New York: Holt, Rinehart, and Winston, 1980.

Corn, Joseph J. *The Winged Gospel: America's Romance with Aviation, 1900–1950*. New York: Oxford University Press, 1983.

Crossfield, A. Scott, with Clay Blair Jr. *Always Another Dawn: The Story of a Rocket Test Pilot*. Cleveland: World, 1960.

Deichmann, Ute. *Biologists under Hitler*. Trans. Thomas Dunlap. Cambridge: Harvard University Press, 1996.

Dempsey, Charles A. *Fifty Years of Research on Man in Flight: Air Force Aerospace Medical Research Laboratory*. Wright-Patterson AFB: Aerospace Medical Research Laboratory, 1985.

Dethloff, Henry C. *Suddenly Tomorrow Came: A History of the Johnson Space Center*. Houston: Johnson Space Center, NASA, 1993.

DeVorkin, David H. *Race to the Stratosphere: Manned Scientific Ballooning in America*. New York: Springer, 1989.

————. *Science with a Vengeance: How the Military Created the U.S. Space Sciences after World War II*. New York: Springer, 1992.

Dick, Steven J. *The Biological Universe: The Twentieth-Century Extraterrestrial Life Debate and the Limits of Science*. Cambridge: Cambridge University Press, 1996.

Dickson, Paul. *Sputnik: The Shock of the Century*. New York: Walker, 2001.

Divine, Robert A. "Lyndon B. Johnson and the Politics of Space." In *The Johnson Years*. Vol. 2: *Vietnam, the Environment, and Science*, ed. Robert A. Divine. Lawrence: University Press of Kansas, 1987.

————. *The Sputnik Challenge*. New York: Oxford University Press, 1993.

Douglas, Deborah G. *United States Women in Aviation 1940–1985*. Washington, D.C.: Smithsonian Institution Press, 1991.

Edelson, Edward. *Healers in Uniform*. Garden City, N.Y.: Doubleday, 1971.

Elliott, Richard G. " 'On a Comet, Always.' A Biography of Dr. W. Randolph Lovelace II." *New Mexico Quarterly* 36 (1966–1967): 351–88.

Engle, Eloise, and Arnold S. Lott. *Man in Flight: Biomedical Achievements in Aerospace*. Annapolis, Md.: Leeward, 1979.

Franklin, Jon, and John Sutherland. *Guinea Pig Doctors: The Drama of Medical Research through Self-Experimentation*. New York: William Morrow, 1984.

Fries, Sylvia Doughty. *NASA Engineers and the Age of Apollo*. Washington, D.C.: NASA, 1992.

Fritzsche, Peter. *A Nation of Fliers: German Aviation and the Popular Imagination*. Cambridge: Harvard University Press, 1992.

Geison, Gerald R., ed. *Physiology in the American Context, 1850–1940*. Bethesda, Md.: American Physiological Society, 1987.

Gimbel, John. "Project Paperclip: German Scientists, American Policy, and the Cold War." *Diplomatic History* 14(3) (Summer, 1990): 343–36.

Grow, Malcolm, and Harry G. Armstrong. *Fit to Fly: A Medical Handbook for Fliers*. New York: D. Appleton-Century, 1942.

Gubitz, Myron B. *Rocketship X-15: A Bold New Step in Aviation.* New York: Julian Messner, 1960.

Guenther, Ben, Jay Miller, and Terry Panopalis. *North American X-15/X-15 A-2.* Arlington, Tex.: Aerofax, 1985.

Haber, Heinz. *Man in Space.* Indianapolis: Bobbs-Merrill, 1953.

———. *The Physical Environment of the Flyer.* San Antonio: Randolph AFB, USAF School of Aviation Medicine, 1954.

Hacker, Barton C., and James M. Grimwood. *On the Shoulders of Titans: A History of Project Gemini.* Washington, D.C.: NASA, Government Printing Office, 1977.

Hartshorne, Edward Yarnall. *The German Universities and National Socialism.* New York: AMS Press, 1981. Reprint, London: Allen and Unwin, 1937.

Hoyt, William Graves. *Lowell and Mars.* Tucson: University of Arizona Press, 1976.

Hunley, J. D., ed. *The Birth of NASA: The Diary of T. Keith Glennan.* Washington, D.C.: NASA, 1993.

International Dachau Committee. *Concentration Camp Dachau, 1933–1945.* Munich: Lipp, 1978.

Kozloski, Lillian D. *U.S. Space Gear: Outfitting the Astronaut.* Washington, D.C.: Smithsonian Institution Press, 1994.

Lambright, W. Henry. *Powering Apollo: James E. Webb of NASA.* Baltimore: Johns Hopkins University Press, 1995.

Lansberg, M. P. *A Primer of Space Medicine.* Amsterdam: Elsevier, 1960.

Lasby, Clarence G. *Project Paperclip: German Scientists and the Cold War.* New York: Atheneum, 1971.

Launius, Roger D. *NASA: A History of the U.S. Civil Space Program.* Malabar, Fla.: Krieger, 1994.

———, John M. Logsdon, and Robert W. Smith, eds. *Reconsidering Sputnik: Forty Years since the Soviet Satellite.* Amsterdam: Harwood Academic, 2000.

———, and Howard E. McCurdy, eds. *Spaceflight and the Myth of Presidential Leadership.* Urbana: University of Illinois, 1997.

Lederer, Susan E. *Subjected to Science: Human Experimentation in America before the Second World War.* Baltimore: Johns Hopkins University Press, 1995.

Levine, Alan J. *The Missile and Space Race.* Westport, Conn.: Praeger, 1994.

Ley, Willy. *Grundriß einer Geschichte der Rakete.* Leipzig: Hachmeister und Thal, 1932.

———. *Mars der Kriegsplanet.* Leipzig: Hachmeister und Thal, 1927.

———, ed. *Die Möglichkeit der Weltraumfahrt.* Leipzig: Hachmeister und Thal, 1928.

———. *Rockets and Space Travel: The Future of Flight beyond the Stratosphere.* New York: Viking, 1947. Rev. and exp. edition of *Rockets: The Future of Travel beyond the Stratosphere.* New York: Viking, 1944.

Lifton, Robert J. *The Nazi Doctors: Medical Killing and the Psychology of Genocide.* New York: Basic Books, 1986.

Link, Mae Mills. *Space Medicine and Project Mercury.* Washington, D.C.: NASA, 1962.

———, and Hubert A. Coleman. *Medical Support of the Army Air Forces in World War II.* Washington, D.C.: Office of the Surgeon General, USAF, 1955.

Logsdon, John M., Dwayne A. Day, and Roger D. Launius, eds. *Exploring the*

Unknown: Selected Documents in the History of the U.S. Civilian Space Program. Vol. 2: *External Relationships*. Washington, D.C.: NASA, 1996.

Logsdon, John M., Linda J. Lear, Jannelle Warren-Findley, Ray A. Williamson, and Dwayne A. Day, eds. *Exploring the Unknown: Selected Documents in the History of the U.S. Civilian Space Program*. Vol. 1: *Organizing for Exploration*. Washington, D.C.: NASA, 1995.

Logsdon, John M., Ray A. Williamson, Roger D. Launius, Russell J. Acker, Stephen J. Garber, and Jonathan L. Friedman, eds. *Exploring the Unknown: Selected Documents in the History of the U.S. Civilian Space Program*. Vol. 4: *Accessing Space*. Washington, D.C.: NASA, 1999.

Lowell, Percival. *Mars and Its Canals*. New York: Macmillan, 1906.

———. *Mars as the Abode of Life*. New York: Macmillan, 1908.

Mack, Pamela, ed. *From Engineering Science to Big Science: The NACA and NASA Collier Trophy Research Project Winners*. Washington, D.C.: NASA, 1998.

Macrakis, Kristie. *Surviving the Swastika: Scientific Research in Nazi Germany*. New York: Oxford University Press, 1993.

Mallan, Lloyd. *Suiting Up for Space: The Evolution of the Space Suit*. New York: John Day, 1971.

Marbarger, John P., ed. *Space Medicine: The Human Factor in Flights beyond the Earth*. Urbana: University of Illinois Press, 1951.

McDougall, Walter A. *The Heavens and the Earth: A Political History of the Space Age*. New York: Basic Books, 1985.

Meeter, George F. *The Holloman Story: Eyewitness Accounts of Space Age Research*. Albuquerque: University of New Mexico Press, 1967.

Merryman, Molly. *Clipped Wings: The Rise and Fall of the Women Airforce Service Pilots (WASPs) of World War II*. New York: New York University Press, 1998.

Neufeld, Michael J. *The Rocket and the Reich: Peenemünde and the Coming of the Ballistic Missile Era*. New York: Free Press, 1995.

Newell, Homer E. *Beyond the Atmosphere: Early Years of Space Science*. Washington, D.C.: NASA, 1980.

Office of History and Research. *Tour of Historic Randolph*. San Antonio: Randolph AFB, Headquarters of Air Education and Training Command, 1996.

Ordway, Frederick I., III, and Mitchell Sharp. *The Rocket Team*. New York: Thomas Y. Crowell, 1979.

Peyton, Green [Green Peyton Wertenbaker]. *Fifty Years of Aerospace Medicine, 1918–1968*. San Antonio: Brooks AFB, School of Aerospace Medicine, 1968.

Pitts, John A. *The Human Factor: Biomedicine in the Manned Space Program to 1980*. Washington, D.C.: NASA, 1985. Reprinted online February 20, 2002. http://www.history.nasa.gov/SP4213/sp4213.htm.

Proctor, Robert N. *The Nazi War on Cancer*. Princeton: Princeton University Press, 1999.

Robie, Bill. *For the Greatest Achievement: A History of the Aero Club of America and the National Aeronautic Association*. Washington, D.C.: Smithsonian Institution Press, 1993.

Robinson, Douglas H. *The Dangerous Sky: A History of Aviation Medicine*. Seattle: University of Washington Press, 1973.

Rothschuh, Karl E. *History of Physiology*. Trans. Guenter B. Risse. Huntington, N.Y.: Krieger, 1973.

Ruff, Siegfried, Martin Ruck, and Gerhard Sedlmayr. *Sicherheit und Rettung in der Luftfahrt*. Koblenz: Bernard und Graefe, 1989.

———, and Hubertus Strughold. *Grundriß der Luftfahrtmedizin*. Leipzig: Johann Ambrosius Barth, 1939, 1942, and 1957.

Ryan, Craig. *The Pre-Astronauts: Manned Ballooning on the Threshold of Space*. Annapolis, Md.: Naval Institute Press, 1995.

Santy, Patricia A. *Choosing the Right Stuff: The Psychological Selection of Astronauts and Cosmonauts*. Westport, Conn.: Praeger, 1994.

Scharr, Adela Riek. *Sisters in the Sky*. Vol. 1: *The WAFs*. Gerald, Mo.: Patrice Press, 1986.

———. *Sisters in the Sky*. Vol. 2: *The WASPs*. Gerald, Mo.: Patrice Press, 1988.

Siddiqi, Asif A. *Challenge to Apollo: The Soviet Union and the Space Race, 1945–1974*. Washington, D.C.: NASA, 2000.

Simon, Leslie E. *German Research in World War II: An Analysis of the Conduct of Research*. New York: John Wiley and Sons, 1947.

Simons, David G., with Don A. Schanche. *Man High*. Garden City, N.Y.: Doubleday, 1960.

Spicker, Stuart F., Ilai Alon, Andre de Vries, and H. Tristram Engelhardt Jr., eds. *The Use of Human Beings in Research: With Special Reference to Clinical Trials*. Dordrecht: Kluwer Academic Publishers, 1988.

Spidle, Jake W., Jr. *The Lovelace Medical Center: Pioneer in American Health Care*. Albuquerque: University of New Mexico Press, 1987.

Strughold, Hubertus. *The Green and Red Planet: A Physiological Study of the Possibility of Life on Mars*. Albuquerque: University of New Mexico Press, 1953.

Sullivan, Walter. *Assault on the Unknown: The International Geophysical Year*. New York: McGraw-Hill, 1961.

Swenson, Loyd S., Jr., James M. Grimwood, and Charles C. Alexander. *This New Ocean: A History of Project Mercury*. Washington, D.C.: NASA, 1966.

Tent, James F. *Mission on the Rhine: Reeducation and Denazification in American-Occupied Germany*. Chicago: University of Chicago Press, 1982.

Thomas, Shirley. *Men of Space*. Vols. 1–4. Philadelphia: Chilton, 1960–1962.

Trischler, Helmut. "Aeronautical Research under National Socialism: Big Science or Small Science?" In *Science in the Third Reich*, ed. Margit Szollosi-Janze, 79–110. Oxford: Berg, 2001.

U.S. Air Force Surgeon General. *German Aviation Medicine, World War II*. Vols. 1 and 2. Washington, D.C.: Department of the Air Force, 1950.

von Diringshofen, Heinz. *Medical Guide for Flying Personnel*. Trans. Velyien E. Henderson. Toronto: University of Toronto Press, 1940.

Ward, Michael P., James S. Milledge, and John B. West. *High-Altitude Medicine and Physiology*. London: Chapman and Hall Medical, 1989.

Weitekamp, Margaret Ann. "The Right Stuff, the Wrong Sex: The Science, Culture, and Politics of the Lovelace Woman in Space Program, 1959–1963." Ph.D. diss., Cornell University, Ithaca, N.Y., May 2001.

West, John B. *High Life: A History of High-Altitude Physiology and Medicine*. New York: Oxford University Press for the American Physiological Society, 1998.

White, Clayton S., and Otis O. Benson Jr., eds. P*hysics and Medicine of the Upper Atmosphere*. Albuquerque: University of New Mexico Press, 1952.

Wilson, Charles L., ed. *Project Mercury Candidate Evaluation Program*. Dayton: Wright-Patterson AFB, Wright Air Development Center, Air Research and Development Command, 1959.

Wilson, J. Tuzo. *IGY: The Year of the New Moons*. New York: Alfred A. Knopf, 1961.

Winter, Frank H. *Rockets into Space*. Cambridge: Harvard University Press, 1990.

Workers of the Writers' Program of the Works Project Administration in the State of Texas, comps. *Randolph Field: A History and Guide*. New York: Devin-Adair, 1942.

INDEX

Pages with illustrations appear in *italic*
typeface.

acceleration, study of: in Germany 39,
60, 68, *84*, 86, 90; in United States, 6,
74, 123–24, 140, 155–57, 161, 169, 192; in
USSR, 249–50*n*53
acclimation/acclimatization, 60, 62–63,
65, 68, 98, 160–61, 169, 228*n*77, 245*n*84
aeroembolism, 28, 29, 60, 62, 70, 93
Aero Medical Association: and ethics,
34; formation of, 12, 32, 221*n*36; and
Lovelace study and, 253*n*9; meetings
of, 107, 167, 178, 197–98, 265; professionalism of aerospace medicine, 4,
54, 67, 121, 149; publication of 39; space
committee of, 150, 239*n*55, 242*n*37
Aeromedical Research Laboratory (at
Wright Field): and BLB mask, 35–36;
during Cold War 105, 121, 133, 139,
173, 182, 190–92, 237*n*27, 259, 264; and
development of aircraft, 75, 76; and
development of medical equipment,
74, 76–78; facilities of, 124; founding
of, 21–22; funding for, 219*n*15; and
LMFI, I, *21*, 40; and Lovelace study,
213; and relationship with the SAM,
123, 125; and space medicine, 124, 127,
137, 138, 147, 152–54, 157, 162–65, *180*,
190–93, 236*n*18; during WWII, 69, 70,
73–79, 88, 186

aeronautical design/engineering:
in Germany, 5, 31, 40, 60; in the
Netherlands, 31; in United States, 31,
152–55, 243*n*41. *See also under* airplanes,
design/engineering of
Air Force Association, 200, 212
air racing and racers, 18, 32, 35, 206, 209,
222*n*44
aircraft equipment, military, 15, 16, 27, 79,
80, 85–86
airline industry: aeromedical research
for, 7, 31, 186; in Germany, 40; in
United States, 11, 31–33
airplanes
aeromedical research platforms: at
Holloman AFB, 244*n*62; in Germany, 45–47, 49–50; in United States,
76–77, 124, 169–72
design/engineering of; pre-WWII, 19,
26–27, 31–32, 60, 73, 75; post-WWII,
89, 124, 140, 169–70; WWII, 85. *See also*
aeronautical design/engineering
experimental: American, 27, 124, 137,
138, 140, 152, 155, 169–72; German,
60, 87, 89, 105, 108
military role of, 11, 60, 79, 105, 137, 170
performance and characteristics of,
18–19, 27, 79, 80, 89, 98, 137, 138
risks associated with: propeller aircraft
11, 16–19, 27, 39, 76–77, 78; jets 60, 70,
80, 89, 123, 124, 125, 152–55, 169–72

airplanes (*cont.*)

specific makes: B-17, 27, 29, 71, 76–77, 78, 80–81, *86*, 220*n*12, 220*n*21, 234*n*57; B-29, 78, 138; Boeing B-307, 32; C-4, 16; C-14, 16; DC-3, 32; Heinkel He-70, 51 and He-178, 89; Henschel Hs-130, 89; Ju-88, 98; Klemm, 47, 89; Messerschmitt Me-163 Komet and Me-262, 89; O-25, 23; O-39, 27; P-16, 13–14, 16; P-51 Mustang, 90; PB-2A, 27; Spitfire, 98; U-2, 173, 186, 246*n*93; Udet U-12 Flamingo, 50, *55;* X-1, 124, 137, 138, 140, 171; X-15, 7, 169–72, 173, *180*, 186, 200, 202

airships, 18, 39, 40, 44, 70, 224*n*17

airsickness, 24, 32, 45, 72, 151

Alpine research, 5, 44, 53, 67, 90, 98

Alps, 5, 37, 44, 53, 62, 90

altitude chamber. *See* low pressure chamber

altitude sickness. *See* specific maladies

American Medical Association, 34, 66, 149

Andes, research in, 31, 35, 132, 134–35, 197

Anfuso, Victor L., 212, 256*n*50

animal subjects testing: and animal rights activists, 243*n*46; bears, 152, 154, 158–59; cats, 243*n*43; dogs 48, 177, 179, 182, 249–50*n*53; insects, 145; pigs, 152, 154; primates, 96, 146, 152, 154–55, 158–59, *179*, 182, 212, 242*n*25; rabbits, 28; rodents, 146–47, 166–61, 216, *181;* small lab animals, 24–25, 95, 146, 153; turtles, 160–61, 244*n*62; unspecified, 73, 94, 124, 140, 249–50*n*53

anoxia, 17, 19, 24, 63, 65–66, 78, 81, 90, 123, 169. *See also* oxygen deprivation/deficiency, acclimation/acclimatization; physiology, high altitude

anthropometry, 74, 75–76, 191

anti-Semitism, 40, 50–53, 56, 88, 91, 92, 94, 228*n*6, 261, 265

Apollo program, 198, 212, 213

Argentina, 63, 114, 160–61, 236*n*21, 244*n*61

Armstrong, Harry G.: and Aero Medical Association, 32–33; appointment to Wright Field, 15–16, 18–19, 21–22; and aviation/aerospace medicine, 16, 26, 80, 105, 107, 108, 124, 126, 149, 178–79; as flight surgeon, 4, 13–18, 23, 29–30, 80, 160, 219*n*10; flying experience of, 12, 13–15, 27, 29–30, 63; as military officer, 15–16, 18–19, 21–22, 23–24, 36, 37–38, 80, 86, 128–29, 264; outspokenness of 15, 21, 26; parachute jump, 29–30; personality of, 16, 29–30, 264, 239*n*64, 264; physical description of, 20, 33; and pilots, 13, 16–17, 19, 28, 220*n*27; and Project Paperclip, 111–14, 117, 118–19, 126, 133; pseudonym of, 16, 218n9; as researcher, 5, 15, 20–22, 23–25, 28–30, 35–36, 38, 78, 123, 236*n*14; and retirement of, 215; at SAM, 124, 126–27, 175, 210, 264; and space medicine, 107, 124, 125, 126–27, 150, 174, 216, 239*n*55; and Strughold, Hubertus, 33, 41, 67, 126; training of 12–13, 1 , 16, 27, 38; and U.S. political system, 40; as writer, 5, 16, 218*n*9; as Wright Lab director, 19–21, 73–74, 80, 123–24, 126, 140, 191, 259, 264, 265–66; youth of, 14

Armstrong, Mary (Mrs. Harry Armstrong), 33, 107, 119

Armstrong, Neil, *180*, 213

Armstrong Line, the, 24, 165

Army Air Forces Aero Medical Center at Heidelberg, 111, 114, 119–20, *131–32*

astronauts: Mercury 7, 204; screening of, 7, 168, 173, 189–93, 200, 202–203, 251*n*78, 251*n*80, 251*n*81, 251*n*82; selection requirements for, 168–69, 187–89, 193–94, 213, 245*n*83; training of, 168, 212–13

astronomy, 141–44, 160

Atlas. *See* missiles

Atomic Energy Commission, 175, 184, 187

Austria, 67, 81, 90, 94–95, 97, 98, 114, 236*n*21, 244*n*61

autoexperimentation. *See* self-experimentation

automobile safety, 140, *163*, 167

aviation medicine: creation of, 11, 12; military, 3, 8, 18, 27, 28, 60, 63, 64, 69; professionalization of, 12, 21–22, 23, 32–33, 34, 54–60, 67–68, 149–50. *See also* space medicine; Aeromedical Research Laboratory

bailouts, 18, 39, *83*, 87, 89–90, 93, 123–24, 156, 162–65, 170. *See also* Armstrong, Harry; Lovelace, W. Randolph; Kittinger, Joe

Balke, Annemarie (Mrs. Bruno Balke), 98

Balke, Bruno: *59*, 62, 63–64, 95, 97–98, 132, 168–69, 228*n*76, 245*n*83, 245*n*84, 254–44*n*33

Balke treadmill test, 193

ballooning, scientific and military, 18, 45–46, 70, 146–47, 159–60, 166, 192, 194, 219*n*10, 244*n*59

balloons, as research platforms, 6, 39, 45–46, 125, 137, 146–47, 152, 159–60, 162–63, 248*n*29

Bauer, Paul, *59*, 118, 228*n*73

Becker-Freyseng, Hermann, 54, 60–61, 64, *82*, 94–95, 97, 118, *132*, 238*n*32, 263

Beckh, Harald von, 114, 160–62, *165*, 182, 236*n*21, 244*n*61, 244*n*62

Beeding, Eli L., 159, *164*

Beischer, Dietrich, 198, 252*n*96

Belgium, 107, 197, 230*n*97

Bell Aircraft (company), 138, 197

bends, the, 28, 70

Benford, Robert J., 236*n*11, 237*n*24, 237*n*28

Benson, Otis O. Jr.: and Aero Medical Association, 149–50; and Paperclips, 133, 257*n*6; at SAM, 73–74, *129*, 177, *181*, 242*n*23; training of, 35, 74, 222*n*42, 230*n*5; and USAF manned space program, 197, 215–16; at Wright Lab, 73–74, 121, 123, 191; during WWII 75, 76, 231*n*12

Benzinger, Theodor Hannes: at AAF Aero Medical Center at Heidelberg, *131*; military service of, 98; as Paperclip, 115; at Rechlin, 40, 59, 63, 95, 115, 227*n*53, 229*n*80, 231*n*16, 233*n*45

Berlin: during WWII, 93, 95, 97, 99–101, 160, 228*n*62, 235*n*65; pre-WWII, 25, 37, 40, 50–54, 63, 67, 229*n*83; post-WWII, 107, 110, 113, 120

Berlin, University of, 5, 60–61, 90, 111, 113

biology and space, 125, 14, 145–46, 160, 198, 246–47*n*10, 249–50*n*53

biophysics and aeromedicine, 73, 74, 124, 145–46, 148–49, 156, 169

BLB. *See* Boothby-Lovelace-Bulbulian mask

blind flying, 18, 32. *See also* radio navigation

Bohr, Niels, 92, 109

Boothby, Walter, 12, 35–36, 134, 221*n*41, 222*n*42

Boothby-Lovelace-Bulbulian (BLB) mask, 35–36, 73

Brauer, Ludolph, 55–56, 228*n*63, 228*n*64

Braun, Wernher von: education of, 121; and Mars, 141; and manned space flight, 6, 105, 121–22, 127–28, *133*, 168, 239*n*61; designs U.S. missiles, 116, 125, 145–46, 148, 178, 186, 216, 246–47*n*10, 247*n*19, 248*n*29; and wartime rocketry, 111

Bronk, Detlev, 112, 197

Brooks Field (**AFB**), Texas, 29, 71, 96–97, 265

Brucker, Wilber M., 185–86, 195–96

Büttner, Konrad, 95, 98–99, 116, 127, *130*, 133, 135, 146, 150, 238*n*38

Cagle, Myrtle "Kay," *205*, 254*n*31

Campbell, Paul, 112–13, 127, 129, 150, 216, 225*n*34, 236*n*14, 242*n*37

Canada, 12, 36–37, 38

Cannon, Walter, 34, 43, 222*n*2, 230*n*5, 231*n*10

CARE packages, 120, 238*n*38

Carlson, Anton, 43, 48–49, 225*n*26, 225*n*27

Carpenter, M. Scott Jr., 194, 212, 250*n*67

[Case] Western Reserve, 47–48, 221*n*41, 226*n*37, 225*n*26

Central Medical Establishment (**CME**), England, 69, 79–81, 85–86, 111

centrifugal forces, 17, 123, 162, 226*n*46. *See also* acceleration, study of; deceleration, study of; G-forces

centrifuges: animal, 51; in Canada, 38; in Germany, 51, 66, 68, 125; invention of 25; at Wright Lab, *21*, 24, 25–26, 74, 78, 124, 191–92

Chicago, Ill., 14–15, 48–49

Chicago, University of, 48–49, 112, 144, 150, 221*n*41, 225*n*26

China, 46–47, 67, 227*n*59

Cincinnati, University of, 38, 76

Civil Aeronautics Authority (**CAA**), 206, 220*n*26

civil aviation, 11–12, 18, 31–32, 185

Clamann, Hans-Georg: at **LMFI** 58, 60–61, 95, 99, 121, 238*n*32; and Nazi Party, 64; papers of, 265; and Project Paperclip, 114; at **SAM**, 146, 168, 176, *181*, 216; training of, 51–52; and United States, 115–18,119, 132, 136; and wartime pressures, 99–100, 100–101

Clamann, Marie (Mrs. Hans-Georg Clamann), 101, 116–18, 132

clothing, 13, 17, 74, 75–76, 77, 85, 124. *See also* pressure suits; protective gear

Cobb, Jerrie: and Lovelace study, 202–206, *204*, *205*, 208–209, 253*n*11, 254*n*20, 254*n*21, 254*n*29, 255*n*40; as pilot, 200–202, 253*n*6; and political lobbying, 210–13, 255*n*42, 256*n*48, 256*n*50

Cochran, Jacqueline (Mrs. Floyd Odlum): and **BLB** mask, 35–36; and Collier Trophy, 35–36; describes Lovelace, 76; and Lovelace study, 200, *203*, 206–207, 209–11, 213, 254*n*20, 254*n*29, 254*n*30; as a pilot, 18, 35, 206, 222*n*44, 254*n*22; and political power, 177, 211, 254*n*26, 256*n*50; and **WASP**, *87*, 211; youth of, 254*n*26

cold: effect on humans, 13–15, 76–77, 87; effect on equipment, 14, 35–36, 75; protection against, 13, 15, 27, 74, 85–86; research on, 39, 74–75, 94–96, 168, 260, 263. *See also* frostbite

Cold War, 70, 110, 122, 128, 173, 194–95, 199, 202, 210–11, 246*n*93

commercial aviation, 11, 31–33, 35, 186. *See also* airline industry

computer technology, 75–76, 190

Congress, U.S., 194, 196; House, 184–86, 211–12, 248*n*29, 256*n*50; Senate, 175, 177, 183–86, 195. *See also* Johnson, Lyndon B.

cosmonauts, 195, 210, 212, 248*n*28, 252*n*2

crashes and crash safety, 17–18, 25, 27, 73, 90, 140, *163*, 221*n*32

Crossfield, Scott, 76, 170–72, 187–88, 193, 197

Dachau, 40, 50, 92–97, 94–95, 122–23, 228*n*62, 233*n*41, 237n24, 260–63

Daisy Track, 158–59, 161, *164*

deafness. *See* hearing

deceleration, study of, 39, 73, 74, 86, 123, 140, 155–56, 161, 162, 169

decompression, explosive, 34–35, 78, 169, 231*n*16

dentistry, 25, 72, 91

Department of Defense (DOD), 148, 178, 183, 184, 185, 186, 194, 195, 196

Deutsche Alpenverein, 62, 63, 229*n*86

Deutsche Versuchsanstalt für Luftfahrt (DVL), 40, *57*, 59–60, 63, 88–89, 90–91, 93–94

Dietrich, Jan, 254*n*31

Dietrich, Marion, 254*n*31

Dill, Bruce, 31, 231*n*10

Diringshofen, Bernd von, 50–51, 90

Diringshofen, Heinz von, 40–41, 50–51, 63, 89–90, 114, 121, 151, 160–61, 226*n*46, 234*n*49

Disney, Walt, 121–22, *133*

Doolittle, James, 18, 32, 186–87, 220*n*27

Dornberger, Walter, 122, 197

Dornier, 40, 87

Drinker, Cecil W. 23, 219*n*17, 230*n*5, 231*n*10

Dryden, Hugh, 185, 248*n*29

Edwards Air Force Base, Calif., 140, 171–72. *See also* Muroc Army Air Base

Einstein, Albert, 92, 109

Eisenhower, Dwight D., 178, 184, 185, 186, 187–88, 194, 196, 199

ejection seats: in Germany, 5, 39, 68, 78, *82*, 87, 89–90, 232*n*25; proposed for

space 165, 243*n*45, 248*n*28; in Sweden, 78; in United States, 6, 73, 78–79, 124, 139, 140, 153, 156–57, 161–62;

engineering, research in, 3, 39, 121–22, 148–49, 151, 184

environment, of space, 125, 146–47, 148–52, 159–60, 162, 191, 197

environmental systems/controls, 176, *180*, 197

Erprobungstelle Rechlin. *See* Rechlin

escape systems. *See also* ejection seats

ethics, 34–35, 40, 64, 108, 122–23, 225*n*27, 228–29*n*78; medical, 34–35, 40, 92, 108, 122–23, 152–53, 232–33*n*36, 237*n*24, 242*n*37, 260–63

exobiology, 6, 105, 141, 143–44, 197–98, 241*n*12, 241*n*13, 241*n*14, 241*n*18

Explorer I (satellite), 176, 246–47*n*10

Farrell, Donald G., 176–77, *181*

Federal Bureau of Investigation (FBI), 135, 240*n*71, 260

Fédération Aéronautique Internationale (FAI), 200, 206–07, 222*n*44, 254*n*22

flak, 80, 235n65

flak suits. *See* protective gear

Flickinger, Don D.: Lovelace study and, 200–202, 206, 213, 254*n*20; and manned space flight 167, 199–200, *201*, 257*n*6; and the Mercury program, 187–88, 193; and MISS program, 180, 182–83, 190–91; parachuting and, 166–67, 245*n*76; retirement of, 216, 245*n*78; as source, 266; during WWII, 166–67

flight suits. *See* pressure suits

flight surgeons: and Aero Medical Association, 150; duties of, 5, 19; hazards of 15, 27–30, 34–35; and pilots, 3, 16–17, 28, 81, 251*n*78; and research, 35, 155, 157, 159–60; training of, 12, 14, 20, 23, 71. *See also* individual flight surgeons flying, physical stresses of: 17–18, 19, 21, 72–73, 80–81, 83, 85–86, 89–90, 123–25, 162. *See also* space flight

flying, psychological stresses of, 17–18, 91, 162, 165

Fort Bliss, Texas, 116, 145–46

France, 42, 66, 78, 97, 206, 230*n*97

Freiburg, University of, 59, 89, 227*n*56, 228*n*67, 229*n*86

Frey, Max von, 43, 44–45, 48, 49, 50, 66, 223–24*n*14, 225*n*28

frostbite, 15, 77, 81, 83, *84,* 85–86, 263

fuel toxicity, 39, 89, 91, 98

Funk, Mary Wallace "Wally" II, *205,* 254*n*31

Gauer, Otto, 54, 90, 115, 123, *132,* 133, 150, 238*n*32, 239*n*50

Gerathewohl, Siegfried, 123, *131,* 150, 151, 232*n*31, 232*n*32, 243*n*43

German American space program, hybridization after WWII: medical, 4, 105, 107, 109–111, 112, 114, 122–23, 145–46, 148, 168, 216, 237*n*28, 260; rocketry, 4, 105, 109–11, 121–23, 145–46, 148, 168

German Aviation Medicine, World War II, 262–63

German scientists, after WWII, 109–11, 111–14, 121–22, 123

Germany
aeronautical engineering/design in, 31, 39–40, 51, *82–84,* 86–89, 110–11, 122, 235*n*73
aftermath of WWII in, *106,* 108–14, 115–16, 119–20, 135–36, 237*n*25, 237*n*28, 238*n*38, 260
aircraft manufacturing in, 18, 40, 47, 44, 84, 87, 89–90, 107
airmindedness in, 40, 44, 224

aviation medicine: pre-WWII, 5, 40–41, 44–45, 50–51, 66–68, 226*n*46, 228*n*63; during WWII, 39–40, 59–60, 63, 78, *82–84,* 88–96, 97–99, 260–63, 229*n*85, 232*n*34, 233*n*41, 233*n*45; post-WWII, 107, 113–14

graduate science and medical education in: Hitler period, 50, 54, 227*n*57; post-WWII, 115–16, 237*n*28, 239*n*50; pre-WWI, 5, 42–43, 47, 220*n*20, 222*n*42, 223*n*8, 223*n*12, 223*n*13, 224–25*n*20, 226*n*37

medical ethics in: Hitler period, 40, 50, 69, 92–97, 122, 232*n*31, 237*n*24, 260–63; Weimar era, 34; WWI, 47, 108

medical licensing in, 43, 50, 63–64

medical research in: pre-WWII, 25, 35, 37, 39–41, 43, 50–51, 53–58, 60–63, 67, 228*n*63; during WWII, 36, 59–60, 63, 68, *83–84,* 86–99, 115, 232*n*34; after WWII, 115, 197, 227*n*57

professional organizations in, 54

remilitarization after WWI, 5, 39, 40–41, 51, 64, 68

sport aviation in, 39, 40, 47

World War II: air war against Britain, 38; flak, 80; invasion of Poland, 67; wonder weapons, 107–108; 69, 70, 76, 79, 82–84, 86–101, 99–101, 160

Gestapo, 55, 92, 228*n*62

G-forces: in airplanes, 18, 87, 200, 243*n*45; experiments with, 34, 50–51, 77, 125, 140, 152–59, *163,* 208; protection against, 74, 90, 170–72; in spacecraft, 168, 169, 183, 192

Glenn, John H. Jr., *182,* 194, 212

Glennan, T. Keith, 187

Gorelick, Sarah, 205, 254*n*31

Göring, Hermann, 39, 40, 51, 63, 68, 88, 224*n*20, 266

Göttingen, University of, 42, 53, 101, 114, 224–25*n*24, 227*n*53, 235*n*73

government spending: in Germany, 3–4, 39, 63–64, 88, 92; in United States, 3–4, 122, 126, 159, 166–67, 184, 207, 219n15, 244n59; after *Sputnik*, 175, 183, 194

Graybiel, Ashton, 128, 255*n*36

Great Depression, 24, 31, 139

Greim, Robert Ritter von, 46–47, 49–50, 51, 224*n*20

Grissom, Virgil I., 194, 210

Grow, Malcolm, 80, 111, 127, 264

Haber, Fritz, 127, *130*, 133, 150, 161, 239*n*57

Haber, Heinz, 124–25, 126–27, *130*, *131*, 133, 145, 150, 174, 176, 239*n*55

Habilitation, 43, 93, 228*n*67, 230*n*91

Hamburg, University of, 50–51, 55, 228*n*63

Harris, Thomas J., 201, 208

Hart, Jane (Mrs. Senator Philip Hart), *205*, 211–12, 254*n*31, 256*n*50

Hartmann, Hans, 53, 62–63, 64, 227*n*53, 227*n*56, 228*n*73, 230*n*96

Harvard: and contract research 121, 220*n*20; department of applied physiology, 23, 219n17; Fatigue Laboratory, 31, 73, 75, 189; instructors, 23, 31, 167, 219n17, 222*n*42, 230*n*5, 231*n*10; Observatory, 142, 197, 241*n*14; Peabody Museum 75–76; step test 193

hearing, 70, 90, 123–24, 191

heart, 24, 33, 48, 65, 93–94, 171, 192, 249–50*n*53

heat, 17–18, 85, 98, 100, 125, 160, 169, 172, 191, 251*n*81

Heidelberg, University of, 105, 111, 114, 115–16, 126, 237*n*25, 237*n*28

Heidelberg AMC. *See* Army Air Forces Aero Medical Center at Heidelberg

Heim, John W. "Bill": appearance, 24; as acting head of Wright lab, 38; collaboration with Armstrong, 22, 23–24, 26, 31, 33, 123; training, 23–24; 220*n*20, 222*n*42, 230*n*5

Heinkel He-70, 51, 87, *84*

Heisenberg, Werner, 64, 228–29*n*78

Henry, James, 138, 146, 157

high-altitude medicine, 4, 24, 34–35, 39, 61, 62–63, 67, 81, 90, 123–25

Himalayas: expeditions to, 35, *59*, 62–63, 67, 134, 215, 227*n*53, 227*n*55, 228*n*73, 230*n*96; journal articles and books about, 118, 227*n*54, 228*n*74, 228*n*75, 228n27; speculation about, 241*n*12

Himmler, Heinrich, 64, 88, 92–95, 262

Hippke, Erich, 41, 51, 60, 67–68, 91, 94–96, 228*n*62

Hitler, Adolf, 39, 40, 46, 50, 68, 88, 96, 101, 229*n*85, 266

Hixson, Jean, 254n31

Holloman, George V., 27, 220*n*26

Holloman AFB, New Mex.: balloon research at, 162–66, 244*n*59; rocket and missile research at, 148; rocket sled research at, 6, 152–59, 166; weightless research at, 160–62, 236*n*21

human-factors research: definition of, 3; interwar years at Wright, 11, 18; and space flight 167, 175, 176, *180*, 182, 187–88, 190, 198; war and, 4; during WWII at Wright, 27, 73; post-WWII at Wright, 123–24, 138; and X-aircraft: 169–72, 173

human-subjects testing: in Germany, 34, 40, 46–47, 49–50, 60–63, 65–66, 69, 92–96, 232*n*29, 232*n*34, 260–63; at Holloman AFB, 152, 154, 155, 157, 159,

human-subjects testing (*cont.*)
159–60, *163, 164;* at SAM, 169; in space-cabin simulator, 176–77; at Wright lab, *21, 22,* 24, 34–35, 76, 78–79, 162–63

Hurrle, Rhea, *205,* 254*n*31

hypoxia. *See* anoxia

ICBMS. *See* missiles

industrial medicine, 16, 187, 218*n*7, 219*n*17

inmates: Allied POWs, 98–99; at Dachau, 94, 95, 233*n*44, 262; "displaced persons," 120; German nationals in United Kingdom, 97; 94; at Nuremberg, 117–18; Paperclips, 115, 117–18, 236*n*19, 237*n*27; as test subjects, in United States, 232–33*n*36

International Geophysical Year, 137, 147–49, *148,* 178, 197, 224–25*n*24, 242*n*33, 246–47*n*10

isolation, 125, 169, 176, 191, 208

Italy, 33, 37, 59, 66, 67, 78, 230*n*97, 266

Ivy, Andrew, 150, 242n37

Japan, 37, 108, 110

jet aircraft, development of: in Germany, 5, 39, 60, 87–90, 109, 123, 236*n*6; in United Kingdom, 109, 236*n*6; in United States, 6, 109, 123, 236*n*6

Johnson, Lyndon B., 7, 173, 175, 183–86, *181,* 194–95, 211

Johnson Space Center, 8, 173

Journal of Aviation Medicine (*JAM*): and aviation, 32, 36, 39, 66, 126, 150, 156, 221*n*32, 265; and space, 168, 178, 196–97

journals, aviation medicine
in Germany, 39, 55–59, 66, 96, 121, 230*n*94, 262
in United States, 32, 36, 39
in USSR, 187
specific titles: *Acta Aerophysiologica,*
56; *American Journal of Physiology,* 66; *Journal of Physiology,* 66; *Journal of the American Medical Association,* 66; *Klinischen Wochenschrift,* 53; *Luftfahrtmedizinische Abhandlung,* 57–58, 227*n*60; *Mitteilung aus dem Gebiete der Luftfahrtmedizin,* 57; *Rivista di Medicina Aeronautica,* 59; *Schriften or Berichte der Deutschen Akademie der Luftfahrtforschung,* 57; *Zeitschrift für Biologie,* 53; *Zeitschrift für Flugtechnik und Motorluftsch-iffahrt,* 56. See also *Journal of Aviation Medicine; Zeitschrift für Luftfahrtmedizin*

Junkers, 40, 87, 89, 127

Jüterbog, 51, 89, 90, 234*n*49

Kaiser Wilhelm Institutes (KWI), 111, 124, 197, 228*n*69

Kennedy, John F., 7, 8, 173, 210, 211, 255*n*40

Kittinger, Joe, 159, 162, 166, 188, 192, 246*n*88, 248*n*28

Klemm, 47, 89

Korean War, 128–29, 213

Leverton, Irene, *205,* 254*n*31

Ley, Willy, *134,* 174

Lilienthalgesellschaft (Lilienthal Organization), 54, 63, 227*n*60

Lindbergh, Charles, 44, 224*n*16, 224*n*18

London, 37, 38, 107, 108, 112, 114

Los Alamos National Laboratory, 171, 190

Lovelace, Mary (Mrs. W. Randolph Lovelace II), 214–15

Lovelace, W. Randolph II: and Aero Medical Association, 150, 253*n*9; and BLB mask, 35–36; and Collier Trophy, 35–36; combat experience of, 78; death of, 214–15; and NASA, 7, 160, 186–87, 193, 197, 253*n*11; and parachute jump, 76–77, *84*, 231*n*13; as a scientist, 121, 241*n*14, 246*n*93; training of, 67, 222*n*42, 230*n*5, 230*n*97, 231*n*10; as Wright lab director, 76, 78 111–12, 186

Lovelace Clinic/Foundation, 128, 134, 173, *180*, 186, 189–90, 193, 202–204, 206–207, 254*n*29

Lovelace study (of women as astronaut candidates): 200, 202–204, 206–11, 213, 253*n*9, 254*n*20, 255*n*36, 255*n*38, 256*n*44. *See also* Lovelace, W. Randolph II

Low, George, 188, 193, 211–12

Lowell, Percival, 141, 241*n*12

Lowell Observatory, 142–43, 144, 241*n*14

low pressure chamber: at CME (England), 81; at Dachau, 92–94, 96; in Germany, 42, 46, 50, 51, 61, 63, 65–66, 67, 68, 228*n*63; at Heidelberg, 111; at SAM, 71, 219*n*13; at Wright, 19–22, 23–24, 28–29, 31–33, 36, 77, 78, 192, 219*n*14

Luft, Alice (Mrs. Ulrich Luft), 97, 119–20, 132, 134, 207

Luft, Friederich "Fred" (son), 97, 132, 134

Luft, Hildegard (sister), 97, 234*n*52

Luft, Mary Muir Wilson (mother), 97, 229–30*n*90, 234*n*52

Luft, Ulrich: and death of Lovelace, 214–26; 228*n*73; at LMFI, 54, 99, 101, 121, 227*n*56, 228*n*77; at Lovelace Clinic, 134–35, 240*n*70, 257*n*6; and Lovelace study, 202–204, 207; and Mercury astronaut selection, 187, 189–90; military service of, 98–99; and mountaineering research, *59*, 67, 90, 132, 134, 227*n*53, and Nazi Party, 64, 229*n*86; and Nuremberg trials, 238*n*32; in Scotland 97; training of, 228*n*67; at

University of Berlin, 111, 113; comes to United States, 115–18, 118–20, 136, 225*n*34, 236*n*15

Luftfahrtmedizinische Forschungsin-stitut (LMFI) [Aviation Medicine Research Institute]: atmosphere of, 66; as educational institute, 227*n*57; founding of, 40–41, 51–52; and journal publishing, 55–58; location of, 53; reputation of, 67; research by *58*, 60–63, 65–66, 230*n*96; staffing of 53–54, 227*n*53, 227*n*56; during WWII, 89, 90, 96, 97, 99–101, 132; after WWII, 113

Lufthansa, 40, 51

Luftwaffe and aeromedical research. *See* Luftfahrtmedizinische Forschungsin-stitut; Jüterbog; Rechlin

Luftwaffe and rearmament after WWI, 40–41, 51, 86, 88

Man in Space Soonest project (MISS), 166, 180, 183, 191

Mars, 126, 141, 141–44, 168, 197, 198, 241*n*12, 241*n*14, 245*n*84

Mauch, Hans, 123, 236*n*18

Mayo Clinic: as research center, 12, 35–36, 75, 77, 121, 189, 197, 221*n*41; as teaching institute, 49, 67, 73, 134, 139, 236*n*15

McClure, Clifton, 160, 161, 192

media, popular, and aerospace medicine, 128, 140, 174, 178, 204–207, 212, 239*n*61, 256*n*57, 256*n*54

Mercury astronaut selection, 3, 171, 173, 188–94, 204, 251*n*78, 251*n*80, 251*n*81, 251*n*82, 251*n*73

Mercury program, 7, 186, 187, 187–89, 193, 200, 203–204, 212–13, 255*n*39

Messerschmitt, 87, 89, 248*n*29

Milch, Erhard, 40, 51, 68, 88, 95–96, 261

military, science research in, 147–48, 173–74. *See also specific projects, labs*

military and civilian relationship, in aerospace, 7, 148, 173, 180, 182–83, 202, 208, 210, 212–13, 255n42

Miller, George, 211, 256n50

Mineola, Long Island, N.Y., 20–21, 32, 35, 48, 225–26n36

missiles: Atlas, 175, 206–207; development of, 5, 107, 184, 220n27; manned, 90, 182, 232n29. *See also* V-1; V-2

moon race, 7, 198, 210–13, 217

Muller, H. J., 128, 141

Munich, University of, 42, 59, 89, 93, 233–34n48

Muroc Army Air Base, 77–78, 124, 137, 138, 142, 154, 165

Murphy's Law. *See* Stapp, John Paul

National Academy of Sciences, 242n33

National Advisory Committee on Aeronautics (NACA): and aviation, 7, 11, 31, 109, 138, 147, 167–69, 180, 220n27, 226n46; becomes NASA, 184, 186

National Aeronautics and Space Administration (NASA): aeromedical capabilities of, 173–74, 187–88; creation of, 173, 183–86, 194; and exobiology, 141; and Lovelace study (women astronauts), 200, 203, 207–13, 253n11; and Paperclips, 122–23; relationship with military, 7, 183–86, 194–96, 198, 215–16, 245n78; and von Braun, Wernher, 122

National Institutes of Health, 145, 188, 246–27n10

National Research Council, 125, 225n26

National Research Laboratory, 145, 148

National Science Foundation, 144, 175, 178, 184, 186, 197

Nazi Party: membership among aeromedical specialists, 63–66, 96, 113,

229n80, 229n86, 237n25, 261; membership among scientists, 50, 51, 54, 58, 68, 92, 122, 225n27, 228–29n78, 230n91; opposition to, 64, 96, 233–34n48, 237n25; policy regarding aeromedicine, 54, 88, 92–93, 112; social policy of, 39, 40, 50, 52, 54, 63–64, 92, 99, 122, 260; sponsorship of research, 40, 57–59, 88, 91, 112, 261

Netherlands, 25, 31, 33, 36, 67, 107, 230n97

Ninety-Nines, the, 201, 206

Nobel Prize, 223n8, 228–29n78, 253n6

Northrup Aircraft, 153, 154, 155

Nuremberg court trials, 82, 92, 95–96, 117–18, 226n47, 228n62, 233–34n48, 242n37, 260–63

Occupation, Allied Zones of, 106, 109, 112, 113, 114, 120, 135

Odlum, Floyd, 206–207, 254n29

Office of Scientific Research and Development, 75, 167

Operation "Lusty." *See* German scientists, after WWII

Opitz, Erich, 54, 63, 67, 90, 101, 238n32

oxygen deprivation/deficiency, 19, 49–50, 56, 58, 60, 76–77, 123–25

oxygen masks/systems/equipment, 19, 20, 27–28, 65, 74–77, 81, 163, 165, 170–71, 245n84. *See also* Boothby-Lovelace-Bulbulian mask

oxygen poisoning, 17, 60–61

Paperclips: and adjustment to America, 118–20, 120, 132–33, 135, 136; and compensation, 115, 117, 120; and emigration to United States, 115–17, 237–38n31; and living conditions, 115, 117, 120. *See also* Project Paperclip

parachuting, 18, 34, 90, 123, 137, 162–65, 213, 231n13, 248n28. *See also* individual jumpers and projects pathology, 59, 227*n*56

Peenemünde, Germany, 6, 111

Pentagon, 37–38, 127

physics and aeromedicine, 3, 73, 74, 145–46, 147, 151, 159, 159–60, 187, 219*n*10

Physics and Medicine of the Upper Atmosphere, 128, 143

physiologists, 71–72

physiology, 42–43, 48–49, 60, 218*n*7, 221*n*41, 222*n*42, 223*n*13, 251*n*80, 251*n*81; exercise, 62, 187; sensory research, 43, 48–49, 72; space, 125

physiology, high-altitude: American research on, 18, 24, 31, 48; Dachau research on, 93–94, 118, 187; German research on, 44–48, 51, 53, 59, 62–63, 67, 90

Pichotka, Joseph, 101, 235*n*71

pilots

military: and gender, 76, 200, 211, 222*n*44, 256*n*52; and relationship with flight surgeons, 3, 17, 19, 28; characteristics of 16–17, 72–73, 167–68, 199, 212; concerns of, 17–18, 19, 21; in United States, 3, 13, 16–17, 28; screening of, 70–71, 72–73, 91, 151, 160, 167–69, 186, 188, 191

racing, 18, 35

suicide, 88, 232*n*29

test: American, 3, 7 18–19, 27, 76; astronauts, *180*, 188, 212, 248*n*28, 248*n*29; German, 98, 224*n*20, 232*n*29; jet 137–38, 155–56, 162–63, 167–68, 170, *180*, 186, 199. *See also* individual test pilots

Poland, 67, 81, 99

Post, Wiley, 18, 219*n*14

pressure suits, 37, 90, 123, 125, 138, 165, 170–71, *180*, 191, 192, 208, 236*n*18

Project Excelsior, 162–65, 166. *See also* parachuting

Project High Dive, 163. *See also* parachuting

Project Man High, 159–60, 166, 248*n*29

Project Paperclip, 6–8, 126, 148–51, 197, 216, 225*n*34, 237*n*27, 257*n*6, 260. *See also* individual Paperclip immigrants

Project Vanguard, 178, 196, 246–47*n*10, 247*n*19

protective gear: temperature, 13–14, 7, 81, 85–86, 74; flak, 80, *85*, 90; G-forces, 90; head injury, 25, 156; pressure, 156, 170–72

psychiatrists and psychiatry, 72–73, 80, 91, 150, 151, 192–93, 251*n*78

psychologists and psychology: and space flight 187, 190, 251*n*78, 251*n*80, 251*n*81; in Germany, 91, 232*n*31; in U.S. military, 3, 16–18, 31, 155, 157

publications, aeromedical, 32, 36, 39. *See also under* journals

Putt, Donald L., 27, 182, 220*n*27

Quarles, Donald A., 185, 195–96

radiation, 39, 171, 186, 197, 243*n*41; cosmic, 124, 125, 144, 145–46, 147–49, 150–51, 160, 169, 197, 219*n*10

radio navigation, 18, 27, 32, 220*n*26.

RAND Corporation, 175, 177

Randolph Field (AFB), Texas, 71, 118, 119, 120, 126, 175, 177

research and development, spending on, 3, 75, 166, 180, 196, 219*n*15

Rascher, Sigmund, 93–95, 233*n*41

Rechlin, 40, 59–60, 88, 90, 133, 232*n*25, 232*n*29, 232*n*34, 233*n*45

Rein, Hermann, 53, 56, 95, 101, 227*n*53, 233*n*45

Reitsch, Hanna, 224*n*20, 232*n*29

respiratory research, 219*n*17, 249–50*n*53

Rockefeller Foundation, 5, 47–49, 67, 224–25*n*24, 226*n*37

rocket-powered aircraft, development of, 5, 6, 39, 87, 90–91, 123, 168, 170

rocketry and rockets, 121–22, 125, 137, 145–46, 147–49, 152, 216, 248*n*28, 249–50*n*53

rocket sleds, 6, 137, 140, *142*, 152, 166, 172

rockoons, 146, 148. *See also* ballooning, scientific and military; balloons, as research platforms; rocketry and rockets

Rocky Mountains, 35, 48, 134–35, 169

Romberg, Hans, *82*, 90, 93–94, 95, 96, 97, 228*n*62, 233*n*41, 233*n*43, 238*n*32

Roosevelt, Franklin D., 36, 67, *75*, 108–109

Rose, Heinrich, 54, 92, 115, 119, *131*, 132, 133, 136

Rosemann, Rudolf, 42, 43

Ruff, Siegfried: and Dachau/Nuremberg *82*, 93–96, 228*n*62, 233*n*41, 238*n*32; at DVL, 41, *57*, 59, 90, 121; at Heidelberg AMC, *132*; military service of, 97; and Nazi party, 63

Russia. *See* Union of Soviet Socialist Republics (USSR)

Sanitätsversuchsgruppe der Aufklärungsgruppe Jüterbog [Medical Research Group of the Jüterbog Reconnaissance Group]. *See* Jüterbog

satellites, 147–49, 173, 174–76, 194, 246–47*n*10, 247*n*19, 248*n*27, 249–50*n*53. *See also* Sputnik

Schäfer, Konrad (also Konrad Schaefer), *82*, 94–95, 99, *132*, 229*n*83, 234*n*49, 238*n*32

Schloss Welkersdorf, 99, 101, 235*n*61

Schmidt, Ingeborg, 54, 92, 115, *131*, 133, 136, 178, 236*n*18, 248*n*26

School of Aviation Medicine (SAM): department of astroecology, 176; department of space medicine, 4, 6, 126–27, *130;* 143–44, 145–46, 197; during Cold War, 112, 115–16, 124, *134*, 154, 175; and Paperclips, 116; and *Sputnik,* 174–75; as teaching institution, 12–13, 259, 128; during WWII, 69, 70, 71–72; after WWII, 98; and Wright Lab, 123

Schriever, Bernard, 196, 220*n*27

Schröder, Oskar, *82*, 95, 112, 226*n*47, 238*n*32

Schwichtenberg, A. H., 189–90, 202–204

scientists: organizations of, 32–33, 67–68; qualities of, 22–23, 64, 60, 153, 156, 237*n*27. *See also* specific individuals

self-experimentation: in aviation medicine, 3, 5, 34–35, 137, *142*, 154–55, 155–59, 167, 231*n*13; in Germany, 5, 65–66, 92, 226*n*46. *See also* individual flight surgeons

Selfridge Field, Michigan, 13, 16, 27, 218*n*9

seawater, desalinization of, 65, 94–95, 99, 263

Shepard, Alan, 7, 171, 194, 210, 216

Simons, David, 157, 159–60, 166, 174, 192, 244*n*59

Slipher, E. C. and V. M., 142, 144

Sloan, Jerri, *205*, 254*n*31

sound barrier, 6, 137, 138, 165, 208, 222*n*44

space
capsules, 149, 151, 168, 183, 255*n*39
colonization of, 6, 105, 168, 174
exploration of, 121–22, 125–26, 127, 141, 148
flight: duration of, 170; risks of, 151–52, 153–55, 165, 168–69, 188, 192
medicine, evolution as discipline, 3, 105, 107, 123, 125–27, 149–50

psychological stresses of, 125, 161, 169–70, 188, 192–93

vehicles, 168, 213

Space Task Group (STG), 187–89, 193

speed, effects of, 123–24, 153, 200

sports medicine. *See* physiology, exercise

Sputnik (*Sputnik I*), 7, 173, 174–77, 178–79, 194–95, 246–47*n*10, 247*n*15, 248*n*27

Sputnik II, 177, 179, 249–50*n*53

SS (Schutzstaffel), 88, 92–94, 229*n*86

Stapp, John Paul: and animal test subjects, 152–54; beliefs of, 129, 163, 165–67, 240*n*5; as flight surgeon, 138, *164;* and funding, 244n59, 244n61; and high-altitude balloon research, 162–67; and Mercury astronaut selection, 7, 188, 91; and Murphy's Law, 140–41; as rocket sled test subject, 6, 137, 140, *142,* 154–58; and space medicine, 174; youth and education of, 138–39, 240*n*2. *See also* Beeding, Eli L.; Daisy Track

Stauffenberg, Claus von, 96, 233–34*n*48

Steadman, Bernice "B," *205,* 254*n*31

Strughold, Hubertus: as author/editor, 58, 97, 115–16, 143, 237*n*24, 262–63; and Dachau/Nuremberg 92, 95–97; and English language, 33, 48; and exobiology, 5, 126, 141–44, *143;* and Nazi Party, 5–6, 51, 54–55, 58, 64–66, 135, 225*n*27, 229*n*86, 234*n*49, 237*n*25, 240*n*71; and space medicine, 107, 124–27, *130,* 150, 176–77, 248*n*26, as instructor, 43–44, 45, 50,115; as LMFI director, 39, 41, 51–52, 53–55, 56–58, 60, 67–68, 89, 95, 99, 101, 107, 113, 126, 227*n*53, 227*n*60, 229*n*83, 229*n*85, 230*n*96, 236*n*19, 238*n*32; military service of, 101; as Paperclip, 105, 113–16, 126, *131,* 135–36, 216; personality of, 33, 49, 216; physical description of, 33, 48; relationship with Harry Armstrong, 33, 114, 126; as researcher, 45–46, 48–50, *55,* 60, 66, 148, 151, 225*n*28, 226*n*40, 236*n*14; religion of, 41, 122; as "Struggie," 49, 115, 226*n*39; at SAM, 124–27, *130,* 174, 176–77, *181,* 197; training of, 5, 41–49, 223–24*n*14, 225–26*n*36, 226*n*37, 226*n*40, 228*n*67; youth of, 41, 44, 223*n*4

Strughold Aeromedical Library, 96–97, *202,* 265

Stumbough, Gene Nora, *205,* 254*n*31

Sweden, 66, 78, 96, 204, 230*n*97

Switzerland, 37, 67, 197, 230*n*97

telemetering (of data), 145–46, 163, 171, 182–83, 190, 249–50*n*53

Tereshkova, Valentina, 212, 252*n*2. *See also* cosmonauts

tolerance level/tolerances, 124, 125, 137, 140, 152–55, 156, 159, 169, 172, 190, 226*n*46. *See also* acclimation/acclimatizaion

Tombaugh, Clyde, 141, 143, 198, 241*n*14

Truman, Harry S, 110, 175, 231*n*9

Udet, Ernst, 46–47, 50, 98

Union of Soviet Socialist Republics (USSR): and Germany, 40, 97, 101, *106,* 114; research in, 7, 18, 33, 111, *130,* 144, 177–79, 246–47*n*10, 248*n*27, 249–50*n*53; space policy of, 7; and United States, 135, 185, 195, 260–61; and women cosmonauts, 200, 212–13, 252*n*2. See also *Sputnik I; Sputnik II*

United Kingdom: and aeronautical/aeromedical research, 33, 37–38, 42, 43, 114, 197, 235*n*73; and CME during WWII, 79–81

United States of America: aeronautical design/engineering in, 31–32, 38, 128, 243*n*41; aviation policy of, 11, 79,

United States of America (*cont.*)
100, 243*n*41; graduate education in
science and medicine, 42, 47, 116, 124,
222*n*42, 223*n*12, 223*n*8, 226*n*37; medical
ethics in, 34–35, 108, 152–54, 232–33*n*36,
243*n*46; social atmosphere of, 116–17,
200, 209, 211–12, 231*n*9, 243*n*46; space
policy of, 7, 105, 121, 148, 180, 183–86,
187, 194–96, 200, 256*n*44; and WWII,
38, 38, 69–86, 100

upper atmosphere, research in, 6, 18, 137,
146–47, 148–49, 186, 197

U.S. Air Force: acceptance of "space,"
127; Air Research & Development
Command, 180; and atomic planes,
243*n*41; manned space program of,
166–67, 167–69, 180, 182–83, 194–98,
199–200, 215–17, 248*n*28; and medical
research, 7, 125, 137, 173; and Southwest
Research Institute, 257*n*6; surgeon
general, 127, 264

U.S. Army: Air Corps, 11, 12, 79, 95,
109–10, 177, 205, 219*n*10, 220*n*26, 263;
Air Forces, 6, 70, 75, 76, 78, 80–81; air
surgeon, 72; Eighth Air Force, 79–80,
86; Fifteenth Air Force, 78, 81, 127; and
missiles, 145, 178, 184, 186, 196, 247*n*19;
Ninth Air Force, 76, 81, 111; and Operation Lusty, 110; Reserves, 76; and
space flight 185, 195–96; Twelfth Air
Force, 81; War College, 116

U.S. Department of Commerce, Aeronautics Bureau, 11, 32, 33

U.S. Justice Department, 261. *See also*
Federal Bureau of Investigation (FBI)

U.S. Navy: and aerospace research, 144,
145, 150, 169, 178; Bureau of Aeronautics, 177; and captured technology, 110;
and Lovelace study, 208–10; Naval
School of Aviation Medicine, 188,

197–98, 255*n*36; and Paperclips, 116

U.S. v. Erhard Milch. See Milch, Erhard;
Nuremberg court trials

U.S. v. Karl Brandt, et al., 82. See
Nuremberg court trials; *individual
defendants*

U.S. War Department, 70, 145

V-1, "buzz bombs," 88, 90–91, 108,
232*n*29, 248*n*29

V-2s, 105, 107–108, 145–49, 152, 157,
241*n*20, 246–47*n*10

Van Allen, James, 128, 147, 177, 246–47*n*10

Vaucouleurs, Gerard de, 141, 197

Versailles (Treaty), 40, 108, 229*n*80. *See
also* Germany, remilitarization after
WWII

vertigo/disorientation, 29–30, 32, 151,
160–61, 170, 182, 190

vision, 24, 39, 50, 54, 65, 72–74, 99, 144,
151–52, 190

war crimes trials, 88, 95–96, 117–18. *See
also* Nuremberg court trials

Webb, James E., 7, 173, *203*, 208, 210–11,
213, 255*n*38, 255*n*39, 255*n*40

weightlessness, 125, 127, 151–52, 160–61,
165, 169, 70, 200, 239*n*50, 244*n*62

Weltz, Georg, 57, 59, 63, *82*, 93, 95

Whipple, Fred, 128, 141, 197

White, Clayton S. "Sam," 128, 134, 214,
240*n*70

Whittingham, Harold, 37, 38

Wiggers, Carl, 43, 47–48, 223–24*n*14,
225*n*26, 225*n*28

windblast, 39, 68, 77, 90, 123–24, 156, 162

women, as astronauts, 7, 200–13, 252*n*2,
254*n*31, 255*n*40, 255*n*42, 256*n*44

Women Airforce Service Pilots (WASP),
76, *87*, 200, 211, 222*n*44, 253*n*3, 256*n*52

Women's Auxiliary Ferrying Squadron (WAFS). *See* Women Airforce Service Pilots

World War I: cutbacks after 4, 11, 15, 18, 32, 37; effects on Germany, 40, 41, 43, 46–47, 224–25n24, 229n80; Germany in 39, 46, 108

World War II: as aeromedical challenge, 5, 69, 76–77, 78, 89–90, 93, 98, 166–67, 260–63; buildup for, 12, 13, 37; casualties, 253n3; strategic planning for, 79, 86; WASP in, 200, 222n44, 253n3; as watershed for aeromedicine, 3–7,

69–70, 75, 107, 110–14, 137, 138, 145, 147

Wright Field (Wright-Patterson AFB), Ohio, 15, 18–19, 25, 27, 37, 116–17, 259

Würzburg, University of, 43, 45, 223–24n14

X-15 program, 169–72, *180*

Yeager, Chuck, 6, 128, 138

Zeitschrift für Luftfahrtmedizin (*ZfL*), 39, 56, 58, 59, 66, 230n94

ISBN 1-58544-439-1